CULTURAL COMPETENCE IN HEALTH EDUCATION AND HEALTH PROMOTION

CULTURAL COMPETENCE IN HEALTH EDUCATION AND HEALTH PROMOTION

Second Edition

Miguel A. Pérez and Raffy R. Luquis

Editors

JOSSEY-BASS™
A Wiley Brand

Cover design by Wiley
Cover image: © CSA Images/Getty Images

Published by Jossey-Bass
A Wiley Brand
One Montgomery Street, Suite 1200, San Francisco, CA 94104-4594—www.josseybass.com

Library of Congress Cataloging-in-Publication Data

Cultural competence in health education and health promotion / Miguel A. Pérez and Raffy R. Luquis. — Second edition.
pages cm
Includes bibliographical references and index.
ISBN 978-1-118-34749-2 (pbk.) — ISBN 978-1-118-45016-1 (epub) — ISBN 978-1-118-34749-2 (pbk.)
1. Transcultural medical care—United States. 2. Minorities—Medical care—United States. 3. Health education—United States. 4. Health promotion—United States. I. Pérez, Miguel A., 1969- editor of compilation. II. Luquis, Raffy R., 1966- editor of compilation.
RA418.5.T73C853 2014
362.1089—dc23

2013027867

SECOND EDITION

PB Printing 10 9 8 7 6 5 4 3 2 1

CONTENTS

We dedicate this publication to our supportive spouses and dedicated children. Helda and Susan, we could not have done this without your support and encouragement. Thanks for being part of our lives.

FOREWORD

For all health educators, regardless of their practice setting, cultural competency is essential for effective practice. With the increasing demographic changes in the US population, the importance of promoting health equity and reducing health disparities, and a greater emphasis on global health, it is important for the profession to have an informative, competency-based, practice-oriented resource for promoting the development and enhancement of skills related to cultural competency. This second edition of *Cultural Competence in Health Education and Health Promotion* meets this need. The book has been organized and written not only to provide the basics in helping prospective health educators develop knowledge and skills related to cultural competency but also to develop the deeper understanding and mastery of more nuanced skills to truly become culturally competent health educators.

Coeditors Miguel A. Pérez and Raffy R. Luquis have organized the content in a format that addresses important health education considerations related to culture, race, and ethnicity, including a clear explanation of the distinction among these three terms. Chapters 1 and 2 present a clear rationale for the importance of cultural competency among health educators, including data related to health status among different cultures, races, and ethnic groups. These chapters also present a description of health disparities among these groups in the United States.

Throughout the book, cultural understanding is promoted through content such as a framework for understanding culture, cultural factors that can affect the practice of health education, and several models for assessing the role of culture in the prevention of disease and the promotion of health. Emphasis is placed on linking cultural understanding to both health education theory and common health education approaches to program planning, implementation, and evaluation. The chapter authors have addressed a wide spectrum of important but often overlooked topics related to cultural diversity, such as the role of place as a social determinant, diversity within individual cultures, the linkage of culture to complementary and alternative medicine, and the importance of awareness and skills related to the role health education plays within the lesbian, gay, bisexual, transgender, and aging communities. It is important to note that the content throughout this book relates directly to the National Commission for Health Education Credentialing, Inc., Areas of Responsibilities for Health Educators.

The book goes far beyond the thorough provision of information. The format of this book is presented in a manner that promotes meaningful application of the content. The objectives listed at the beginning of each chapter provide direction for both instructors and students. Following the presentation of the content, each chapter provides a conclusion, points to remember, and key terms, features that enable students to review, organize, and analyze their understanding of the content within the chapters. In addition, each chapter includes a case study that applies the chapter content to a hypothetical health education scenario. Beyond the case studies, the content of the book sets the stage for further activities within and outside the classroom that will engage students in meaningful learning activities emphasizing critical thinking and authentic application of the knowledge and skills addressed in the chapters.

From my perspective as a university faculty member and department chair, I see this book as an excellent resource for both instructors and students in undergraduate or graduate courses in which cultural competency is an important topic. I certainly see it as a primary textbook in classes that focus on cultural competence in health education and promotion. Because of the applied nature of this book to health education practice and the essential nature of cultural competency to all that we do as health educators, I also see it as a supplementary textbook in classes that address planning, implementation, and evaluation in health education and health promotion.

While I consider this book to be an outstanding textbook for undergraduate and graduate professional preparation classes, it is also an excellent addition to the professional library of health education practitioners regardless of practice setting. Chapter 12 addresses the need for cultural competence among practicing health educators. The chapter authors identify tools that can be used to assess the cultural competence of organizations involved in health education. One recommendation in the chapter is that organizations provide ongoing cultural and linguistic training to health educators. *Cultural Competence in Health Education and Health Promotion* could serve as an excellent resource for such training.

Health education and health promotion will never realize its full potential until skilled practitioners are able to consistently develop and implement programs that meet the needs and maximize the assets of individuals and communities representing all cultures. To do this, we must ensure that our professional preparation programs help prospective professionals develop the knowledge, understanding, and skills that are essential for cultural competency. In addition, health educators engaged in professional practice must maintain their competencies as communities continue to be enriched through increasingly diverse populations. I believe that *Cultural Competence in Health Education and Health Promotion* will serve as a valuable resource as we move forward to meet this challenge.

David A. Birch, PhD, MCHES
Professor and Chair
Department of Health Science
The University of Alabama
Tuscaloosa, Alabama

PREFACE

Welcome to the second edition of *Cultural Competence in Health Education and Health Promotion*. This textbook is designed to assist you as you explore the interaction between culture, attitudes, and behaviors and their application to health education programs and strategies. The chapters focus on examining selected health indicators of underrepresented groups, discuss best practice models for cultural competence training, and provide strategies for reaching diverse populations while avoiding generalizations and stereotypes based on race, ethnicity, gender, and selected social issues. While no publication can guarantee the reader "cultural competence," the chapters in this publication are designed to assist on the road to this lofty goal.

This textbook is unique in that it focuses on issues of cultural and linguistic competency as they influence the health education and health promotion field. Each chapter is written by and for health education academicians and practitioners. Each author presents a thorough examination of the literature and research about the impact of culture, race, and ethnicity on health disparities, health equity, communication, beliefs systems, education strategies, and other factors essential to have a complete understanding of cultural and linguistic competency. This edition has been expanded in several ways to provide both students and practitioners with a better understanding of cultural and linguistic competency within health education and health promotion. All chapters have been revised or expanded to reflect up-to-date information on cultural and linguistic competency health education—including the revised CLAS standards released in late April 2013. Each of the chapters provides key terms and a case study (except for Chapter 12) for students and practitioners to apply the concepts discussed.

This textbook contains twelve chapters that center on the common theme of learning and understanding different cultures. Chapter 1, "Implications of Changing US Demographics for Health Educators," provides current information on demographics and descriptions of the profiles of major ethnic and racial populations in the United States. New to this edition, Chapter 2, "Diversity and Health Education," focuses on concepts of diversity, race, ethnicity, and culture. Also new to this edition, Chapter 3, "Health Disparities and Social Determinants of Health: Implications for Health Education," addresses social determinants of health and their influence over health and health disparities in the United States. Chapter 4, "Complementary and Alternative Medicine in Culturally Competent Health Education," provides an overview of the principles involved in the practice of complementary healing, alternative medicine, and holistic health. The completely revised Chapter 5, "Spirituality and Cultural Diversity," provides information on religious and spiritual trends in the United States and their influence on health and well-being. Chapter 6, "Health Education Theoretical Models and Multicultural Populations," describes and provides examples of how to apply two theoretical models and two assessment frameworks that address the role of culture in the prevention of disease and promotion of health. Chapter 7, "Planning, Implementing, and Evaluating Culturally Appropriate Programs," has been revised to focus on factors to consider when developing health education programs for culturally diverse individuals and groups. Chapter 8, "Culturally Appropriate Communication," has been revised to include the health communication model, the importance of verbal and non-verbal communication across different groups, and strategies for how to incorporate linguistic competency into health education and health promotion. New to this edition, Chapter 9, "Foundations for Health Literacy and Culturally Appropriate Health Education Programs," provides a definition of health literacy, its importance to health education, and the relationship between health literacy and cultural competence. Both Chapter 10, "The Aging US Population: An Increasing Diverse Population," and Chapter 11, "Culture and Sexual Orientation," provide an exploration of issues affecting two unique cultural groups and the role of health educators and practitioners in addressing their respective needs. Finally, Chapter 12, "Cultural Competency and Health Education: A Window of Opportunity," provides some final thoughts on the importance of cultural and linguistic competence and discusses how to integrate these concepts into health education and health promotion programs.

The authors and the editors of *Cultural Competence in Health Education and Health Promotion* intend that this second edition will continue to fulfill the current and future needs in cultural and linguistic competency for both professional preparation and the development of health education and promotion programs by educators and practitioners. Join us in what we hope will be a lifelong journey toward cultural competence.

THE EDITORS

Miguel A. Pérez is a health educator who specializes in international health and applied research, adolescent health issues, and cultural competence. In 2001, he received a Fulbright Award to teach at the Universidad El Bosque in Bogota, Colombia. In 2005, he was a Fulbright senior specialist scholar in public/global health at the Nelson Mandela Metropolitan University, South Africa. In 2006, he was a Fulbright senior specialist scholar in public/global health at the Universidad del Norte in Barranquilla, Colombia. Most recently he has worked in developing health promotion training programs in the Dominican Republic and Thailand. He has been the chairperson of the Department of Public Health at Fresno State since 2008. Pérez received his doctorate from Penn State University and is a fellow with the former American Association for Health Education and with the Research Consortium of the American Alliance for Health, Physical Education, Recreation, and Dance.

Raffy R. Luquis is an associate professor and the program coordinator of the health education master's degree in the School of Behavioral Sciences and Education at Penn State Harrisburg. He earned his PhD in health science at the University of Arkansas and his MS in health education and his BS in science at the Pennsylvania State University. His primary teaching and research interests are multicultural health, cultural competency in health promotion, community health, program evaluation, and human sexuality. He has numerous refereed publications and more than fifty national, regional, and state presentations. He is a fellow of the former American Association for Health Education and the Research Consortium of the American Alliance for Health, Physical Education, Recreation, and Dance. He earned the master certified health education specialist credential from the National Commission for Health Education Credentialing in 2011.

THE CONTRIBUTORS

Joan E. Cowdery is a faculty member and program coordinator for the Health Education program in the School of Health Promotion and Human Performance at Eastern Michigan University, Ypsilanti. Her research experience includes the use of innovative technologies, including tailoring and virtual worlds, to encourage healthy behavior change in diverse populations. She received her PhD in health education and health promotion from the University of Alabama and the University of Alabama-Birmingham School of Public Health, where her dissertation research focused on quality of life in women living with HIV.

William H. Dailey Jr. is a gerontology lecturer in the Department of Public Health and the Department of Social Work/Gerontology at Fresno State and also teaches at Fresno City College as a faculty member in the Social Sciences Department. He also works with Farley, his guide dog. William earned his doctorate of education focusing on the area of educational leadership and change in dealing with disabilities related to aging issues at Fielding Graduate University. His doctoral dissertation focuses on the collaborative limitations, perceptions, and interactions among practitioners to meet the needs of an increasing elder population. Dailey was appointed as a delegate to the White House Conference on Aging held in December 2005 in Washington, DC. He continues to collaborate with the California delegation on key aging issues. His research interests include the role of grandparents in raising their grandchildren, aging and disability issues facing elders, alternative housing and transportation issues, and LGBT elders.

Alba Lucia Diaz-Cuellar is assistant professor of health promotion in the School of Health and Human Services—Department of Community Health at National University. She has more than twenty-five years of experience in public health and education fields, working with diverse communities of all ages and ethnic backgrounds. She is an active member of the United Nations Children's Fund, which she served as director of health and education programs in Africa (Guinea Bissau, Nigeria, South Africa), Southeast Asia (Thailand, Myanmar), and Latin America (Bolivia, Peru, Ecuador, Colombia, and Venezuela). In addition to teaching and research, she conducts short-term consultancies with the United Nations on worldwide projects on peace processes, the reduction of education and health disparities, and the elimination of extreme levels of poverty. Her research interests include the interconnections of politics, power, and poverty, with special emphasis on social justice, indigenous health, international migration, community organizing, and community empowerment. Her most recent research has focused on the area of health promotion and disease prevention, particularly health education and health advocacy. The core of her community-based research lies in the investigation of the impact of grassroots interventions, the use of community-based health educators (indigenous *promotoras)* for the dissemination of the concept of the Ulysses syndrome at national and international levels.

Suzanne F. Evans serves as core faculty and the School of Education online coordinator at Pacific Oaks College in Pasadena, California. Prior to joining Pacific Oaks, she served as an associate professor in the School of Health and Human Services at National University. As a member of the full-time graduate faculty, she taught in the community health, public health, and health education programs. She previously taught in the School of Education in teacher education, special education, reading, and curriculum development. Because of her belief that scholarship is an integral aspect of the role of professional educators, her research agenda and scholarship activities have focused on culture-centered education, culturally proficient practices, the value and utilization of multicultural literature, professional development with teachers in the use of transformative and culturally responsive pedagogy, and stress and resilience.

Bertha Felix-Mata completed a bachelor's degree in psychology at California State University, Fresno. She earned a master's degree in public health with emphasis in behavioral sciences and health education at the University of California Los Angeles and a doctorate in education from Fielding Graduate University, School of Educational Leadership and Change. She has assumed key leadership roles in seeking and obtaining program funds to provide access to health care and educational programs specifically addressing disadvantaged populations. She volunteers as a speaker and volunteer board member for various organizations. Felix-Mata has served as adjunct professor for Fresno State University, where she taught in the department of Chicano Latino studies, women's studies, and the Health Science Department. Her lifelong community service has been recognized by the California State Legislature with the 2000

Woman of the Year Award for Community Services, the 2000 Educator of the Year Award, presented by the League of United Latin American Citizens, and the Administrator of the Year in 2011 by the Association of Mexican American Educators.

Emogene Johnson Vaughn is a professor in the Department of Health, Physical Education and Exercise Science at Norfolk State University, Norfolk, Virginia. Her teaching interests are in the areas of personal health and online instruction. Other responsibilities have included serving as a wellness coordinator and coordinating the health education service course. Her ongoing interests are in the evaluation of teen pregnancy prevention programs with the Virginia Department of Health.

Vickie D. Krenz is professor of public health at California State University, Fresno, where she has been a faculty member for twenty-two years. Currently she serves as the director of the master of public health program and is a former chair in the department. She is a well-known evaluator in the area of tobacco prevention and has received national recognition for her work in this area. She holds a bachelor's degree in religious studies, a master's degree in philosophy and religion, and a master of science in public health. She earned her PhD in health education at the University of Utah, Salt Lake City. She has served as vice president for the Southwest District for the American Association for Health, Physical Education, Recreation, and Dance.

Helda Pinzon-Perez, a native of Colombia, is a professor and director of the master of public health program at Fresno State. Her research interests are centered on multicultural issues in health care, international health, and holistic health. She teaches courses related to cultural competence and alternative medicine, as well as research methods. She holds master's degrees in public health and is a family nurse practitioner as well as a certified nurse educator.

D. Kay Woodiel is a professor and graduate coordinator for the health education program in the School of Health Promotion and Human Performance at Eastern Michigan University (EMU), Ypsilanti. Her research interest areas include cultural competence, health disparities, and LGBT health. She received her PhD in health science from the University of Arkansas, where her dissertation research focused on the mental health of mental health care professionals. She served as the director of diversity and community involvement at EMU for five years and has received the Ron Collins Distinguished Faculty Award for Service.

Kara N. Zografos is an associate professor in the Department of Public Health at Fresno State, where she also serves as undergraduate advisor for the community health option of the public health major. She teaches periodically for the School of Public Health at Loma Linda University. She has taught and written about diseases including asthma, protective alcohol-use behaviors among college students, and religion and health. She earned her DrPH in health education from Loma Linda University, her MPH in health promotion from California State University, Fresno, and her BS in health science from California State University, Fresno.

ACKNOWLEDGMENTS

We thank each of the contributors to this book for their dedication to the field of health education and for sharing their knowledge, experiences, and expertise in the chapter they developed. We extend our appreciation as well to the staff at Jossey-Bass for their careful review and assistance in the development of this book. Proposal reviewers Kathleen G. Allison, Denise Britigan, Bonnie Chakravorty, Quynh Dang, Heather Diaz, Amy Hammock, Cynthia Hatcher, Nishele Lenards, Kimberly Parker, Lori Pelletier, Augusta Villanueva, Ashley Walker, Charles M. Ware, Karen Winkler, and Kathleen J. Young provided valuable feedback on the original book proposal. Denise Britigan, Bonnie Chakravorty, and Kimberly Parker also provided thoughtful and constructive comments on the complete manuscript.

We dedicate this work to the countless individuals who have helped us along the way and have encouraged us to pursue our dreams. Special thanks to our families who through their support, understanding, and patience have made this dream a reality. We love you!

M.A.P.
R.R.L.

CHAPTER 1

IMPLICATIONS OF CHANGING US DEMOGRAPHICS FOR HEALTH EDUCATORS

Miguel A. Pérez
Raffy R. Luquis

The 1985 *Secretary's Report on Black and Minority Health* for the first time authoritatively documented the health disparities that different population groups in the United States experience (US Department of Health and Human Services, 1998). This seminal report provided the basis for the Healthy People initiative, which has established ambitious health benchmarks to be achieved at the end of their respective time frames (US Department of Health and Human Services, 2011).

Healthy People 2020 establishes the current national health targets, with four overarching goals to be achieved by the end of the decade (see box 1.1). Achieving these goals depends on collaboration among sundry segments of society to ensure that Americans not only have access to superior health care services but also incorporate preventive measures, including health education, into their daily lives.

The goals established by Healthy People 2020 require an understanding of *demographic shifts* and their impact on the health status of selected population segments. This chapter explores the impact of demographic changes on preparing a culturally competent health education workforce. It also provides a brief description of relevant cultural characteristics of each of the major ethnic groups in the United States.

LEARNING OBJECTIVES

After completing this chapter, you will be able to

- **Identify the four overarching goals in Healthy People 2020.**
- **Explain the demographic changes and population trends in the United States.**
- **Describe selected characteristics of the major racial and ethnic groups in the United States.**
- **Discuss challenges and opportunities for health educators.**

demographic shifts
Statistical changes in the socioeconomic characteristics of a population or consumer group.

BOX 1.1 HEALTHY PEOPLE 2020 OVERARCHING GOALS

- Attain high-quality, longer lives free of preventable disease, disability, injury, and premature death.
- Achieve health equity, eliminate disparities, and improve the health of all groups.
- Create social and physical environments that promote good health for all.
- Promote quality of life, healthy development, and healthy behaviors across all life stages.

Demographic Shifts

Demographic Characteristics

Data from the 2010 decennial census show that 308,745,538 resided in the United States in 2010 (US Census Bureau, 2011a) with steady population increases expected until 2050 (see table 1.1). Moreover, the Census Bureau projects that the nation will become more diverse and the majority of the population will be concentrated in urban areas, continuing a trend that started in the late nineteenth century.

Table 1.1 Projections of the Population and Components of Change for the United States, 2015–2050

Year	Population	Numeric Change	Percent Change
2015	325,540	3,117	0.97
2020	341,387	3,196	0.95
2025	357,452	3,217	0.91
2030	373,504	3,206	0.87
2035	389,531	3,209	0.83
2040	405,655	3,240	0.81
2045	422,059	3,315	0.79
2050	439,010	3,450	0.79

Source: US Census Bureau (2008a).

Note: Resident population as of July 1 for each year. Numbers in thousands.

race
The categorization of parts of a population based on physical appearance due to particular historical social and political forces

ethnicity
Pertaining to or characteristic of a people, especially a group (ethnic group) sharing a common and distinctive culture, religion, language, or the like

Race and Ethnicity

Census data project a continuing diversification of the US population in terms of *race* and *ethnicity* (see table 1.2). In fact, the Agency for Healthcare Research and Quality projects that members of underrepresented groups

Table 1.2 Projections of the Population by Sex, Race, and Hispanic Origin for the United States, 2015–2050 (in thousands)

Sex, Race, and Hispanic Origin	2015	2020	2030	2040	2050
One race	319,105	333,913	363,621	392,875	422,828
White	256,306	266,275	286,109	305,247	324,800
Black	42,137	44,389	48,728	52,868	56,944
AIAN	3,472	3,759	4,313	4,875	5,462
Asian	16,527	18,756	23,586	28,836	34,399
NHPI	662	734	885	1,048	1,222
Two or more races	6,435	7,474	9,883	12,781	16,183
Race alone or in combination:					
White	261,922	272,835	294,881	316,707	339,441
Black	44,906	47,748	53,519	59,454	65,703
AIAN	5,463	5,907	6,770	7,654	8,592
Asian	18,952	21,586	27,352	33,722	40,586
NHPI	1,325	1,480	1,814	2,181	2,577
Not Hispanic	267,828	275,022	287,573	297,432	306,218
One race	262,309	268,648	279,243	286,782	292,876
White	203,208	205,255	207,217	206,065	203,347
Black	39,916	41,847	45,461	48,780	51,949
AIAN	2,548	2,697	2,946	3,157	3,358
Asian	16,141	18,308	22,991	28,064	33,418
NHPI	497	541	628	716	803
Two or more races	5,519	6,374	8,329	10,650	13,342
Race alone or in combination:					
White	208,014	210,838	214,599	215,604	215,411
Black	42,267	44,697	49,518	54,339	59,318
AIAN	4,194	4,445	4,874	5,256	5,633
Asian	18,289	20,801	26,266	32,252	38,644
NHPI	1,051	1,158	1,375	1,600	1,827
Hispanic	**57,711**	**66,365**	**85,931**	**108,223**	**132,792**
One race	56,795	65,265	84,377	106,092	129,951
White	53,098	61,020	78,892	99,183	121,453
Black	2,221	2,543	3,267	4,088	4,995
AIAN	924	1,062	1,367	1,717	2,104
Asian	387	448	595	772	981
NHPI	165	193	257	332	419
Two or more races	916	1,100	1,553	2,131	2,841
Race alone or in combination:					
White	53,908	61,997	80,282	101,103	124,030
Black	2,639	3,051	4,002	5,115	6,385
AIAN	1,269	1,462	1,896	2,399	2,959
Asian	664	785	1,086	1,470	1,942
NHPI	274	322	439	581	750

Source: US Census Bureau (2008b).

Note: Hispanic may be of any race. AIAN: American Indians or Alaska Natives. NHPI: Native Hawaiian and other Pacific Islander.

are expected to make up more than 40 percent of the US population by 2035 and 47 percent by 2050 (Brach & Fraser, 2000). The shifts in the ethnic and racial distribution and the age distribution of the US population denote an urgent need for health educators to develop culturally appropriate programs (Luquis & Pérez, 2005, 2006; Luquis, Pérez, & Young, 2006; Pérez, Gonzalez, & Pinzon-Pérez, 2006).

The 2000 Census marked a shift in how ethnic and racial data are collected. The Census Bureau introduced a larger pool of options, which allowed individuals to select more than one ethnic or racial background. Although controversial, this measure allows the identification of individuals of mixed descent.

Foreign Born and Immigrant

According to the American Community Survey Five-Year Estimates (2006–2010), 12.7 percent of the US population, or some 38,675,012 people, were foreign born; that is, they were residents who were not US citizens at birth (US Census Bureau, n.d.). This category includes legal permanent residents (immigrants), temporary migrants (such as students), humanitarian migrants (refugees), naturalized US citizens, and persons illegally present in the United States (US Census Bureau, 2006). The remainder of the US population was born in one of the fifty states (85.9 percent) or Puerto Rico (1.3 percent).

The American Community Survey Five-Year Estimates (2006–2010) show that the majority of the foreign-born population, excluding those born at sea, came from Latin America (see table 1.3).

Approximately 72 percent of foreign-born individuals are legal immigrants, with over a third (37 percent) being naturalized citizens. It is estimated that some 8 million foreign-born individuals were unauthorized

Table 1.3 World Region of Birth of Foreign-Born Population in the United States, 2010

	Estimate	Percent
Europe	4,847,078	12.5%
Asia	10,747,229	27.8
Africa	1,466,454	3.8
Oceania	214,809	0.6
Latin America	20,565,108	53.2
North America	834,095	2.2

Source: US Census Bureau (n.d.).

immigrants in 2010, marking a decrease from a peak of 8.4 million in 2007 (Hoefer, Rytina, & Baker, 2011; Passel & Cohn, 2011).

Language

Almost 80 percent of the US population 5 years and older speaks only English (US Census, n.d.). Of those who speak a language other than English at home, 8.7 percent report speaking it "less than well." (See table 1.4 for a list of the major languages spoken in the United States.)

California has the largest percentage of residents who speak a language at home other than English (40.8 percent), followed by New Mexico (36.0 percent) and Texas (32.5 percent) (US Census Bureau, n.d.).

Table 1.4 Languages Spoken in the United States, 2010

Language	Percent
English	79.9%
Spanish	12.5
Other Indo-European	3.7
Asian and Pacific Islander	3.1
Other	0.8

Source: US Census Bureau (n.d.).

The Elderly

The median age in the United States in 2010 was 37 years of age; however, the fastest-growing age group is those age 65 and older (table 1.5). In fact, demographers estimate that the number of individuals in this age category will more than double by the middle of this century (US Census Bureau, 1995, 2010b). (See table 1.5 for age distribution in the United States in 2010.)

Table 1.5 Projections of the Population by Selected Age Groups for the United States, 2015–2050

Sex and Age	2015	2020	2030	2040	2050
45 to 64 years	83,911	84,356	84,296	92,000	98,490
65 years and over	46,837	54,804	72,092	81,238	88,547
85 years and over	6,292	6,597	8,745	14,198	19,041
100 years and over	105	135	208	298	601

Source: US Census Bureau (2010b).

The elderly population is characterized by several factors, including more females than males (57 percent and 43 percent, respectively, in 2010). Not surprisingly, as the population shifts, the elderly population is also expected to become more racially and ethnically diverse. The proportion of elderly in each of the four major racial and ethnic groups—white, black, American Indian and Alaska Native, and Asian and Pacific Islander and in the Hispanic-origin population—is expected to increase substantially during the first half of this century.

Gender

In 2010, 50.8 percent of the US population were females and 49.2 percent were males. Similarly, in 2010, 85.9 percent of females and 84.6 percent of males had obtained a high school diploma, and 27.5 percent of females and 28.5 percent of males had obtained a baccalaureate degree (US Census, 2010b).

Sexual Orientation

Gates (2011) has estimated that 3.5 percent of adults in the United States, or some 9 million people, self-identify as gay, lesbian, or bisexual. Moreover, approximately 0.3 percent of the population classify themselves as transgendered. These findings support several studies that have estimated that 5 to 10 percent of the US population is lesbian, gay, bisexual, or transgender (National Coalition for LGBT Health and Boston Public Health Commission, 2002). Nonetheless, it is important to understand that the estimate that 10 percent of men are gay and 5 percent of women are lesbian is based on Kinsey Institute data, which may not accurately represent the percentage of LGBT individuals in the population (Gay and Lesbian Medical Association and LGBT health experts, 2001).

Although the US Census Bureau asks respondents to identify their race and ethnicity, it does not ask about sexual orientation. The census, however, does ask several questions about respondents' household composition by marital status and gender of partner (table 1.6).

A review of 2010 census data by demographers at the Williams Institute of the University of California, Los Angeles School of Law (Gates & Cooke, 2011) indicates that there are 646,464 same-sex couples in the United States, or 5.5 per 1,000 households. The same analysis shows that 51 percent of females in same-sex couples and 49 percent of males in similar relationships classify themselves as spouses.

The relative lack of definite data on the size of this population and the fear that many LGBT people, especially youths, have concerning revealing their sexual identity make reliable data difficult to obtain (Perrin, 2002; RAND, 2010). This lack of information makes it increasingly difficult to develop, implement, and evaluate effective health education programs for this population group.

Table 1.6 Households and Household Type by Sex of Partner, 2010

	Estimate	Percent
Total households	116,716,292	100
Family households	77,538,296	66.4
Male householder	52,964,517	45.4
Female householder	24,573,779	21.1
Nonfamily households	39,177,996	33.6
Male householder	18,459,253	15.8
Male householder living alone	13,906,294	11.9
Female householder	20,718,743	17.8
Female householder living alone	17,298,61	14.8

Source: US Census (2010a).

People with Disabilities

According to the US Centers for Disease Control and Prevention (2011) some 71.4 million adults have experienced difficulty with at least one basic action (e.g., hearing) or a limitation on complex activity (e.g., difficulty with physical functioning). Table 1.7 shows some of the most common forms of disability experienced by Americans.

Table 1.7 Disabilities Experienced by US Adults, 2009

Disability	Number (Percent)
Hearing difficulty	37.1 million (16.2%)
Vision difficulty	21.5 million (9.4%)
Difficulty walking a quarter mile or unable to do so o	16.7 million (7.3%)
Difficulty with any physical functioning	35.8 million (15.6%)

Source: Centers for Disease Control (2011).

The data show disparities in disabilities by age and race/ethnicity (table 1.8). These differences may be exacerbated by cultural factors, lack of access to health care, or inability to follow medical directives.

According to Altman and Bernstein (2008), a person's disability or limitation has a direct impact on his or her perceived health status and ability to enjoy life. They note as well that disabilities and other limitations have an impact on a person's emotional status and self-rated health status (Altman & Bernstein, 2008).

Table 1.8 Percentage of Adults with Disabilities by Age and Ethnicity, 2009

	18 to 64 Years	65 Years and Older
Whites	24.4%	58.9%
African Americans	27.5	57.7
American Indian/Alaska Natives	31.1	61.7
Asians	12.9	43.2
Native Hawaiians/Pacific Islander	[a]	[a]
Two or more races	37.2	56.2
Hispanics/Latinos	19.8	56.2

Source: US Department of Health and Human Services (2011).

[a] Data are unavailable.

Demographics of Racial and Ethnic Groups

The following section provides a brief overview of the demographic characteristics of the major ethnic and racial groups in the United States. These descriptions do not, of course, apply to every individual who identifies as a member of a particular population group; significant differences exist within every racial and ethnic group. Rather, they offer overarching generalizations about the characteristics that members of each group share.

African Americans

African Americans, or blacks, are defined as persons whose lineage includes ancestors who originated from any of the black racial groups in Africa. Contrary to popular belief, African Americans make up a diverse group that encompasses individuals of African descent, Caribbean descent, and South American descent. African Americans are the second largest racial group in the United States, with approximately 42.0 million people, or 14 percent of the population. The majority of this population (38.9 million) identified as black alone, and the rest reported black in combination with one or more other races (US Census Bureau, 2011b). In addition, the black alone or in-combination population experienced a higher growth (15 percent) than the total population (10 percent) from 2000. The majority of people who reported they were black and one or more other races identified themselves as black and white (59 percent). This combination constituted the largest increase in the multiple-race black population.

According to the 2010 Census, 55 percent of the African Americans/black alone or in combination population reside in the South (US Census

Bureau, 2011b). In addition, this population represents over 50 percent of the total population in the District of Colombia and over 25 percent of the population in six states: Mississippi, Louisiana, Georgia, Maryland, South Carolina, and Alabama. The ten states with the largest African American population were New York (3.3 million), Florida (3.2 million), Texas (3.2 million), Georgia (3.1 million), California (2.7 million), North Carolina (2.2 million), Illinois (2.0 million), Maryland (1.8 million), Virginia (1.7 million), and Ohio (1.5 million).

In comparison with the non-Hispanic white population, the African American population has a higher proportion of younger people, its members are less likely to be married, and a large proportion of its households are maintained by women (US Census Bureau, 2010c). In 2010, approximately 82 percent of African Americans aged 25 and older had completed high school, and 18 percent had attained a bachelor's degree or higher level of education (US Census Bureau, 2010c), yet these percentages are lower than the percentages obtained by their non-Hispanic white counterparts.

Moreover, African Americans are more likely to be employed in service, sales, production, and related occupations (US Census Bureau, 2010c). Consequently, in 2010, the average African American family median income was less than the non-Hispanic white family median income ($32,068 versus $54,620), the unemployment rate was twice that of non-Hispanic whites, and almost one-third were living at the poverty level (Office of Minority Health, 2012).

In 2010, 44 percent of African Americans had employer-sponsored health insurance, and 28 percent relied on Medicaid, that is, public health insurance. These figures were lower than those for the non-Hispanic white population. According to the Office of Minority Health (2012), the death rate for African Americans in 2007 was higher than that for non-Hispanic whites for heart disease, stroke, cancer, asthma, influenza and pneumonia, diabetes, HIV/AIDS, and homicide. Finally, the life expectancy for African Americans is four years shorter than the life expectancy for the rest of the US population.

Hispanics

Hispanics are the largest minority group and one of the fastest-growing population groups in the United States.[1] In this group are all those of Cuban, Mexican, Puerto Rican, South or Central American, or other Spanish culture or origin, regardless of race. In 2010, 50.5 million people of Hispanic/Latino origin were living in the United States, which accounted for 16 percent of the total population (US Census, 2011c). Between 2000 and 2010, the Hispanic population grew at four times the rate of the total population, and estimates are that by 2050, they will account for 30 percent of the total population

(US Census Bureau, 2008b). Although Hispanics share a number of cultural characteristics, the many groups that make up this population are also in many ways culturally and socially variant. For example, although a majority of Hispanics speak Spanish and follow the Roman Catholic faith, they speak their common language in many different dialects and practice their common religion with many spiritual variations (Marin & Marin, 1991).

In 2010, among Hispanic subgroups, Mexicans ranked as the largest, at 63 percent of the Hispanic population, followed by Puerto Ricans, Central and South Americans, and Cubans (US Census Bureau, 2011c). Hispanics were more likely to live in the West (41 percent) and South (36 percent) and to reside in central cities within metropolitan areas (US Census Bureau, 2011c). Over 50 percent of the Hispanic population lived in three states: California, Florida, and Texas.

Hispanics are younger on average than non-Hispanic whites, with approximately one in three being under the age of 18 and with a median age of 27.3 years. The average age for the non-Hispanic white population was 40.3 years in 2010 (US Census Bureau, 2011c). In 2010, nearly three-quarters of Hispanics were US citizens, with three in five having been born in the United States. Three-quarters of Hispanics spoke Spanish at home, and one-third spoke English less than very well (US Census Bureau, 2010c).

In 2010, Hispanic households were more likely to be family households (78 percent) than were non-Hispanic white households (66 percent). While husband-wife families composed 50 percent of the households, one in five households was maintained by a woman with no husband present (US Census Bureau, 2010c). Moreover, approximately 62 percent of Hispanics aged 25 and older had graduated from high school and 13 percent had attained a bachelor's degree or higher level of education.

Hispanics were much more likely than non-Hispanic whites to be unemployed or to work in service, construction, and production jobs. Hispanics were also more likely to have a lower median income level and to live in poverty than non-Hispanic whites were (US Census Bureau, 2010c). In 2010, about 25 percent of Hispanics, in comparison to 10 percent of non-Hispanic whites, were living at the poverty level (US Census Bureau, 2010c). Moreover, Hispanics had the highest uninsured rates (31 percent) of any other racial or ethnic group in the United States. Still, the uninsured rate varied by Hispanic subgroup, with the Mexican and Central and South American subgroups having higher percentages of people without health insurance than the Puerto Rican and Cuban subgroups do (Office of Minority Health, 2012).

Hispanic health is influenced by factors such as the language barrier, lack of access to preventive care, and lack of health insurance. The leading causes of illness and death among Hispanics are heart disease, cancer, unintentional injuries (accidents), stroke, and diabetes. In addition, Hispanics are significantly affected by asthma, chronic obstructive pulmonary disease, HIV/AIDS, obesity, suicide, and liver disease (Office of Minority Health, 2012).

Asians

The Asian population in the United States encompasses many groups that differ in language and culture (US Census Bureau, 2012b). "Asian" refers to people who have their origins in the Far East, in Southeast Asia, or on the Indian subcontinent, including people from Cambodia, China, the Philippines, India, Japan, Korea, Malaysia, Pakistan, and Vietnam (Reeves & Bennett, 2003). According to the 2010 Census, 14.7 million people reported Asian alone as their race, and 2.6 million reported Asian in combination with one or more races. Thus, 5.6 percent (17.3 million) of the people living in the United States were identified as Asian, with Chinese (23 percent), Asian Indians (19 percent), and Filipinos (17 percent) accounting for about 60 percent of this population (US Census Bureau, 2012b). Moreover, the Asian population had grown more than four times faster than the US population as a whole since 2000 (US Census Bureau, 2012b). A recent report by the Pew Research Center (2012) described Asian Americans as "the highest-income, best-educated and fastest-growing racial group in the US, with Asians now making up the largest share of recent immigrants" (para. 1); it thus surpassed the Hispanic population as the largest group of new immigrants. Finally, in 2010, almost three-fourths of the Asian population resided in ten states: California (5.6 million), New York (1.6 million), Texas (1.1 million), New Jersey (0.8 million), Hawaii (0.8 million), Illinois (0.7 million), Washington (0.6 million), Florida (0.6 million), Virginia (0.5 million), and Pennsylvania (0.4 million) (US Census Bureau, 2012b).

The Asian population is younger on average than the non-Hispanic white population. In 2010, Asians had a median age of 35.6, about seven years younger than non-Hispanic whites (US Census Bureau, 2010c). Moreover, Asians were more likely than non-Hispanic whites to be married (58 percent) and to live in family households (74 percent), with a higher percentage of households maintained by married couples (60 percent). Although more than two-thirds of Asians were US citizens, either through birth or naturalization, approximately 67 percent were foreign born (US Census Bureau, 2010c). Most important, about 63 percent of foreign-born Asians arrived in the United States after 1990, and about 77 percent spoke a language other than English at home. Moreover, the proportion of those 5 years of age and older who spoke a language other than English at home varied among Asians: 55 percent of Vietnamese, 43 percent of Chinese, 22 percent of Filipinos, and 22 percent of Asian Indians (Office of Minority Health, 2012)

When it comes to education, approximately 85 percent of Asians twenty-five years and older had at least a high school diploma, and 50 percent had attained a bachelor's degree or higher level of education (US Census Bureau, 2010c). However, the educational level varied among Asians; for example, 73 percent of Taiwanese have attained a bachelor's degree (Office of Minority Health, 2012). Moreover, Asians were more likely to be employed in management, professional, and related occupations than were non-Hispanic whites—48 versus 40 percent, respectively. Nevertheless, the proportions of Asians employed in this sector fluctuated from 19 percent among Laotians to 67 percent among Asian Indians (Office of Minority Health, 2012). In 2010, the median income for Asian households was almost $13,000 higher than the median income for white non-Hispanic households ($67,142 versus $54,168). Still, about 12 percent of Asians lived below the poverty level, compared to 11 percent of non-Hispanic whites (US Census Bureau, 2010c).

In 2010, a high percentage of Asians (69 percent) had private health insurance coverage, but that also varied by subgroup. Private insurance coverage ranged from 79 percent among Filipinos to 48 percent among Hmong. Similarly, the uninsured status varied from 11 percent among Filipinos to 20 percent among Vietnamese (Office of Minority Health, 2012). It is also significant to note that Asian women had the highest life expectancy of any other racial and ethnic group in the United States, and Chinese women had the longest life expectancy among all the Asian subgroups. Still, Asians contend with several factors affecting their health, including infrequent medical visits and language and cultural barriers (Office of Minority Health, 2012). Finally, Asians are at higher risk than others for cancer, heart disease, stroke, unintentional injuries, diabetes, chronic pulmonary disease, hepatitis B, HIV/AIDS, smoking, tuberculosis, and liver diseases.

Native Hawaiian and Other Pacific Islanders

Native Hawaiian and other Pacific Islander (NHPI) refers to people who are natives of Hawaii and other Pacific islands, including people of Polynesian, Micronesian, and Melanesian backgrounds (US Census Bureau, 2012c). They differ in language and culture across many subgroups. According to the 2010 US Census Bureau estimate, close to 1.2 million Native Hawaiians (540,000) and Pacific Islanders (685,000) were residing in the United States in that year. Over 50 percent resided in two states: California and Hawaii (US Census Bureau, 2012c). In addition, the Native Hawaiian, Samoan, and Guamanian or Chamorro were the first, second, and third-largest NHPI groups in the United States.

In 2010, the median age for this group was 16 years less than the median age of non-Hispanic whites (26.2 versus 42.1). Seventy-six percent of the population was under the age of 44, with nearly 35 percent under the age of 18 (US Census Bureau, 2010c). In addition, approximately 43 percent of NHPI aged 15 years and older were married, compared to 53 percent of the non-Hispanic white population. The majority of NHPI households were families (74 percent), with 50 percent maintained by married couples. Almost 84 percent of the NHPI were US citizens by birth or by naturalization, and 91 percent of them spoke only English at home or spoke English very well (US Census Bureau, 2010c).

When it came to education, a high percentage of NHPI had graduated from high school (88 percent), and 20 percent had attained a bachelor's degree or higher level of education (US Census Bureau, 2010c). In 2010, almost 28 percent were employed in sales or office occupations, and 28 percent were employed in management, professional, and related occupations. The median household income for NHPI of $52,364 was similar to that for non-Hispanic whites. Still, 17 percent of Pacific Islanders were living under the poverty level, compared to 9 percent of non-Hispanic whites (US Census Bureau, 2010c).

In 2010, almost 61 percent of NHPI had private insurance and 28 percent relied on public insurance (Office of Minority Health, 2012). Data on the health status of this population showed that NHPI have higher rates of smoking, alcohol consumption, and obesity than other racial and ethnic groups do. Some leading causes of morbidity and mortality among this group are cancer, heart disease, unintentional injuries (accidents), stroke, diabetes, hepatitis B, HIV/AIDS, and tuberculosis (Office of Minority Health, 2012).

American Indians and Alaska Natives

In 2010, the US Census Bureau reported over 5 million people were American Indians or Alaska Natives (AIAN), entirely or in combination, representing slightly more than 1.7 percent of the US population. This group is made up of people who have their origins in any of the original peoples of North, Central, and South America and who maintain tribal affiliation or community attachment. In 2010, AIAN other than those living in Alaska were most likely to live in one of ten states: California, Oklahoma, Arizona, Texas, New York, New Mexico, Washington, North Carolina, Florida, and Michigan (US Census Bureau, 2012a). Moreover, the majority of the AIAN alone-or-in-combination population (78 percent) lived outside of AIAN reservation with the largest AIAN population. Among American Indians, Cherokee, with 15 percent of the population, was the largest tribal grouping, followed by Navajo (15 percent). Among Alaska Natives, the Yupik and the Inupiat groups were the two largest tribal subgroups (US Census Bureau, 2012a).

In 2010, American Indians and Alaska Natives were younger than non-Hispanic whites, with a median age of 30.2 years. American Indians and Alaska Natives aged 15 and older were less likely to be married than non-Hispanic whites (36.8 and 53 percent, respectively). Approximately 65 percent of American Indian and Alaska Native households were family households, with 39 percent maintained by married couples (US Census Bureau, 2010c). Although only 6 percent of American Indian and Alaska Native grandparents lived in the same household as their grandchildren, a large percentage of them (49 percent) were responsible for the care of the grandchildren. Finally, approximately 79 percent of American Indians and Alaska Natives aged 5 and older spoke only English at home (US Census Bureau, 2010c).

Information on educational attainment showed that approximately 80 percent of American Indians and Alaska Natives aged 25 and over had at least a high school diploma, and 17 percent had attained a bachelor's degree or higher level of education (US Census Bureau, 2010c). Those aged 16 and older were employed in a variety of occupations, including 28 percent in management, professional, and related occupations; 24 percent in sales and office occupations; and 23 percent in service occupations (US Census Bureau, 2010c). Still, the median household income of $36,623 for these two groups was $17,000 less than the median household income for non-Hispanic white households. Thirty percent of American Indians and Alaska Natives lived below the poverty level, and 24 percent had no health insurance coverage (US Census Bureau, 2010c).

There are 565 federally recognized American Indian and Alaska Native tribes and more than 100 state-recognized tribes (Office of Minority Health, 2012). Federally recognized tribes receive health and educational assistance from the Indian Health Service, a governmental agency that operates a comprehensive health service delivery system for 1.9 million American Indians and Alaska Natives who reside mainly in reservations and rural communities. The Indian Health Service funds thirty-four urban Indian health organizations, which operate at forty-one sites located in cities throughout the United States and provide medical and dental services; community services; alcohol and drug abuse prevention, education, and treatment services; mental health services; nutrition education; and counseling (Office of Minority Health, 2012). Nonetheless, American Indians and Alaska Natives frequently face issues such as cultural barriers, geographical isolation, inadequate sewage disposal, and low incomes that prevent them from receiving high-quality medical care. In addition, they are disproportionately affected by heart disease, cancer, unintentional injuries (accidents), diabetes, stroke, mental health issues, suicide, obesity, substance abuse, sudden infant death syndrome, teenage pregnancy, liver disease, and hepatitis (Office of Minority Health, 2012).

White

According to the Census Bureau, *white* "refers to a person having origins in any of the original peoples of Europe, the Middle East, or North Africa" (US Census Bureau, 2011d, p. 2). This encompasses individuals who self-identified as Caucasian, Irish, German, Polish, Arab, Lebanese, Algerian, and Moroccan among others.

The white population is the largest racial group in the United States, with approximately 223.6 million people, or 72 percent of the total population in 2010. However, that number includes members of the Hispanic population who self-identified as white. When this is taken into consideration, the white, non-Hispanic, population accounted for approximately 196.8 million, or 64 percent of the population, in 2010 (US Census Bureau, 2011d). This population showed the lowest growth in the previous decade, which, coupled with the great growth in other racial and ethnic groups, resulted in a decline in the proportion of the total population. Sixty percent of the white population lived in the South and Midwest; the four states with the largest white population were California, Texas, Florida, and New York.

The white population is older than the other racial and ethnic groups, with a median age of 39.2 years. In 2010, 66 percent of the white households were family households, with 51 percent in a married couple family (US Census Bureau, 2010c). Moreover, approximately 88 percent of white population aged 25 and older had graduated from high school, and 30 percent had attained a bachelor's degree or higher level of education.

In 2010, the majority of the white population (63 percent) was employed in management, business, sciences, arts, sales, and office occupations. As a result, the median household income of $52,347 was higher than the median household income of African American, Hispanic, and American Indian/Alaskan Natives (US Census Bureau, 2010c). Seventy percent of the white population had private health insurance, and the overall poverty rate was less than 13 percent. Finally, the top five causes of death for the white population are heart disease, cancer, chronic lower respiratory disease, stroke, and unintentional injuries (Heron, 2012).

Ethnic and Racial Group Stereotypes and Health Education

Health educators should not use the general characteristics we set out in the previous section to make generalizations or create stereotypes of individuals from those groups. In addition, health educators must determine if an individual fits the cultural characteristics of the group rather than use a stereotype (Fleming, 2006; Purnell, 2005). Stereotypes create myths that can influence how health educators view and think about certain racial and ethnic groups based on their religion, gender, occupation, or nationality (Temple, 2001). For example, a health educator could make the generalization that all Hispanic individuals practice the Catholic faith; hence, there is no need to educate them about contraception because this would go against their religious beliefs. This health educator would be stereotyping the individual based on one cultural characteristic of this population and would fail to address the individual's need.

Health educators can avoid stereotyping in these ways:

- Learn the characteristics of the different racial and ethnic groups and acknowledge the diversity within each group.
- Become aware of how they ask questions of the individual when addressing his or her needs.
- Educate others on how stereotypes affect the process of health education.
- Create a safe environment in which individuals feel free to discuss any health issue or concern without making judgments based on their racial and ethnic background.

Healthy People 2020 and Health Education

Healthy People 2020 is based on the previous Healthy People initiatives, with "a renewed focus on identifying, measuring, tracking, and reducing health disparities through determinants of health approach" (US Department of Health and Human Services, 2011). More important, Healthy People 2020 expanded on the previous goals by stating four new overarching goals (these are set out in box 1.1). As part of Healthy People 2010, the document focused on two important concepts: health equity and the social determinants of health. The US Department of Health and Human Services (2010) defined *health equity* as

> the attainment of the highest level of health for all people. Achieving health equity requires valuing everyone equally with focused and ongoing societal efforts to address avoidable inequalities, historical and contemporary injustices, and the elimination of health and health care disparities. (para. 1)

While efforts to achieve health equity have focused primarily on disease or illness and on health care, the absence of disease is not the same as good health. Thus, health educators need to understand the complexity of the relationship of health, biology, behaviors, health services, socioeconomic status, physical environment, discrimination, racism, literacy level, and legislative policies. These factors that influence individual or population health are known as *determinants of health*. Social factors, policymaking, health services, individual behaviors, and biology and genetics are determinants of health (US Department of Health and Human Services, 2011). Thus, in order to decrease health disparities and promote health equity, health educators must develop interventions that address multiple determinants of health. The authors of the following chapters discuss the factors of and strategies to address health disparities among different ethnic and racial groups.

Conclusion

Members of underrepresented groups face a number of barriers to obtaining optimal health. Health educators must work in conjunction with health care professionals not only to improve the health status of these groups but also to attempt to decrease the adverse health consequences for this population of the kinds of socioeconomic factors discussed in this chapter and also of events like the Tuskegee syphilis experiment, which willfully misled and denied available treatment to low-income African Americans in Tuskegee, Alabama. Health educators must be cognizant of the differences existing between and among ethnic and racial groups in the United States. The following chapters discuss many ways of reaching out to these diverse populations.

Points to Remember

- Demographic shifts in the US population involving race, ethnicity, age, and sexual orientation make it imperative for health educators to learn how to deliver high-quality and culturally appropriate health education and prevention programs.
- An accurate understanding of the needs of different ethnic and cultural groups will go a long way toward achieving the goal of reaching diverse groups with prevention programs.

Case Study

Almost all health promotion planning models require the collection of demographic data for the populations to be served. Using US Census Bureau data, create a demographic profile for the county in which you reside. Be sure to collect the following information:

1. Total population
2. Age distribution
3. Sex distribution
4. Ethnic and racial composition
5. Educational level
6. Socioeconomic characteristics
    a. Family incomes
    b. Occupational categories
    c. Estimated level of unemployment
    d. Poverty ratios
7. Health characteristics
    a. Vital statistics (numbers and rates of births and deaths)
    b. Incidence and prevalence of diseases (morbidity)
    c. Leading causes of death (mortality)
8. Any other data you consider important for understanding the population in your county.

KEY TERMS

Demographic shift

Ethnicity

Race

Note

1. The term *Hispanic* is used in this textbook as defined by the US Census Bureau. The term *Latino* is sometimes used synonymously to define this population group.

References

Altman, B., & Bernstein, A. (2008). *Disability and health in the United States, 2001–2005*. Hyattsville, MD: National Center for Health Statistics.

Brach, C., & Fraser, I. (2000). Can cultural competency reduce racial and ethnic disparities? A review and conceptual model. *Medical Care Research and Review, 57*(Suppl. 1), 181–217.

Centers for Disease Control and Prevention. (2011). *Disability and functioning (adults)*. Retrieved from http://www.cdc.gov/nchs/fastats/disable.htm

Fleming, W. C. (2006). Myths and stereotypes about Native Americans. *Phi Delta Kappan, 88*(3), 213–217.

Gates, G. (2011). *How many people are lesbian, gay, bisexual, and transgendered?* University of California, Los Angeles School of Law. Retrieved from http://williamsinstitute.law.ucla.edu/wp-content/uploads/Gates-How-Many-People-LGBT-Apr-2011.pdf

Gates, G., & Cooke, A. (2011). *United States Census snapshot: 2010*. Los Angeles: University of California, Los Angeles School of Law. Retrieved from http://williamsinstitute.law.ucla.edu/wp-content/uploads/Census2010Snapshot-US-v2.pdf

Gay and Lesbian Medical Association and LGBT health experts. (2001). *Healthy People 2010 Companion Document for Lesbian, Gay, Bisexual, and Transgender (LGBT) Health*. San Francisco: Gay and Lesbian Medical Association.

Heron M. (2012). *Deaths: Leading causes for 2008*. National Vital Statistics Reports, 60(6). Hyattsville, MD: National Center for Health Statistics. Retrieved from http://www.cdc.gov/nchs/data/nvsr/nvsr60/nvsr60_06.pdf

Hoefer, M., Rytina, N., & Baker, B. C. (2011, February). *Estimates of the unauthorized immigrant population residing in the United States: January 2010*. Retrieved from http://www.dhs.gov/xlibrary/assets/statistics/publications/ois_ill_pe_2010.pdf

Luquis, R., & Pérez, M. A. (2005). Health educators and cultural competence: Implications for the profession. *American Journal of Health Studies, 20*(3), 156–163.

Luquis, R. R., & Pérez, M. A. (2006). Cultural competency among school health educators. *Journal of Cultural Diversity, 13*(4), 217–222.

Luquis, R., Pérez, M. A., & Young, K. (2006). Cultural competence development in health education professional preparation programs. *American Journal of Health Education, 37*(4), 233–241.

Marin, G., & Marin, B. V. (1991). *Research with Hispanic populations*. Thousand Oaks, CA: Sage.

National Coalition for LGBT Health & Boston Public Health Commission. (2002, June 28). *Double jeopardy: How racism and homophobia impact the health of black and Latino lesbian, gay, bisexual, and transgender (LGBT) communities*. Retrieved from http://www.lgbthealth.net/downloads/research/BPHCLGBTLatinoBlackHealthDispar.doc

Office of Minority Health. (2012). *Data and statistics*. Retrieved from http://www.minorityhealth.hhs.gov/templates/browse.aspx?lvl=1&lvlID=2

Passel, J. S., & Cohn, D. (2011, February). *Unauthorized immigrant population: National and state trends, 2010*. Washington, DC: Pew Hispanic Center.

Pérez, M. A., Gonzalez, A., & Pinzon-Pérez, H. (2006). Cultural competence in health care systems: A case study. *Californian Journal of Health Promotion, 4*(1), 102–108.

Perrin, E. (2002). *Sexual orientation in child and adolescent health care.* New York, NY: Kluwer Academic/Plenum.

Pew Research Center (2012). *The rise of Asian Americans.* Retrieved from http://www.pewsocialtrends.org/2012/06/19/the-rise-of-asian-americans/

Purnell, L. D. (2005). The Purnell model for cultural competence. *Journal of Multicultural Nursing and Health, 11*(2), 7–15.

RAND. (2010). Few lesbian, gay, bisexual teens tell their doctor their sexual orientation, RAND study finds. Retrieved from http://www.rand.org/congress/newsletters/health/2007/03/sexuality_teens.html

Reeves, T., & Bennett, C. (2003). The *Asian and Pacific Islander population in the United States: March 2002* (Current Population Reports, Series P20–540). Washington, DC: US Census Bureau.

Temple, M. (2001). Creating awareness of the relationship between racial and ethnic stereotypes and health. *Journal of School Health, 71*(1), 42–43.

US Census Bureau. (1995). *Statistical brief: Sixty-five plus in the United States.* Retrieved from http://www.census.gov/elderlyissues.

US Census Bureau. (2006). *2005 American Community Survey.* Retrieved from http://factfinder.census.gov/servlet/ADPTable?_bm=y&-geo_id=01000US&-ds_name=ACS_2005_EST_G00_&-_lang=en&-_caller=geoselect&-format=

US Census Bureau. (2008a). *Projections of the population and components of change for the United States: 2010 to 2050.* Retrieved from http://www.census.gov/population/www/projections/summarytables.html

US Census Bureau. (2008b). *Projections of the population by sex, race, and Hispanic origin for the United States: 2010 to 2050.* Retrieved from http://www.census.gov/population/www/projections/summarytables.html

US Census Bureau. (2010a). *Households and families: 2010.* Retrieved from http://factfinder2.census.gov/faces/tableservices/jsf/pages/productview.xhtml?pid=DEC_10_SF1_QTP11&prodType=table

US Census Bureau. (2010b). *Selected population profile in the United States 2008–2010 American Community Survey 3-year estimates.* Retrieved from http://factfinder2.census.gov/faces/tableservices/jsf/pages/productview.xhtml?pid=ACS_10_3YR_S0201&prodType=table

US Census Bureau, (2010c). *Selected population profile in the United States 2010 American Community Survey 1-year estimates.* Retrieved from http://factfinder2.census.gov/faces/nav/jsf/pages/searchresults.xhtml?refresh=t

US Census Bureau. (2011a). *State and county quick facts.* Retrieved from http://quickfacts.census.gov/qfd/states/00000.html

US Census Bureau. (2011b). *The black population: 2010.* Retrieved from http://www.census.gov/prod/cen2010/briefs/c2010br-06.pdf

US Census Bureau. (2011c). *The Hispanic population: 2010.* Retrieved from http://www.census.gov/prod/cen2010/briefs/c2010br-04.pdf

US Census Bureau. (2011d). *The white population: 2010.* Retrieved from http://www.census.gov/prod/cen2010/briefs/c2010br-05.pdf

US Census Bureau. (2012a). *The American Indian and Alaska Native population: 2010.* Retrieved from http://www.census.gov/prod/cen2010/briefs/c2010br-10.pdf

US Census Bureau. (2012b). *The Asian population: 2010.* Retrieved from http://www.census.gov/prod/cen2010/briefs/c2010br-11.pdf

US Census Bureau. (2012c). *The Native Hawaiian and Other Pacific Islander population: 2010.* Retrieved from http://www.census.gov/prod/2001pubs/c2kbr01–14.pdf

US Census Bureau. (n.d.). *Selected social characteristics in the United States 2006–2010 American Community Survey 5-Year Estimates.* Retrieved from http://factfinder2.census.gov/faces/tableservices/jsf/pages/productview.xhtml?pid=ACS_10_5YR_DP02&prodType=table

US Department of Health and Human Services (1988). *Report of the Secretary's Task Force on Black and Minority Health.* Washington, DC: Author.

US Department of Health and Human Services. (2011). *About Healthy People.* Retrieved from http://healthypeople.gov/2020/about/default.aspx

CHAPTER 2

DIVERSITY AND HEALTH EDUCATION

Alba Lucia Diaz-Cuellar
Suzanne F. Evans

Significant demographic changes taking place in the United States are having a direct impact on health education and public health. Data from the US Census Bureau (2010) show that minority populations grew dramatically, from 20 percent to 58 percent, between 1980 and 2010. Traditionally the United States has been known for its *diversity* based on an influx of individuals from all over the world. In our modern world, however, there is much cultural dissonance. We have only to think of how complicated things become in a nation of immigrants such as ours. We are all Americans, yet in many ways we are a diverse society; we do not all speak the same language or eat the same foods. What we do have in common, besides our essential humanity, is our acknowledgment of the existence of other *cultures* around us. In other words, we share our diversity, and that has become a hallmark of our culture (Jervis, 2011).

This diversity extends into health education and public health. Indeed "other" cultures perhaps are not so far removed from our daily lives as they were not so long ago. Health education teachers increasingly need to find ways of talking about culture that take into account the multicultural classroom or community in which they teach. This requires a different kind of sensitivity, different tools, and different approaches. The shrinking globe means that we have to find ways of discussing differences that include the "different" in the discussion (Jervis, 2011).

Ramsey (2004) points out how educators can sometimes use the different cultural elements found in their

LEARNING OBJECTIVES

After completing this chapter, you will be able to

- Compare and contrast the concepts of diversity, race, ethnicity, and culture.
- Delineate key racial and ethnic groups in the United States: African Americans/blacks, Asians/Pacific Islanders, Native Americans and Alaska Natives, whites, and Hispanics/Latinos.
- Identify cultural practices among various groups.
- Identify the importance of the identification of the Ulysses syndrome in newly arrived members of ethnic minority communities and its relevance to health education.
- Define principles and practices of cultural competence.
- Discuss cultural nuances and relevance to particular groups.
- Recognize the significance of cultural competency and its importance to health care organizations and public health education.

diversity
A dynamic philosophy of inclusion based on respect for cultures, beliefs, values, and individual differences of all kinds.

cultures
Defined by the National Center for Cultural Competence (2002) as "an integrated pattern of human behavior that includes thoughts, communications, languages, practices, beliefs, values, customs, courtesies, rituals, manners of interacting and roles, relationships and expected behaviors of a racial, ethnic, religious, or social group; and the ability to transmit the above to succeeding generations."

own groups as starting points to discuss the basic concepts of culture: language, intergenerational transmission, cultural artifacts, and others. She also draws attention to the discontinuities, both linguistic and behavioral, that recent immigrants from other cultures have experienced. The unconscious reactions of peers and professionals to unfamiliar behaviors of individuals can also be stressful. Health educators often misinterpret the behaviors of immigrants (Jervis, 2011).

Diversity in American society has made it necessary to understand the health care and health promotion needs of various groups in an effort to provide optimal services and to understand health-seeking behaviors, attitudes, cultural nuances, and perceptions about health. Health educators must understand cultural nuances, cultural beliefs and values, and treatment-seeking behaviors in order to provide the best service to a diverse population. Addressing these factors will lead to overcoming barriers to care among racial and ethnic minorities and succeeding in offering high-quality services that can lead to the elimination of racial and ethnic disparities.

Our future depends on our ability to embrace and value diversity and dismantle all forms of ethnic oppression and discrimination. Taking positive stances on issues of diversity requires that we raise awareness of how racism exists and works. Aware of the suffering that cultural exploitation, social injustice, and cultural oppression cause, new generations of health educators need to be committed to practice respect and generosity in their thinking, speaking, and acting.

Defining Diversity, Race, Ethnicity, and Culture: Implications for Health Education

Diversity

ethnicity
Pertaining to or characteristic of a people, especially a group (ethnic group) sharing a common and distinctive culture, religion, language, or the like.

race
The categorization of parts of a population based on physical appearance due to particular historical social and political forces.

Diversity is a dynamic philosophy of inclusion based on respect for cultures, beliefs, values, and individual differences of all kinds. It respects and affirms the value in differences in *ethnicity* and *race*, gender, age, sexual orientation, socioeconomic status, linguistics, religion, politics, and special needs (Betancourt, Green, & Carrillo, 2002). It is also viewed as a commitment to understanding and appreciating the variety of characteristics that make individuals unique, promoting an atmosphere that embraces and celebrates individual and collective achievement (University of Tennessee Libraries Diversity Committee, 2003).

A new vision for diversity is needed that also examines not only the typical racial/ethnic or gender composition of a population, but also how different groups perceive and interact with the environment, political and ideological beliefs, and equity in access to opportunities and care (Clayton-Pedersen, Parker, Smith, Moreno, & Teraguchi,

2007). Paying attention to diversity is necessary in order to prepare all members of our society to seek common goals of a democratic society (Betancourt et al., 2002).

Within the realm of diversity are the distinctions of majority and minority groups. *Majority population* refers to the group with the larger percentage of the total population, with the remaining groups viewed as minorities. A minority group tends to be a group living within a society that is disadvantaged in terms of power, control of their own lives, and wealth. The dominant group within a social system has more power, control, and wealth (Hammond & Cheney, 2009). There are a number of ways the dominant group can treat its minority groups, including marginalization, the purposeful and at times subtle mistreatment of minority group members that leaves them out of most of the opportunities of society, often resulting in deprivation and exclusion (Hammond & Cheney, 2009).

Race

Historically, *race* refers to "biological variation including phenotypical differences in stature, skin color, hair color, facial shape and other inherited characteristics that may or may not be mutually exclusive in each individual" (University of Wisconsin-Fox Valley, 2006). Racial features are genetic and inherited and include elements such as skin color, hair color and texture, eye color, and susceptibility to specific diseases.

Society tends to assign people to racial categories not because of science or fact but because of opinion and social experience. "Race is an unscientific, societally constructed taxonomy that is based on an ideology that views some human population groups as inherently superior to others on the basis of external physical characteristics or geographic origin" (Williams, Lavizzo-Mourey, & Warren, 1994, p. 26). In reality, then, race is primarily, though not exclusively, a socially constructed category (Anderson & Taylor, 2009). It is not the biological characteristics alone that define racial groups, but how groups have been treated historically and socially. A race that powerful groups in society label as inferior is often singled out for differential and unfair treatment (Bamshad & Olson, 2003; Jervis, 2011).

Although the concept of race is socially meaningful, it is of limited biological significance. "Racial or ethnic variations in health status result primarily from variations among races in exposure or vulnerability to behavioral, psychosocial, material, and environmental risk factors and resources" (Williams et al., 1994, p. 26).

Another emerging category of racial identification is biracial or multiracial. In the 2010 US Census, approximately 9 million individuals, or 2.9 percent of the population, self-identified as multiracial. *Multiracial* is defined as persons who identify as belonging to two or more races. Rockquemore and Brunsma (2008) identify four major variations on biracial identity: the transcendent identity, which consciously denies having any racial identity; the singular identity, which identifies as either black or white rather than biracial; the border identity, which encompasses socially accepted racial categorizations of black and white; and the protean, which involves multiple identities based on contexts. Biracial or multiracial identity is a personal choice that has important consequences for social relationships between groups and in institutional infrastructures like health care (Makalani, 2001).

Ethnicity

Ethnicity is conceptually different from race and refers to people, their religion, languages, traditions, and heritage (Hammond & Cheney, 2009). *Ethnicity* refers to "a group or individual's concept of cultural identity which includes a wide variety of learned behaviors that a human being uses in his or her natural and social environment to survive, which may result in cultural demarcation between and within societies" (University of Wisconsin-Fox Valley, 2006, p. 1). People generally begin with identifying their membership with an ethnic group and then explaining their ethnicity as the relationship to a particular ethnic group. Wan and Vanderwerf (2009) state, "It is more helpful, we believe, to begin with ethnicity itself, viewing it as a sense of solidarity shared between people (usually related through real or fictive kinship) who see themselves as distinct and different from others" (p. 1). In other words, ethnicity refers to people who share common cultural characteristics and ethnic identity; they feel a sense of oneness and a shared fate. Ethnicity thus connotes shared cultural traits and a shared group history. Some ethnic groups also share linguistic or religious traits, and others share a common group history but not a common language or religion (Beyer, 2010).

An ethnic group consists of people who share a common orientation toward the world, whose members identify with each other on the basis of a real or a presumed common genealogy or ancestry, and who are perceived by others as having a distinctive culture (Hammond & Cheney, 2009). Ethnic groups distinguish themselves differently from one time period to another. They have a consciousness of their common cultural bond and typically seek to define themselves, but they also are defined by the stereotypes of dominant groups. An ethnic group does not exist simply because of the common national or cultural origins of the group, however. It develops because of their unique historical and social experiences, which become the basis for the group's ethnic identity. As a land of immigrants, the United States is home to many ethnic groups, perhaps more than are in any other nation (see chapter 1 for a discussion on the different racial and ethnic groups). Immigrants bring with them the special features of their cultures of origin and strive to maintain cultural ties to their places of origin while at the same time becoming American. We speak of Italian American, Irish American, and Jewish American cultures, for example. These ethnic groups form subcultures within the (larger) American culture.

According to the Office of Minority Health and Health Disparities (2009) and the US Census (2010), the non-Hispanic white population is still the largest major race and ethnic group in the United States, but it is growing at the slowest rate (Humes, Jones, & Ramirez, 2011). The Hispanic and Asian populations have grown considerably due to relatively higher levels of immigration. The US Office of Management and Budget's standards mandate that race and Hispanic origin (ethnicity) are separate and distinct concepts (Humes, et al., 2011). Latino/Hispanics are defined as persons of Mexican, Puerto Rican, Cuban, Central or South American, or other Spanish culture or origin regardless of race. As Ada and Beutel (1993) indicated, neither of these terms corresponds to or defines "the ever changing complexities inherent in the reality" of this heterogeneous population. "Hispanic" is an ethnicity rather than a race, and people who identify their origin as Latino may be of any race. Hispanic can be further classified by nationality, an identity that can be defined by a person's place of legal birth or citizenship status. Native Americans and Alaska Natives (labeled as American Indians by the Office of Management and Budget) are identified as indigenous to the United States or having origins in any of the original peoples of North America. Asian Americans and Pacific Islanders are persons having origins in any of the original peoples of the Far East, Southeast Asia, the Indian subcontinent, or the Pacific Islands. Asian Americans and Pacific Islanders are grouped not by language but because they arrived from Asia: Vietnam, Indonesia, India, Japan, Korea, China, Philippine Islands, and Samoa.

Culture

Culture is a concept that has many meanings. From a behavioral perspective, it is essential for the existence of a society and is an integral part of every society (Tylor, 1871). Through culture, people interact with others in the society. Culture comprises values and beliefs (Kroeber & Kluckholn, 1952); it is learned, shared, and transmitted from one generation to the next (Beyer, 2003; Chamberlain, 2005; Linton, 1945); and it helps organize and interpret life (Gordon, 1964). It includes thoughts, styles of communicating, ways of interacting, views on roles and relationships, values, practices, and customs (Robins, Fantone, Hermann, Alexander, & Zweifler, 1998; Donini-Lenhoff & Hendrick, 2000). It also includes a number of additional influences and factors, such as socioeconomic status, physical mental ability, sexual orientation, and occupation (Betancourt et al., 2002). According to Cross, Bazron, Dennis, and Isaacs (1989), culture has an impact on our lives: it determines on the most fundamental level the way in which we perceive our world, how we assign meaning to what we see, and how we respond to it. People of one culture share a specific language, traditions, behavior, perceptions, and beliefs. Culture gives them an identity, which makes them unique and different from people of other cultures.

Culture is therefore an organic concept that is evolving constantly. A clear definition comes from the National Center for Cultural Competence (2012), which defines *culture* as "an integrated pattern of human behavior that includes thoughts, communications, languages, practices, beliefs, values, customs, courtesies, rituals, manners of interacting and roles, relationships and expected behaviors of a racial, ethnic, religious or social group; and the ability to transmit the above to succeeding generations."

Banks and Banks (2001) have identified culture as having two distinct sections: macroculture and microculture. Macroculture is our common values and beliefs from living in the same country; microculture is the culture that specific group members share. The goal is to function successfully within both of these cultures (Banks & Banks, 2001). Within this context, culture affects every aspect of our lives. However, most people are so entrenched in their own culture that they do not recognize that other people live according to the norms of their own culture too (Brislin, 2000).

Our understanding of our own culture and cultures other than our own has an impact on how we interact with people not of our culture. Limited understanding, for example, can lead us to make mistaken assumptions and judgments and place unclear expectations on others. Much of what causes conflict or confusion occurs when people of different cultures interact with no awareness of the difference between their cultures. Cultural misunderstandings and conflicts arise mostly out of culturally shaped perceptions and interpretations of each other's cultural norms, values, and beliefs. Ethnocentrism is a negative result of culture and occurs when a person comes to believe that his or her culture is superior to all other cultures.

Although "culture is a shared set of belief systems, values, practices and assumptions which determine how we interact with and interpret the world," it is often not discussed. It can be said that "culture is like air: it surrounds us, we breathe it, and it gives us life, but we are unaware of it until we are thrust into an environment where it is different" (Roat, Gheisar, Putsch, and SenGupta, 1999, pp. 157–158). According to Kaminsky (2002), culture is like an iceberg where nine-tenths of culture is out of conscious awareness. We can therefore talk about two main layers of culture: the objective or visible layer, which includes aspects such as language, food, clothing, and customs, and the hidden, or subjective, deep part of culture that is grounded in values, cultural assumptions, nonverbal communication, thought patterns, and cognitive perceptions.

Usually people who settle in other nations adopt aspects of the dominant culture while at the same time striving to preserve their own as well. Often the individual adoption of cultural norms and values is influenced by one's degree of acculturation or assimilation: "Acculturation is the acquisition of a new cultural identity without ridding oneself of elements of the first culture, while assimilation occurs when the new culture is incorporated and the first one is lost or given up" (Roat et al., 1999, p. 168).

Cultural Practices and Their Impact on Health Education Strategies and Outcomes

A person's cultural background provides the foundation for his or her health beliefs and practices. While there are some behaviors which can be found in all cultures, their interpretations and applications vary from one culture to the next. A person's cultural practices are also influenced by his or her acculturation level. This section explores the implication of cultural practices as they pertain to the development and implementation of health education strategies.

Cultural Universals

Certain elements of culture are universal: certain behavioral traits and patterns are shared by all cultures around the world. For instance, all cultures classify relations based on blood relations and marriage, differentiate between good and bad, have some form of art, use jewelry, classify people according to gender and age, and so on (Kartha, 2011).

Dominant Culture

Just as cultures share many universal elements, they also differ on many dimensions, and these differences in basic values can result in cross-cultural miscommunication and strife. The culture of the dominant culture or group in power often dictates the accepted values. According to Samovar, Porter, and McDaniel (2013), dominant cultures use a variety of methods to consolidate their power, including fear, money, and force. White men, they argue, create the dominant culture in the United States. Although white men no longer represent a majority of US society, they are in enough powerful positions to continue to establish the mainstream culture.

Lynch and Hanson (1998) suggest that some of the values contained within the dominant culture of the United States include the importance of individualism and privacy; informality in interaction with others; an emphasis on the future, time, and punctuality; a high regard for achievement, work, and material acquisition; and competition. These values often conflict with other cultural groups that may instead value tradition, cooperation, tranquility, enjoyment of life, family obligation, and a present worldview.

Values Framework

Brown and Laundrum-Brown (1995) listed a number of areas of difference among cultures:

- Psychobehavioral modality (being or becoming)
- Axiology (interpersonal values such as competition or cooperation, direct or indirect communication, emotional constraint or expression, seeking help, or saving face)
- Ethos (beliefs in independence or interdependence, allegiance to self or family, harmony and respect or control and dominance)
- Epistemology or ways of learning (cognitive processes or affective domain)
- Logic or reasoning processes (circular or linear)
- Ontology, or the nature of reality (spiritual or objective)
- Concept of time (cyclical or event or clock based)
- Concepts of self (individual or collective self)

In 1987, Ho extended this thinking by examining the paradigms of people of color (Asian Americans, Native Americans, African Americans, and Latinos) in contrast to those of white European Americans in the areas of work/activity, concept of self, time orientation, nature and environment, and human nature. He found that people of color tend to live in harmony with nature, whereas European Americans see humans as superior and preferring mastery over nature. In work and activity, European Americans, Asian Americans, and African American were more doing oriented, while Native Americans and Latinos were characterized as "being to becoming" (Diller & Moule, 2005). European Americans are oriented to the future, while Latinos and Asians have a past-present orientation, and Native Americans and African Americans have a present orientation. In personal relationships, European Americans have an individualistic focus compared to the collectivist focus of the other groups (Ho, 1987; Banks & Banks, 2001). Finally, in the area of human nature, Ho found that European

Americans and African Americans view people as both good and bad, while the other three groups view humans as inherently good.

Another way to explore cultural differences is to examine the concepts representative of all cultures, which include silence versus talk and space and proximity (Mehrabian, 1972; Kimmel, 1978). Silence, for example, is interpreted differently depending on the culture. Silence in many Asian cultures may be interpreted as a dignified expression (Sue & Sue, 1990), "a desire to continue speaking after making a particular point" (Sue & Sue, 1977, p. 427), or a sign of respect to elders (Sue & Sue, 1977). In Latin American indigenous communities, silence is an expression of the beauty of being able to "have a dialogue with one's heart," to examine what is being said, and to reflect before responding. Most members of the European American culture feel uncomfortable with silence, and even children are encouraged to enter freely into adult conversations, to ask many questions, and to be assertive—behaviors that members of traditional cultures see as abrupt and disrespectful (Jensen, 1985). As health educators, it is important to understand the different interpretations and to be aware that silence or indirectness does not mean that persons of other cultures do not understand what is being said, but may be more accurately seen as signs of respect. Many cultural norms support indirectness as respectful behavior.

Levels of personal and interpersonal space are determined by cultural backgrounds (Susman & Rosenfeld, 1982). Hall (1976) identified four interpersonal distances zone characteristics of US culture: intimate, personal, social, and public. In the European American culture, individuals tend to be more comfortable when others stand far than when they stand too close (Goldman, 1993). Furthermore, in many cultures all over the world, personal space can be seen in terms of dominance and social status. The issues of proximity and space may lead to misunderstandings and confusion when people from different cultures interact. For example, members of some ethnic groups or cultures, where close proximity is the norm, may interpret the distance put by a European American health educator as a sign of coldness, rejection, or arrogance (Sue & Sue, 1977). It is important for health educators to understand these different interpretations and to be aware that silence or indirectness does not mean that persons of other cultures do not understand what is being said; rather, their silence may be more accurately seen as a sign of respect. Many cultural norms support indirectness as respectful behavior.

Levels of personal and interpersonal space are determined by cultural backgrounds (Susman & Rosenfeld, 1982). Hall (1966) identified four interpersonal distance zone characteristics of US culture: intimate, personal, social, and public. In the European American culture, individuals tend to be more comfortable when others stand far from them than when they stand too close (Goldman, 1993). Furthermore, in many cultures all over the world, personal space can be seen in terms of dominance and social status. The issues of proximity and space may lead to misunderstandings and confusion when people from different cultures interact. For example, members of some ethnic groups or cultures, where close proximity is the norm, may interpret the distance a European American health educator stands from them as a sign of coldness, rejection, or arrogance (Labarca, 2012).

Culture and Health

Health is defined by cultures as a group's view of the physical, mental, emotional, and social components required for a person to be considered healthy (Cushner, 2002; Giger & Davidhizar, 1991). It is therefore culturally defined, and certain health behaviors exist among cultures that should be explored (Rose, 2011). Various groups often share specific views of health and illnesses (Giger & Davidhizar, 1991). Accordingly, different cultural groups tend to have different health treatment options.

For example, although European Americans cannot be viewed as one culture and people, but a loosely associated series of subcultures, generalized beliefs nevertheless can be attributed to them (Smedley, Stith, & Nelson, 2002). European Americans tend to value individualism and independence; they are future oriented; they value practicality, efficiency, and promptness; they respect the intrinsic value of work; and they support competition (Stratishealth, 2012). Most European Americans also favor traditional Western medicine. They tend to practice preventive medicine, yet also suffer from a rise in rates of chronic diseases and diseases related to obesity. A small trend by European Americans to integrate a more holistic mind-body-spirit approach of care has begun.

For Asians/Pacific Islanders, the extended family has significant influence, particularly the oldest male in the family, who is often the decision maker and spokesperson. Maintaining harmony is an important value for Asian families and results in an avoidance of conflicts and direct confrontations. Because of these traits, Asians/Pacific Islanders tend not to disagree with the recommendations of health care professionals but nevertheless may not follow treatment recommendations (McLaughlin & Braun, 1998).

Hispanics as an ethnic group vary greatly in terms of race, religion, and national origins, which results in distinct cultural beliefs and customs. Nevertheless, some common characteristics include the respect of older family members, who are often consulted on important matters involving health and illness. There is a tendency to believe that illness is God's will or the result of divine intervention for previous or current sinful behaviors. Due to ties to indigenous cultures, some Hispanic patients may prefer the use of home remedies or folk healers (McLaughlin & Braun, 1998).

Similar to Hispanics, many African Americans place a great deal of importance on the family and church. The wide use of extended kinship bonds, which includes grandparents, aunts, uncles, and cousins, often determines the relationship with health care providers. In many cases, a key family member is consulted on important health-related decisions, and the church is an important support system (McLaughlin & Braun, 1998).

Like other ethnic groups, Native Americans place great value on family and spiritual beliefs. Generally Native American groups believe in being oriented in the present and valuing cooperation. However, the most relevant belief in terms of health care is their belief that a state of health exists when a person lives in total harmony with nature. As a result, illness is viewed as an imbalance between the ill person and natural or supernatural forces. Many contemporary Native Americans still use a medicine man or woman, known as a shaman (McLaughlin & Braun, 1998).

These examples of beliefs highlight the need to understand the effects of culture on health and health care. A framework for examining generally accepted values and health beliefs of specific groups is provided in table 2.1. We caution readers to view these profiles of groups as guidelines to avoid adding further to stereotypes. According to Diller and Moule (2005), "While in certain situations learning about a particular local community or cultural group can be helpful, a closer examination of the definition of culture highlights that these efforts—when broadly applied—are reductionist and can lead to stereotyping and oversimplification of culture" (p. 181).

Describing this general cultural framework of commonly held values within which some cultural groups operate provides a starting place for *cultural competence*. Within each group are subgroups and variations in cultural norms. A key aspect of cultural competency is understanding the nuances or subtle differences between cultures (Rose, 2011). It is therefore best to always work with people from an individual perspective (Masson, 2005).

cultural competence
The capacity to work effectively across racial, ethnic, and linguistically diverse groups.

Cultural Groups

Culture is a very important aspect and significant part of our lives, personally and professionally, and a crucial factor for ensuring effective and efficient services to our communities. Health educators who are inexperienced and new to the field may assume that certain behaviors are universal and have the same meaning. This may create major problems for culturally different communities. Therefore, to become culturally competent means learning about and understanding the particular needs of various ethnic groups.

The 2010 US Census listed fifteen racial categories, with the option of self-identifying as a multiracial category: white, black or African American, Native American or Native Alaskan, Asian Indian, Korean, Chinese,

Table 2.1 A Framework for Understanding Culture

	African Americans	Native Americans	Hispanic/Latino	Asian	Pacific Islanders	European American	Middle East
Health perspective	Harmony Illness stems from sin	Harmony with nature Illness stems from disharmony	Health is a gift from God	Harmony Balance	Harmony Traditional medicine	Biomedical	Based on good and evil
Pyschobehavioral activity	Action oriented	Being	Being	Action oriented	Being	Action oriented	Becoming
Axiology	Cooperation Direct communication Help orientation	Cooperation Indirect communication Save face	Cooperation Indirect communication Help orientation	Cooperation Indirect communication Save face	Cooperation Indirect communication Help orientation	Competition Direct communication Help orientation	Cooperation Direct communication Save face
Ethos	Independent Respect elders Strong kinship bonds Equalitarian family	Interdependent Respect elders Noninterference Extended family	Interdependent Respect elders Authority based Extended family Patriarchal	Interdependent Respect goal oriented Authority based Extended family Patriarchal	Interdependent collectivist Respect elders Extended family Patriarchal	Individuality Self-motivated Goal oriented Nuclear family	Interdependent Respect elders Authority based Patriarchal
Epistemology	Cognitive Kinesthetic	Affective Spatial	Cognitive Irrational	Cognitive Traditional	Affective	Cognitive and affective Easy to change	Cognitive Traditional
Logic	Linear	Circular	Circular	Circular	Circular	Linear	Linear
Ontology	Religious focus	Spiritual	Religion Fatalism	Spiritual	Spiritual	Religious	Religious
Concept Of time	Present	Cyclical Present	Past and present	Present	Past and present	Linear Future focus Punctuality	Past and present
Concepts of self	Collectivist Extended family	Collectivist Extended family	Collectivist Extended family	Collectivist Extended family	Collectivist Extended family	Individual Nuclear Family	Collectivist Extended family
Nature and environment	Connected with	Connected to and with nature Harmony	Connected to nature	Harmony with nature—yin/yang	Connected	Separate from nature Attempt to control	Connected
Human nature	Good and bad	Good	Good	Good	Good	Good and bad	Good and bad
Proximity	Close proximity	Close proximity	Close proximity	Close proximity	Close proximity	Close proximity	Close proximity
Silence versus talk	Active talk High volume	Silence	Silence	Silence	Talk	Talk	Silence

Japanese, Vietnamese, Filipino, Native Hawaiian, Samoan, Guamanian, other Pacific Islander, other Asian, and other races. One important US ethnic classification is Hispanic, a category that the US Census Bureau developed to describe people of "Latin" origin and their descendants (US Census Bureau, Population Division, 2003). The US Census Bureau indicates that "'Hispanic or Latino' refers to a person of Cuban, Mexican, Puerto Rican, South or Central American, or other Spanish culture or origin regardless of race" (Humes, Jones, & Ramirez, 2011, p. 3). As a categorical classification, Hispanic is at best an ambiguous one because there are nineteen countries between Mexico and South America (including a few Spanish-speaking island nations) and one country in Europe (Spain) that could be a nation of origin for Hispanic persons and their ancestors (Hammond & Cheney, 2009). Therefore, assuming that all US Hispanics are homogeneous is a mistake. According to the federal statistical system, race and Hispanic origin are two separate concepts. People who are Hispanic may be of any race, and people in each racial group may be either Hispanic or not Hispanic (US Census Bureau, 2003). Similarly, there is only one Middle Eastern ethnic group listed in the census data: Arabs. According to the census guidelines, Arabs are supposed to check white as their race or can write in "Arab" or their chosen ethnicity, although they are still counted officially as white. The Office of Management and Budget has established definitions for racial and ethnic groups. (See chapter 1 for a discussion on the definitions for ethnic groups in the United States.)

Immigrants and Migrants

When examining cultural groups, it is important to determine whether an individual is a migrant, first-generation immigrant, or refugee; the length of time he or she has lived in the country; and the reason precipitating the immigration. Determining the reason for migration may determine the immigrant's emotional state, resiliency levels. and ability to navigate the stressful changes, his or her acceptance into the new country, and whether she or he is allowed to stay. According to the International Organization for Migration (2004), an immigrant is a nonnational who moves into a country for the purpose of settlement. Migrants move to a country other than that of their usual residence for a period of at least one year, so that the country of destination becomes their new country of usual residence. Migrant populations are highly diverse; they originate from different regions of the world; represent many cultures and languages; and have differing migration patterns, legal status, and reasons for migrating. Their education levels and occupations range from manual laborers who may be illiterate to highly skilled professionals. Not surprisingly, this diversity translates into different health profiles for subpopulations of migrants (UN Statistics Division, 2013).

A population that merits discussion are undocumented immigrants. Kosoko-Lasaki, Cook, and O'Brien (2009) noted that 350,000 undocumented immigrants entered the United States in 2004: 81 percent were from Latin America, 9 percent from China, 6 percent from Europe and Canada, and 4 percent from Africa and other countries. Of this group, children under 18 years of age accounted for 17 percent of the undocumented populations in 2004.

Stages of Adjustment to the New Country

Unique among all groups are those categorized as newcomers. To some extent, all newcomers proceed through specific stages of adjustment as they strive to integrate into a new culture (Atkinson, Morten, & Sue, 1989; Cushner, 2002; Trifonovitch, 1977):

- *Honeymoon/euphoria stage.* Newcomers enter this phase at the time when the new intercultural experience appears to be exactly what they had hoped for.
- *Conformity stage.* As the newcomers encounter cultural differences and begin to adjust to the physiological and psychological changes that occur in them, they attempt to fit into the dominant group. They begin to experience increased tension and frustration.
- *Dissonance stage.* As the tensions and frustrations escalate due to the cultural differences and inability to be of the dominant group, individuals move into the stage of dissonance. This is a critical stage as ethnocentric reactions emerge and subjective cultural factors collide (Trifonovitch, 1977).
- *Resistance and immersion stage.* This reactive stage is characterized by either hostility or withdrawal from relationships and interactions. In the hostility reaction, individuals respond with anger toward the oppression and racism they had experienced from the dominant culture. Or they react with withdrawal from interactions with the dominant group and an emerging identification with their own group.
- *Introspection stage.* The migrants now begin to develop a deeper sense of self and support for the minority group. They develop a concern and empathy toward their own self and others of the same minority group (Atkinson et al., 1989).
- *Integrative awareness stage.* The newcomers have developed a selective appreciation of and trust toward some of the members of the dominant

group. This stage is considered a relief phase, accompanied by humor and joy as individuals begin to understand subjective cultural aspects. In this stage, also known as the stage of home or adaptation, they are able to interpret and interact from their own cultural perspective and that of the dominant group of the new country (Atkinson et al,, 1989; Cushner, 2002)

People travel through these stages in multiple ways and at varying time frames. Most require sufficient time to move through the stages and understand the subjective cultural changes in enough depth to live effectively.

It is essential that health educators understand this process of expecting that families and individuals will experience numerous changes and reactions that may impede their learning and full functioning.

The Special Challenges of Undocumented Immigrants

Health educators working with undocumented immigrants face challenges that are different from those they experience when working with documented migrants. First, the levels of stress that undocumented migrants face are higher. They live with the constant fear of deportation and being separated from their family. In addition, their status makes them vulnerable to exploitation.

A study of 416 documented and undocumented Mexican and Central American immigrants living in two major cities in Texas examined the differences between documented and undocumented Latino immigrants in three immigration-related challenges: separation from family, traditionality, and language difficulties. Results indicated that although undocumented immigrants reported higher levels of the immigration challenges of separation from family, traditionality, and language difficulties than documented immigrants did, both groups reported similar levels of fear of deportation (Arbona et al., 2010). Often the awareness of their vulnerability leads them to keep a low profile with authorities, which includes health care workers. Undocumented migrants often do not report any injustices (e.g., from legal authorities, landlords, and employers) or seek medical care because of their fear of being reported. Only when there is trust between an educator and migrant might he or she express that fear and disclose details about his or her predicaments.

To develop that trust, health educators must understand the stages of an immigrant's journey to adaptation in a new country and acknowledge the multiple and chronic stressors associated with the immigrant experience. They must attain "an ethno-relative perspective, an expectation that one will have significant adjustments to make when living and working with others as well as an ability to understand components of one's own and others' subjective culture" (Cushner, 2002, p. 88).

The Ulysses Syndrome

Migration is a complex undertaking that has profound human impacts. Since the second half of the twentieth century, the migration rate has soared and become largely characterized by the movement of lower-income individuals seeking prosperity or safety to wealthier countries (Achotegui, 2009). For millions of individuals, emigration presents stress levels that are so intense that they exceed the human capacity of adaptation. Immigrants become highly vulnerable to a syndrome characterized by chronic and multiple stress that has become known as the *Ulysses syndrome*. Ulysses refers to the Greek hero in Homer's *The Odyssey* who spent ten years living in a distant land facing countless adversities and another ten seeking to return to his home. The significance of Ulysses' story is such that the term *odyssey* is defined in multiple languages and multiple cultures around the world as a complex and treacherous journey marked by many changes.

Ulysses syndrome
A series of symptoms that affects migrants confronted with multiple and chronic levels of stress.

This syndrome is an emerging health concept in the context of globalization in which the living conditions of a large majority of immigrants have deteriorated dramatically. The Ulysses syndrome focuses on often misunderstood psychosocial challenges, including varied forms of recurring and protracted stress that immigrants experience in leaving their home country and adapting to a different environment. The key contribution of this concept is its elucidation of the direct correlation between the extreme levels of stress and the onset of psychological and psychosomatic symptoms.

Newly arrived migrants face a number of stressors:

- Social isolation, loneliness, and forced separation, especially when an immigrant leaves behind his or her spouse or young children
- A sense of despair and failure of the migratory goals and absence of opportunity
- Survival factor, that is, finding food and shelter
- The afflictions caused by the physical dangers of the journey undertaken and the typical coercive acts associated with journeys by groups that extort and threaten the migrants
- Discriminatory attitudes in the receiving country, including, in the case of undocumented immigrants, a constant fear of detention and deportation (Achotegui, 2009)

This combination of loneliness, the failure to achieve one's objectives, and experiences of extreme hardships and fear forms the psychological and psychosocial basis of the Ulysses syndrome.

As new immigrants deal with these factors, they move through seven levels of grief (Achotegui, 1999):

1. Grief for the family and loved ones
2. Grief due to encountering a different language and the subsequent inability to communicate needs, feelings, and ideas
3. Grief for culture, especially customs, sense of time, religion, and values
4. Grief for homeland, landscape, the light, the temperature, colors, and smells
5. Grief for social status
6. Grief in relationship to the peer group along with prejudices, xenophobia, or racism
7. Grief due to risk regarding physical integrity such as dangers in the migratory journey, dangerous jobs, or changes in diet

These seven levels of grief can be lived in a simple, complicated, or extreme way as the response to the migrant's efforts to adapt to the new environment (Achotegui, 2012).

Since the mid-1990s, an element of oppression and marginalization has especially hit immigrants from Latin America as the result of an increasing anti-immigrant sentiment across the United States. The expansion of border and interior enforcement operations by the US government and the movement of regulatory power over immigration to local governments have had dramatic economic, social, and psychological effects on immigrants, their families, and the communities where they live and work. These measures have hit anyone who may be identified as an immigrant from Latin America. Trust between the police and the community is eroding, and accusations of racial profiling and civil rights violations seem to be on the increase. Fearing apprehension and deportation, undocumented and legal immigrants sometimes are afraid to leave home, drive their cars, or go out in public (Hagan, Castrom, & Rodriguez, 2010).

Health Problems That Migrants Experience

As they undergo these various levels of grief, the lives and livelihoods of these first-generation migrants often experience health problems that arise as a result of the migratory and adaptation processes. The health effects are multiplied because the stressors are intense, multiple, and chronic; appear out of their control; occur with little social support; and result in symptoms such as sadness, recurrent nervousness, irritability, migraines, weariness, insomnia, fatigue, and gastric and osteophysical complaints. The stressful experiences during migration and the experience of becoming a racial/ethnic minority, subject to discrimination and racial conflict with other groups, damages the mental health of migrants and appears to have long-lasting effects on their mental health (Ornelas & Perreira, 2013). The health system often does not provide adequately for these patients because their problem is dismissed as being trivial or their condition is not adequately diagnosed.

In the United States, biomedical approaches view these symptoms not as a reactive response to the predicaments met by the newcomers but as signs of depression. First-generation immigrants are treated as being depressive or psychotic with a series of treatments that may turn into additional stressors. It is of paramount importance to understand that the symptoms these immigrants suffer pertain to the mental health sector of health care, which is broader than the psychopathology. Table 2.2 highlights how understanding the Ulysses syndrome forms a gateway between mental health and mental disorder.

Table 2.2 Understanding the Ulysses Syndrome

Mental Health	Ulysses Syndrome	Mental Disorder
Mental health is a state of well-being in which an individual realizes his or her own abilities, can cope with the normal stresses of life, can work productively, and is able to make a contribution to his or her community. In this positive sense, mental health is the foundation for individual well-being and the effective functioning of a community.	A series of symptoms that affects migrants confronted with multiple and chronic levels of stress. Note that if they are offered a job or an opportunity to move out of these levels of stress, they respond positively and take the opportunity. Therefore, they are not "depressed." The objective of intervention would be to avoid the worsening conditions, so that they do not suffer a standard mental disorder.	A mental disorder or mental illness is a psychological or behavioral pattern generally associated with subjective distress, anxiety, depression, or disability that occurs in an individual and is not part of normal development or culture. Such a disorder may consist of a combination of affective, behavioral, cognitive, and perceptual components.

Source: Schoeller-Diaz (2012).

Developing Standard Diagnostic Criteria

Standard diagnostic criteria applied to members of different cultural groups pose various levels of discriminatory practices. While in ethnomedicine the existence of the spiritual world is widely considered, standard diagnoses fail to capture the knowledge, attitudes, practices, values, and beliefs of those from other cultural groups. The diagnosis of depression fits into a particular Western medical and cultural model, which reduces the psychosocial problem to that of an individual who in the diagnosis is abstracted from a socioeconomic content and then held solely responsible for his or her mental well-being (Foucault, 2005).

Health educators who are working with migrant and refugee populations in the United States need to advocate for a sociocultural approach using culturally sensitive health educators alongside indigenous linguistically and culturally competent community health educators, or *promotoras*, to help newly arrived migrants who are experiencing the Ulysses syndrome. It is imperative that the health issues related to high levels of stress associated with immigration be addressed. The World Health Organization (2011) highlights this need: "In a world defined by profound disparities, migration is a fact of life and governments face the challenge of integrating the health needs of migrants into national plans, policies and strategies, taking into account the human rights of these individuals, including their right to health."

The concept of the Ulysses syndrome poses a powerful challenge to dominant approaches. It is a nonclinical and more comprehensive assessment of the plight of newly arrived immigrants who suffer from chronic and multiple stress syndrome. This calls for prevention at both the individual and community levels. With the culturally and linguistically appropriate approaches that community health workers (CHWs), *promotoras*, and culturally competent health educators use, immigrants are made aware of the importance of keeping strong ties with their language and culture, which are the most empowering factors in their overall well-being (Diaz-Cuellar, 2007). The CHWs and *promotoras*, many of whom have been immigrants themselves, play a vital role in supporting those going through the migratory process and help them achieve their goals without compromising their health (Ramos, Hernández, Ferreira-Pinto, Ortiz, & Somerville, 2006; Waitzkin et al., 2006). Based on their own experiences, CHWs can fortify the personal resilience of newly arrived migrants by employing techniques from their common culture to alleviate grief and generate a sense of empowerment (Schoeller-Diaz, 2012).

This social support becomes increasingly important in maintaining the mental and physical health of immigrants and their communities. Migrants who lack health support are exposed to a higher risk of developing severe mental disorders (Achotegui, 2012).

Although second-generation immigrants in the United States are more likely to achieve higher earnings than first-generation immigrants and are less likely to live in poverty (US Census Bureau, 2010), better health does not always follow. For example, depression in Latinos is highly correlated with the numbers of years they have spent in the United States. Latinos have strong family bonds that help them move forward in life in spite of their economic difficulties, fewer years of education, and lower socioeconomic status. However, as Latino immigrants acculturate, they have increasing difficulty in maintaining those family connections, the children begin to lose their cultural connection in favor of developing an American lifestyle, stress levels rise, and the incidence of illness increases (Chang, Garcia, Huang, & Maheda, 2010).

Building social cohesion in communities is essential to maintaining better health. Social support has a protective effect in preventing or decreasing the risk of development of illness, especially in second-generation immigrants confronted with acculturation and the impact of oppression and marginalization (California Newsreel and Vital Pictures, 2008; Marmot & Wilkinson, 2006).

Cultural Competence Principles and Practices in Diverse Settings

This section explores some principles related to service delivery to culturally diverse populations.

Cultural Competence

Cultural competence is based on the core principles of culture: that culture is a predominant force in people's lives, people are served in varying degrees by the dominant culture, they have personal identities and group identities, diversity within cultures is vast and significant, and each group has unique cultural needs that cannot be met within the boundaries of the dominant culture. Cultural competence manifests in individuals, communities, schools, and organizations and occurs developmentally in all settings. The role of health educators is to help individuals and entities move forward to higher levels of cultural competency. Health educators in fact have a responsibility to become culturally competent themselves (Luquis & Pérez, 2003).

Cultural competence is a set of congruent behaviors, attitudes, and policies that come together in a system or among professionals, enabling effective work to be done in cross-cultural situations (Roat et al., 1999). To be culturally competent, health educators need to be aware of their own cultural identity, cultural values, and cultural assumptions and determine how their identity and value orientation might affect their professional practice and relationship with other health educators from different ethnic groups. "Competence implies having the capacity to function effectively as an individual within an organization and society within the context of the cultural beliefs, behaviors, and needs presented by their communities" (Roat et al., 1999, p. 161).

Cultural competence is having the capacity to function effectively within the context of clients' cultural beliefs, behaviors, and needs of and establishing relationships with individuals and family before, during, and after care. Communication is essential, but it can be inhibited by language barriers, literacy levels, and cultural beliefs and alternative health beliefs or practices. Since cultural competence is a developmental process, it requires an understanding of several key social determinants: socioeconomic status and its impact on health disparities from a racial and ethnic vantage point; understanding treatment-seeking behaviors based on diversity and cultural nuances specific to cultural and ethnic groups; and taking into account that a lack of linguistic competence can be a barrier to providing optimal health care (Chamberlain, 2005).

Cultural and linguistic competence is a necessary response to the increasing ethically, culturally, and linguistically diverse populations and changing immigrant patterns in the United States. It is as well a tool to eliminate long-standing disparities in the health status of people of diverse backgrounds while helping to improve the quality of care and health outcomes. "Quite simply, health care services that are respectful of and responsive to the health beliefs, practices and cultural and linguistic needs of diverse patients can help bring about positive health outcomes" (US Department of Health and Human Services, 2012, p. 23).

Cultural Competence in Diverse Settings

Health educators are expected to work in diverse settings, including the community at large, schools, churches, clinics, and businesses, and with families and individuals, and must possess cultural competence to navigate the needs within those settings. They must examine how they address issues of diversity—a multiplicity of ethnicities, worldviews, lifestyles, and learning styles—and develop strategies that will increase their effectiveness. To reduce racial and ethnic disparities, health educators must help promote awareness about disparities among the general public, health care providers, insurance companies, and policymakers

Health educators work in communities. In this setting, they use programs and resources that address the cultural values, beliefs, and practices of various groups. Within the community setting, health educators must develop a pedagogy that bridges past experiences with the present and the future (Marbley, Bonner, McKissack, Henfield, & Watts, 2007). For example, they should be aware of potential mistrust by older African American males for testing and treatment based on memories of the invasive procedures done as part of the Tuskegee syphilis study.

A key strategy is to work with experts in the community CHWs, for example, acting as cultural bridges between communities and institutions.

They are trained to deal with the health problems of community members and work in close collaboration with health services. According to the World Health Organization and Global Health Workforce Alliance (2006), CHWs serve as connectors between health care consumers and providers to promote health among groups that traditionally lack access to adequate care. By identifying community problems, developing innovative solutions, and translating them into practice, "CHWs/Promotoras can respond creatively to local needs and achieve dramatic improvements by reaching the `hard to reach' community members and linking them to resources and advocating on their behalf" (Diaz-Cuellar, 2007, p. 197).

Two major settings within the community are schools and religious institutions. Within school settings, health educators must work collaboratively with teachers and within the policies and procedures of the school (McAllister & Irvine, 2000). Working within religious institutions also requires that health educators learn about various religious and spiritual beliefs and practices about health and healing. It may also require them to suspend their personal beliefs to work effectively with religious groups.

Health educators also may work directly with individuals and families and are often confronted with the dilemma of working with individuals and families who hold views in opposition to their own (Vaughn, 2008). Being culturally competent in this setting means listening to families and incorporating their views and beliefs into a collaborative solution to their health and lifestyle issues.

Finally, health educators are working more in businesses, hospitals, and college or university settings. Each poses challenges, including addressing the needs of multiple age groups, cultures, and education levels within multiple ethnic and cultural groups in one environment. Health educators must be able to relate to these diverse populations with acknowledgment, appreciation, and respect. They must also take into account differences in communication, life view, experience, and biases as they plan and then implement services and programs. In these settings, they must also balance the needs of the organization and administration with best practices in health education and promotion.

Cultural Competence: Working across Cultures

Cross-Cultural and Intercultural Competence

Intercultural competence and *cross-cultural competence* are interchangeable terms and can be defined as a complex set of cognitive, affective, and behavioral skills and characteristics that supports effective and appropriate interaction in a variety of cultural contexts, especially with those who are linguistically and culturally different from oneself (Bennett, 2011; Fantini, 2006). It is the ability to step beyond one's own culture and function with other individuals from linguistically and culturally diverse backgrounds.

Intercultural competence has been widely researched and explored. Ruben (1976) identified seven dimensions of intercultural competence: display of respect for other individuals, the ability to respond in a non-judgmental way, multiple orientations to knowledge, empathy, flexible and harmonizing behavior, management of interactions based on needs of others, and tolerance for ambiguity. The Developmental Model of Intercultural Sensitivity (DMIS) (Bennett, 1993; Paige, Jacobs-Cassuto, Yershova, & DeJaeghere, 2003) is used to explain how individuals respond to cultural differences and how their responses evolve. This model consists of six stages grouped into three ethnocentric stages (the individual's culture is the central worldview) and three ethnorelative stages (the individual's culture is one of many equally valid worldviews). The ethnocentric stages are denial of differences, defense with negative stereotyping and superiority of one's own culture, and minimization of differences. The ethnorelative stages of development lead to an acceptance of the cultural context of actions and have three phases: acceptance and respect of cultural differences, adaptation of a frame of reference to other cultural viewpoints, and integration of other worldviews into one's own. These six stages constitute a continuum from least culturally competent to most culturally competent, and they illustrate a dynamic way of modeling the development of intercultural competence (Intercultural Competence Assessment Project, 2007; Sinicrope, Norris, & Watanabe, 2007).

Hammer, Bennett, and Wiseman (2003) highlight a major distinction between intercultural sensitivity and intercultural competence: intercultural sensitivity is "the ability to discriminate and experience relevant cultural differences," whereas intercultural competence is "the ability to think and act in intercultural appropriate ways" (p. 422). Therefore, a key aspect of intercultural competence is "the ability to function in a manner that is perceived to be relatively consistent with the needs, capacities, goals, and expectations of the individuals in one's environment while satisfying one's own needs, capacities, goals, and expectations" (Ruben, 1976, p. 336). The acquisition of such competencies is important for personal enrichment, the ability to communicate well, and for providing health educators the capabilities necessary for promoting successful collaboration across cultures.

Cultural understanding comes through "dialogue," (Freire, 1987). Dialogue, according to Freire, should be based on mutual respect and the sharing of power among participants. One needs one's own cultural lenses to be able to have that "dialogue." In this dialogue, the worlds of the parties meet and partly overlap, forming the space where meaning is created and knowledge is generated (Ringe, 2008). To have a fruitful dialogue takes courage because it means making oneself vulnerable and putting one's own framework to question. The implications for health education practice are obvious. A culturally competent health educator has a constantly inquisitive and self-critical mind, is able to generate a wide repertoire of responses (verbal and nonverbal) consistent with the lifestyles and values of culturally different communities, and can build bridges between cultures by going beyond the obvious, visible, and surface of his or her own worldview.

Linguistic Competence

Linguistic competence refers to understanding the fact that many people in the United States do not speak English or have limited English proficiency and seek health care in environments where their predominant language is not spoken (Rose, 2011). The National Center for Cultural Competence (Goode & Jones, 2004) defined *linguistic competence* as "the capacity of an organization and its personnel to communicate effectively, and convey information in a manner that is easily understood by diverse audiences including persons of limited English proficiency, those who have low skills or are not literate, and individuals with disabilities."

There is a need for linguistic competence in health care and public health to ensure effective communication and optimal care take place.

Cultural Competence Continuum

Cultural and linguistic competence can be taught and learned and requires a commitment to individual personal growth. Challenging one's social conditioning and cultural incompetence is the essence of cultural competence as a dynamic developmental process (Goode & Jones, 2004). The core principles already noted are embedded at the six levels of the cultural competence continuum: cultural destructiveness, cultural incapacity, cultural blindness, cultural precompetence, cultural competence, and cultural proficiency. The cultural competence continuum, which is not intended to be viewed in a linear fashion, enables health care educators and public health entities to determine their level of cultural competence and what steps should be considered to achieve cultural proficiency.

Cultural Destructiveness

This first level, cultural destructiveness, is focused on seeing differences and stomping them out. Any perceived or real differences from the dominant mainstream culture are punished or suppressed and viewed as destructive to cultures and the individuals within these cultures. At this level, it is assumed that one's race or culture is superior and other cultures are subhuman, and one focuses on eliminating other cultures. In essence, it is using one's power to eliminate the culture of another. Examples range from genocide to exclusion of a group within a health education curriculum.

Cultural Incapacity

The second stage of cultural incapacity involves seeing the differences and viewing them as wrong. It is based on a belief in the superiority of one's own culture and in behavior that disempowers other cultures.

At this stage, cultural differences are neither punished nor supported, and no attention, time, teaching, or resources are devoted to understanding and supporting cultural differences. Individuals believe in the superiority of their own culture and behaving in ways that disempower another's culture. For example, they may support a disproportionate allocation of resources to certain groups, expect "others" to change, exclude groups from the health curriculum, or support a lack of an equal representation of staff and administrators who reflect the diversity in the community. The system remains extremely biased and may convey subtle messages to people of color that they are not valued or welcome.

Cultural Blindness

In this third stage, individuals see the differences in other cultures but act as if they do not. They do not recognize the cultural differences among and between cultures and act as if the differences do not matter or are inconsequential. They devote no resources, attention, or time to understanding cultural differences, which severely limits their ability to work effectively with a diverse population. For example, educators may experience discomfort in noting differences in cultures or believe their program does not need to focus on cultural issues because they see no diversity in groups. They believe that everyone learns in the same way and that they are not prejudiced. Culturally blind agencies are characterized by the belief that the dominant culture's traditional approaches are universally applicable and no changes or adaptations are needed.

Cultural Precompetence

By the cultural precompetence stage, there is recognition of the differences but an inadequate response to redress nonliberating structures, teaching practices, and inequities. Here individuals have an awareness of the limitations of their skills or an organization's practices when interacting with other cultural groups. For example, the health educator might delegate diversity work to others or use a quick fix, a packaged short-term program, or a single activity during Black History month–and believe he or she is responding well to the diversity.

Cultural Competence

In this fifth stage, individuals see the differences and understand the effects of the differences. They now interact with other cultural groups using the five essential elements of cultural proficiency, assessing culture, claiming the differences and valuing diversity, reframing the differences or managing the dynamics of difference, adapting to the differences and diversity, and changing practices for differences. They have learned to value and respect cultural differences and attempt to find ways to celebrate, encourage, and respond to differences within and among themselves while they pursue knowledge about social justice, privilege, and power relations in our society. The culturally competent educator seeks advice and consultation from the minority community. These educators now support ongoing education of self and others, model behaviors that look at another's perspective through another lens, and serve as advocates for all constituencies. There is continuing self-assessment regarding culture, careful attention to the dynamics of difference, and the use of multiple adaptations to better meet the needs of minority populations.

Cultural Proficiency

The final stage of cultural proficiency encompasses seeing differences and responding positively and in an affirming manner. Individuals focus on esteeming culture, knowing how to learn about individual and organizational culture, and interacting effectively in a variety of cultural environments. They recognize and respond to cultural differences and successfully redress nonliberating structures, teaching practices, and inequities. Here health educators support personal change and transformation, serve in alliances for groups other than their own, differentiate the needs of all learners, and incorporate the community in planning and implementing appropriate programs and services.

The Ongoing Journey

Cultural competency is an ongoing journey that can be led by health educators who use the cultural knowledge, prior experiences, and performance styles of diverse learners to make learning appropriate and effective for them. The degree of cultural competence a health educator achieves is based on his or her own growth in attitudes, policies, and practice. Attitudes change to become less ethnocentric and biased, policies change to become more flexible and culturally impartial, and practices become more congruent with the culture of the client.

Culturally competent educators (Gay, 2000):

- Acknowledge the legitimacy of the cultural heritages of different ethnic groups as worthy content
- Build bridges of meaningfulness
- Use a wide variety of instructional strategies connected to different learning styles
- Recognize and use learners' culture and language in instruction
- Respect learners' personal and community identities
- Acknowledge learners' differences as well as their commonalities
- Promote equity and mutual respect among learners
- Motivate learners to participate actively in their learning

According to Robins et al. (2011), there are six essential elements of culturally proficient instructors:

- Assessing culture by being aware of their own culture
- Valuing diversity by developing a community of learning with students
- Managing the dynamics of difference by appreciating the power of conflicts
- Resolving the conflicts
- Adapting to diversity by committing to continuous learning
- Institutionalizing cultural knowledge by working to influence public health organizations and systems

Cultural Resistance and Barriers

Culturally proficient health educators see the process of teaching and learning from the social context of the learners. They can also identify the barriers that each student faces and address the conditions that produce these barriers.

Nevertheless, there are multiple barriers to cultural proficiency. According to Robins, Lindsey, Lindsey, and Terrell (2011) most barriers derive from the following assumptions:

> (1) all people have access to knowledge, skills, and attitudes in the same manner and quality; (2) all people in the classroom or training room relate to everyone else the way they related to the instructor when he or she was a learning; (3) it doesn't matter whether the students are members of a historically entitled population (e.g. propertied white men) or of a historically oppressed group; (4) it doesn't matter whether the students are successful in this society or are less so . . .; and (5) the

> instructor has tremendous power and equal potential for influence over all the learners in the environment, regardless of the students' background or experiences or current situation. (p. 75)

There are a number of barriers to cultural competence. A major one is a sense of entitlement and unawareness of the need to adapt. Another is content or curriculum that projects only one cultural experience, segregates diversity as a separate course, does not customize materials for the needs of a group of learners, or contains inappropriate policies and practices. The delivery of instruction that emphasizes lower-order thinking skills is another. The expectations of the educator may often be a barrier if those expectations and preconceptions are based on stereotypical views of learners. Finally, culturally inadequate resources that continue and maintain inappropriate policies and practices and biased management practices that assume some cultural groups do not care about learning and subsequently result in a lack of services serve as barriers to cultural competence. It is imperative that in their practice, health educators recognize, examine, and attempt to eliminate these barriers.

Conclusion

Understanding diversity and developing cultural competence is a long-term and ongoing process. To be culturally competent, individuals need to learn about themselves, understand the community, and learn how to treat each person as a unique individual who is not necessarily representative of his or her whole group. Health educators need to examine the specific cultural values of groups as well individual information about a person's status as a newcomer, immigrant, or refugee. This delicate balance, not easy to learn, is essential to building a culturally competent framework from which to address the needs of multicultural communities in the United States. It is our best hope for a better future.

Integrating cultural proficiency practices into the individual practices of health educators and public health organizational policies is a call to action. When an individual adopts cultural proficiency, the essential elements become his or her standard practice. People and their organizations become culturally proficient when they practice specific strategies and behaviors consistently (Robins et al., 2011).

Cultural proficiency is an inside-out approach that begins by learning about oneself. Consequently, educators who are working to become culturally proficient must continue to learn, seeking information about the people they teach and integrating the culture and context of people with whom they work. One of the most difficult parts of this growth is processing one's own issues regarding power and oppression. This involves developing the capacity to confront personal issues with power and oppression, recognizing these issues and processing feelings, acknowledging biases and prejudices, and drawing new conclusions about oneself (Robins et al., 2011). In addition, health educators need specific skills and techniques to manage the dynamics of difference to facilitate effective cross-cultural communication and develop facilitation skills to foster healthy communication, encourage critical reflection, and engage with the learners as a community of practice.

Points to Remember

- Diversity refers to the makeup of a given population: its ethnic and racial backgrounds, age, physical and cognitive abilities, family status, sexual orientation, socioeconomic status, religious and spiritual values, and geographic location.
- Culture is an integrated pattern of human behavior that includes thoughts, communications, languages, practices, beliefs, values, customs, roles, relationships, and expected behaviors of a racial, ethnic, religious, or social group and the ability to transmit these patterns to succeeding generations.
- There are both cultural universals and many dimensions along which cultures differ. The dominant culture often dictates the paradigm of accepted values that include psychobehavioral modality; ethos; epistemology; logic or reasoning processes; ontology or the nature of reality; concepts of time and time orientation, of self, of nature and environment, and of human nature; paralanguage; proximity; high or low context; and nonverbal behavior.
- Although the US Census lists fifteen racial categories, there are generally accepted values of specific groups. Within each group are subgroups and variations in cultural norms. Health educators must explore newcomer, refugee, and immigrant status and treat each person individually.
- The Ulysses syndrome focuses on often misunderstood psychosocial challenges, including varied forms of recurring and protracted stress, experienced by immigrants in their departure from the home country and their adaptation to a different environment. The syndrome forms the gateway between mental health and mental disorder.
- Cultural competence is a set of congruent behaviors, attitudes, and policies that come together in a system or among professionals, enabling effective work to be done in cross-cultural situations. It is a developmental process and requires an understanding of several key social determinants. Cultural competency is one of the main ingredients in closing the disparities gap in health care.

- The cultural proficiency continuum is based on the core principles of cultural competence. Those principles are embedded in the six levels of the cultural proficiency continuum. The benefits of using the cultural competence continuum is that it enables health care educators and public health entities to determine their level of cultural competence and what steps to consider to achieve cultural proficiency.
- Integrating cultural proficiency practices into the individual practices of health educators and public health organizational policies is a call to action. People and their organizations become competent when they practice specific strategies and behaviors consistently.
- Cultural proficiency is an inside-out approach that first involves learning about oneself. Educators who are working to become culturally proficient must continue to learn, seeking information about the people they teach and integrating the culture and context of people with whom they work. It is essential that health educators maintain neutrality and acceptance when working with clients/patients who have viewpoints opposed to their own health educator.

Case Study

Judith, a healthy young woman from Latin America, migrated to the United States with her husband. They were fueled by the dream of offering a better future to their two young daughters, whom they left in their home country with Judith's family members. Shortly after arriving, Judith began experiencing nervousness, migraines, fatigue, and severe gastric pain. She was seen by an English-speaking general and primary physician, who, without providing her with any form of health education in her native language (a brochure, flyer, booklet, or basic information), prescribed her an antidepressant for the treatment of major depressive disorder, obsessive-compulsive disorder, and resistant depression. The medication did not alleviate her symptoms, which in fact stemmed from homesickness because her six-month-old son and two-year-old daughter were not with her. Rather, it worsened the initial condition and had undesirable side effects, including increased irritability, impulsive behavior, and negative thoughts.

1. What might be some cultural frameworks under which Judith operates?
2. What stressors has she experienced?
3. How does Judith's case fall within the Ulysses syndrome?
4. What problems does this case highlight?
5. What could you do as a health educator to assist Judith?

KEY TERMS

Cultural competency
Culture
Diversity
Ethnicity
Race
Ulysses syndrome

References

Achotegui, J. (1999). Los duelos de la migración: una perspectiva psicopatológica y psicosocial. In E. Perdiguero and J. M. Comelles (comp.) *Medicina y cultura* (pp. 88–100). Barcelona, Spain: Editorial Bellaterra.

Achotegui, J. (2009). *Emigrar en el siglo XXI: Estrés y duelo migratorio en el mundo de hoy. El Síndrome del inmigrante con estrés crónico y múltiple-Síndrome de Ulises.* Llançá, Spain: Editions El Mundo de la Mente.

Achotegui, J. (2012). *How to assess stress and migratory mourning. Scales for risk factors in mental health. Application to stress and migratory mourning. The Ulysses Scale.* Llançá, Spain: Ediciones El Mundo de la mente.

Ada, A. F., & Beutel, D. (1993). *Participatory research as a dialogue for social action.* Unpublished manuscript, University of San Francisco.

Anderson, M. L., & Taylor, H. F. (2009). *Sociology: The essentials.* Belmont, CA: Thomson Wadsworth.

Arbona, L., Olivera, N., Rodriguez, N., Hagan, J., Linares, A., & Wiesner, M. (2010). Acculturative stress among documented and undocumented Latino immigrants in the United States. *Hispanic Journal of Behavioral Sciences, 32*(3). Retrieved from http://www.mendeley.com/catalog/acculturative-stress-among-documented-undocumented-Latino-immigrants-united-states/

Atkinson, D. R., Morten, G., & Sue, D. W. (1989). A minority identity development model. In D. R. Atkinson, G. Morten, & D. W. Sue (Eds.), *Counseling American minorities* (pp. 35–52). Dubuque, IA: W. C. Brown.

Bamshad, M., & Olson, S. (2003). Does race exist? (2003). *Scientific American 5*(8), 78–85. Retrieved from http://schools.tdsb.on.ca/rhking/departments/science/bio/evol_pop_ dyn/does_race_exist.pdf

Banks, J., & Banks, C. (2001). *Multicultural education: Issues and perspectives.* Boston, MA: Allyn and Bacon.

Bennett, J. M. (1993). Toward ethno relativism: A developmental model of intercultural sensitivity. In R. M. Paige (Ed.), *Education for the intercultural experience* (pp. 1–71). Yarmouth, ME: Intercultural Press.

Bennett, J. (2011, February 20–23). *Developing intercultural competence for international education faculty and staff.* Paper presented at the Association of International Education Administrators Conference, San Francisco, CA. www.aieaworld.org

Betancourt, J. R., Green, A. R., & Carillo, E. J. (2002). *Cultural competence in healthcare: Emerging frameworks and practical approaches.* New York, NY: Commonwealth Fund.

Beyer, C. K. (2003). An investigation of multicultural transformation: Success of culturally diverse students in integrated school. *International Journal of Diversity in Organizations, Communities and Nations, 3,* 445–446.

Beyer, C. K. (2010). Innovative strategies that work with nondiverse teachers for diverse classrooms. *Journal of Research in Innovative Teaching, 3,* 114–124.

Brislin, R. (2000). *Understanding culture's influence on behavior.* Fort Worth, TX: Harcourt.

Brown, M. T., & Laundrum-Brown, J. (1995). Counselor supervision: Cross cultural perspectives. In J. P. Ponterotto, J. M. Casas, L. A. Suzuki, & G. M. Alexander (Eds.), *Handbook of multicultural counseling.* Thousand Oaks, CA: Sage.

California Newsreel and Vital Pictures (Producer). (2008). *Unnatural causes—is inequality making us sick?* [DVD] Available from http://www.unnaturalcauses.org/

Chamberlain, S. P. (2005). Recognizing and responding to cultural differences in the education of culturally and linguistically diverse learners. *Intervention in School and Clinic, 40* (4), 195–211.

Chang, D., Garcia, M., Huang, S., & Maheda, P. (2010). *The effect of assimilation on depression rates among generations of Latino immigrants.* Paper presented at Stanford Medical Youth Science Program 2010 Summer Residential Program. Retrieved from .http://smysp.stanford.edu/documentation/research Projects/2010/effectsOfAssimilationAmongLatinoImmigrants.pdf

Clayton-Pedersen, A. R., Parker, S., Smith, D. G., Moreno, J. F., & Teraguchi, D. H. (2007). *Making a real difference with diversity: A guide to institutional change.* Washington, DC: Association of American Colleges and Universities Press.

Cross, T., Bazron, B., Dennis K., & Isaacs, M. (1989). *Towards a culturally competent system of care.* Washington, DC: Georgetown University Child Development Center.

Cushner, K. (2002). *Human diversity in action: Developing multicultural competencies for the classroom* (2nd ed.). New York: McGraw-Hill.

Diaz-Cuellar, A. L. (2007). *The effectiveness of indigenous community health workers: International perspective.* Doctoral dissertation, University of San Francisco, CA.

Diller, J. V., & Moule, J. (2005). *Cultural competence: A primer for educators.* Belmont, CA: Thomson Wadsworth.

Donini-Lehnoff, F. G., & Hedrick, H. L. (2000). Increasing awareness and implementation of cultural competence principles in health professional education. *Journal of Allied Health, 29*(4), 241–245.

Fantini, A. E. (2006). *Exploring and assessing intercultural competence.* Retrieved from http://www.sit.edu/publications/docs/feil_research_report.pdf

Foucault, M. (2005). *El poder psiquiátrico*. Buenos Aires: Fondo de Cultura Económica.

Freire, P. (1987). *Pedagogy of the oppressed*. New York, NY: Continuum.

Gay, G. (2000). *Culturally responsive teaching: Theory, research, and practice*. New York, NY: Teachers College Press.

Giger, J. N., & Davidhizar, R. E. (1991). *Transcultural nursing, assessment and intervention*. St. Louis, MO: Mosby Year Book.

Goldman, A. (1993). Implications of Japanese total quality control for Western organizations: Dimensions of an intercultural hybrid. *Journal of Business Communication, 30*(1), 29–47.

Goode, T., & Jones, W. (2004). Increasing awareness and implementation of cultural competence principles in health professions education. *Journal of Allied Health, 29*(4), 241–245.

Gordon, M. (1964). *Assimilation in American life*. New York: Oxford University Press.

Hagan, J., Castrom B., & Rodriquez, N. (2010). The effect of US deportation policies on immigrant families and communities: Cross-border perspectives. *North Carolina Law Review, 88*. Retrieved from http://www.nclawreview.org/documents/88/5/hagan.pdf

Hall, E. (1976). *Beyond culture*. Garden City, NY: Anchor Press.

Hammer, M. R., Bennett, M. J., & Wiseman, R. (2003). Measuring intercultural sensitivity: The intercultural development inventory. *International Journal of Intercultural Relations, 27*, 421–443.

Hammond, R., & Cheney, P. (2009). *Intro to Sociology*. Freebook source. Retrieved from http://freebooks.uvu.edu/SOC1010/

Ho, M. (1987). *Family therapy with ethnic minorities*. Newbury Park, CA: Sage.

Humes, K., Jones, N., & Ramirez, R. (2011). *Overview of race and Hispanic origin: 2010 Census briefs*. Retrieved from www.census.gov/prod/cen2010

Intercultural Competence Assessment Project. (2007). Intercultural competence assessment. Retrieved from http://www.incaproject.org/index.htm

International Organization for Migration. (2004). *International migration law n°1—Glossary on migration*. Retrieved from http://www.iom.int/cms/en/sites/iom/home/about-migration/facts—figures-1.html

Jensen, A. R. (1985). The nature of the black-white difference on various psychometric tests: Spearman's hypothesis. *Behavioral and Brain Sciences, 8*(2), 193–253.

Jervis, N. (2011). *What is culture?* China Institute. Retrieved from http://emsc32.nysed.gov/ciai/socst/grade3/whatisa.html

Kaminsky, L. (2002). *Diverse teams for diverse people with diverse health issues: Malkam cross cultural training manual*. Office for Health Management. Retrieved from. https://pnd.hseland.ie/download/pdf/evpaper_kaminsky.pdf

Kartha, D. (2011). *What is culture?* Retrieved from http://www.buzzle.com/articles/what-is-culture.html

Kosoko-Lasaki, S., Cook, C., & O'Brien, R. (2009). *Cultural proficiency in addressing health disparities.* Sudbury, MA: Jones & Bartlett.

Kroeber, A. L., & Kluckholn, C. (1952). *Culture: A critical review of concepts and definitions.* Cambridge, MA: Peabody Museum.

Labarca, C. (2012). *Coursework for Familias Sanas y Activas.* San Diego: San Diego Prevention Research Center.

Linton, R. (1945). *The cultural background of personality.* New York, NY: Appleton-Century.

Luquis, R. R., & Pérez, M.A. (2003). Achieving cultural competence: The challenges for health educators. *American Journal of Health Education, 34* (3), 131–138.

Lynch, E. W., & Hanson, M. J. (1998). *Developing cross-cultural competence: A guide for working with young children and their families.* Baltimore, MD: Brookes.

Makalani, M. (2001). A biracial identity or a new race? The historical limitations and political implications of a biracial identity. *Souls: A Critical Journal of Black Politics, Cultural and Society, 3*(4), 83–112.

Marbley, A. F., Bonner, A., McKissack, S., Henfield, M. S., & Watts, L. M. (2007). Interfacing culture specific pedagogy with counseling: A proposed diversity training model. *Multicultural Education, 19*(3), 8–16.

Marmot, M., & Wilkinson, R. G. (2006). *Social determinants of health.* London: Oxford University Press.

Masson, V. (2005). Here to be seen: Ten practical lessons in cultural consciousness in primary healthcare. *Journal of Cultural Diversity, 12*(3), 94–98.

McAllister, G., & Irvine, J. (2000). Cross cultural competency and multicultural teacher education. *Review of Educational Research, 70*(1), 3–24.

McLaughlin, L., & Braun, K. (1998). Asian and Pacific Islander cultural values: Considerations for healthcare decision-making. *Health and Social Work, 23* (2), 116–126.

Mehrabian, A. (1972). *Nonverbal communication.* Chicago, IL: Aldine-Atherton.

Mehrabian, A. (1978). How we communicate feelings nonverbally. *Psychology Today.* Recording No. 20170. New York: Ziff Davis.

National Center for Cultural Competence of Georgetown University. (2012). *Foundations of cultural and linguistic competence.* Retrieved from http://www11.georgetown.edu/research/gucchd/nccc/foundations/index.html

Office of Minority Health and Health Disparities. (2009). *Black or African American populations.* Retrieved from http://www.cdc.gov/omhd/Populations/BAA/BAA.htm

Ornelas, I. J., & Perreira, K. M. (2013). *The role of migration in the etiology of depression among Latino immigrant parents.* Retrieved from http://paa2011.princeton.edu/papers/110066

Paige, R. M., Jacobs-Cassuto, M., Yershova, Y. A., & DeJaeghere, J. (2003). Assessing intercultural sensitivity: An empirical analysis of the Intercultural Development Inventory. *International Journal of Intercultural Relations, 27,* 467–486.

Ramos, R. L., Hernández, A., Ferreira-Pinto, J. B., Ortiz, M., Somerville, G. G. (2006). Promovision: Designing a capacity-building program to strengthen and expand the role of promotores in HIV prevention. *Health Promotion Practice, 7*(4), 444–449.

Ramsey, P. G. (2004). *Teaching and learning in a diverse world: Multicultural education for young children.* New York, NY: Teachers College Press.

Ringe, H. A. (2008). *Participatory action research: Cultural perspectives.* Master's thesis, Free University, Amsterdam, Holland.

Roat, C. E., Gheisar, B., Putsch, R., & SenGupta, I. (1999). *Cross cultural health care. Bridging the gap: A basic training for medical interpreters.* San Francisco, CA: SFCC Press.

Robins, K. N., Lindsey, R. B., Lindsey, D. B., & Terrell, R. D. (2011). *Culturally proficient instruction: A guide for people who teach.* Thousand Oaks, CA: Corwin Press.

Robins, L., Fantone, J., Hermann, J., Alexander, G., & Zweifer, A. (1998). Improving cultural awareness and sensitivity training in medical school. *Academic Medicine, 73*(10), S31-S34.

Rockquemore, K., & Brusma, D. (2008). *Beyond black: Biracial identity in America.* Boston, MA: Rowman & Littlefield.

Rose, P. R. (2011). *Cultural competency for health administration and public health.* Sudbury, MA: Jones and Bartlett.

Ruben, B. D. (1976). Assessing communication competency for intercultural adaptation. *Group and Organization Studies, 1*(3), 334–354.

Samovar, L. A., Porter, R. E., McDaniel, E. R. (2013). *Communication between cultures.* Boston, MA: Wadsworth.

Schoeller-Diaz, D. (2012). *Hope in the face of displacement and rapid urbanization. A study on the factors that contribute to human security and resilience.* Cambridge, MA: Harvard University Press.

Sinicrope, C., Norris, J., & Watanabe, Y. (2007). Understanding and assessing intercultural competence. *Second Language Studies, 26* (1), 1–58.

Smedley, D., Stith, A., & Nelson, A. (Eds.). (2002). *Unequal treatment: Confronting racial and ethnic disparities in health care.* Washington, DC: Institute of Medicine, Academies of Science Press.

Stratishealth. (2012). *Culture care connection.* Bloomington, MN. Retrieved from http://www.culturecareconnection.org/matters/index.html

Sue, D. W., & Sue, D. (1977). Barriers to effective cross-cultural counseling. *Journal of Counseling Psychology, 24,* 420–429.

Sue, D. W., & Sue, D (1990). *Counseling the culturally different: Theory and practice* (2nd ed.) New York, NY: Wiley.

Susman, N. M., & Rosenfeld, H. M. (1982). Influence of culture, language, and sex on conversational distance. *Journal of Personality and Social Psychology, 42*(1), 66–74.

Trifonovitch, G. (1977). Cultural leaning/cultural teaching. *Educational Perspectives, 16*(4), 18–22.

Tylor, E. B. (1871). *Primitive culture and anthropology.* Cambridge: Cambridge University Press.

United Nations Statistics Division. (2013). *International migration.* Retrieved from http://unstats.un.org/unsd/demographic/sconcerns/migration/

University of Tennessee Libraries Diversity Committee. (2003). *What is diversity?* Retrieved from http://www.lib.utk.edu/diversity/diversity_definition.html

University of Wisconsin-Fox Valley. (2006). *An anthropological view of ethnicity and race.* Retrieved from http://www.uwfox.uwc.edu/academics/depts/ant/perspective.html

US Census Bureau. (2010). *Census redistricting data (Public Law 94–171) summary file—technical documentation.* Retrieved from www.census.gov/prod/cen2010/doc/pl94–171.pdf

US Census Bureau, Population Division, Social and Demographic Statistics. (2003). *US Census Bureau guidance on the presentation and comparison of race and Hispanic origin data.* Retrieved from http://www.census.gov/population/www/socdemo/compraceho.html

US Department of Health and Human Services, Health Resources and Services Administration. (2000). *Transforming the face of health proficiency competence education: The role of the HRSA Centers of Excellence.* Washington, DC: Bureau of Health Professions, Division of Health Careers Diversity and Development.

US Department of Health and Human Services, Office of Minority Health. (2012). *What is cultural competency?* Retrieved from http://minorityhealth.hhs.gov/templates/browse.aspx?lvl=2&lvlID=11

Vaughn, I. J. (2008). Cultural competence and health education. In M A. Pérez & R. R. Luquis (Eds.), *Cultural competence in health education and health promotion* (pp. 43–66). San Francisco, CA: Jossey-Bass.

Waitzkin, H., Getrich, C., Heying, S., Rodriquez, L., Parmar, A., Willging, C., . . . Santos, R. (2006). Promotoras as mental health practitioners in primary care: A multi-method study of an intervention to address contextual sources of depression. *Journal of Community Health*, 36(2), 316–331.

Wan, E., & Vanderwerf, M. (2009). A review of the literature on ethnicity, national identity and related missiological studies. *Global Missiology English, 3*(6). Retrieved from http://ojs.globalmissiology.org/index.php/english/article/view/194

Williams, D. R., Lavizzo-Mourney, R., & Warren, R. C. (1994). The concept of race and health status in America. *Public Health Report, 109* (1), 26–41.

World Health Organization. (2011). *Health of migrants: The way forward.* Presentation at Summer Institute of Migration and Health, University of California, Berkeley.

World Health Organization and Global Health Workforce Alliance. (2006). *Scaling up saving lives: Task Force for Scaling Up Education and Training for Community Health Workers.*

CHAPTER 3

HEALTH DISPARITIES AND SOCIAL DETERMINANTS OF HEALTH: IMPLICATIONS FOR HEALTH EDUCATION

Kara N. Zografos
Miguel A. Pérez

LEARNING OBJECTIVES

After completing this chapter, you will be able to

- Define health disparities
- Discuss health disparities within the context of Healthy People 2020
- Explain the social determinants of health
- Discuss health disparity morbidity data by age, gender, and ethnicity/race

The implementation of preventive strategies, along with advances in medical technology, has resulted in improved life expectancy for most Americans. Despite improved health outcomes and increased life expectancies, the nation's health status will not reach an optimal level while health disparities continue to exist (Centers for Disease Control, 2009a). The Centers for Disease Control (2011a) defines *health disparities* as "preventable differences in the burden of disease, injury and violence, or opportunities to achieve optimal health experienced by socially disadvantaged racial, ethnic, and/or other population groups and communities" (para. 1). The National Institutes of Health (2010) defines the term in this way: "the differences in the incidence, prevalence, mortality, and burden of diseases and other adverse health conditions that exist among specific population groups in the United States" (para. 1).

The elimination of health disparities is a national priority established by the Healthy People initiatives. Healthy People 2020 considers health disparities and the excess mortality and morbidity associated with them as high-priority areas (Healthy People, 2010a). In 2000, Congress called for the establishment of the National Center on Minority Health and Health Disparities within the National Institutes of Health (NIH) and the development of a strategic plan to address the poor health status of minorities, low-income individuals, and those living in rural areas. The NIH now ranks health disparities third among its top five priorities (National Institute on Minority Health and Health Disparities, 2009).

This chapter describes health disparities and social determinants of health, including implications for health education, and reviews *health disparity* morbidity data by age, gender, and ethnicity/race. It concludes with suggestions on how to work with diverse groups of individuals and a brief case study that provides a hands-on opportunity for learners in a classroom or small group setting to practice critical thinking skills in helping a member of a minority group without health insurance.

health disparity
Differences in the incidence and prevalence of health conditions and health status between groups based on race/ethnicity, socioeconomic status, gender, disability status, or a combination of these factors.

Health Equality

Health equality refers to a person's ability to attain his or her full health potential without interference from his or her social position or ethnic/racial background (Whitehead & Dahlgren, 2007). The World Health Organization (WHO, 2008) has identified poverty, food insecurity, social exclusion and discrimination, poor housing, unhealthy early childhood conditions, and low occupational status as proxy determinants of most diseases, deaths, and health inequalities between and within countries.

Health inequality is a term that is often used interchangeably with the term *health disparities* in the scientific and economic literature to refer to summary measures of population health associated with individual or group-specific attributes such as income, education, or race/ethnicity. Health disparities result from various factors, including poverty, environmental threats, inadequate access to health care, individual and behavioral factors, educational inequalities, or any combination of these factors (CDC, 2011b). Poverty, a condition of insufficient resources for meeting basic needs of food, shelter, and clothing, is considered the single most substantial source of health disparities in the United States and is typically operationalized through the construct of socioeconomic status (Pettit & Nienhaus, 2010). According to House and Williams (2000), *socioeconomic status* refers to "an individual's position in a system of social stratification that differentially allocates the resources that enable an individual to achieve health or other desired goals" (p. 83).

International evidence shows that those with higher levels of education live longer, have better health, and pursue healthier lifestyles since educational level influences job placement, income, and access to health-related information and resources. The 2009 Commission to Build a Healthier America report suggests that at almost all educational levels, non-Hispanic white adults do better than all other racial and ethnic groups (Robert Wood Johnson Foundation, 2009). Although there is evidence of a relationship between these factors, the exact causes of health disparities are not completely understood. The Institute of Medicine (IOM), in its *Unequal Treatment* report (2002b), stated that "the sources of these disparities are complex, are rooted in historic and contemporary inequities, and involve many participants at several levels, including health systems, their administrative and bureaucratic processes, utilization managers, health care professionals, and patients" (p. 1).

Recent demographic changes, including an increase in the number of individuals belonging to minority racial and ethnic populations, an increase in the number of foreign-born residents, and an increase in the number of residents who do not speak English as their primary language, make it imperative that public health professionals and practitioners learn more about health disparities (US Census Bureau, 2012). Many of the existing strategies to address health disparities—specifically those that focus on only health education, health promotion, and improving access to health care by providing health insurance to the uninsured—are inadequate. For instance, Sudano and Baker (2006) found that health disparities for African Americans and Hispanics were largely attributable to income and education, and not merely individual behavior and limited access to health care. Health educators are encouraged to gain a clearer understanding of the causes for disparities, including the impact of differences in social determinants of health, in order to more effectively address those issues. In addition, it is suggested that health educators become more involved in health policy activities, including formulating health policies and engaging in political processes to determine these policies (Price, McKinney, & Braun, 2011).

Morbidity Indicators for Selected US Population Groups

The Healthy People 2020 leading health indicators are current public health issues that will result in future public health problems if left unaddressed. The selection process for these indicators was similar to the extensive collaboration efforts used to develop Healthy People 2020 and included participation by federal and nonfederal scientists, researchers, and health professionals. Reductions in the leading causes of preventable deaths and major illnesses would occur if these indicators were properly addressed, specifically those related to tobacco, health disparities, and overweight and obesity (Healthy People, 2010b). The following discussion highlights some of the morbidity indicators not mentioned elsewhere in this chapter.

Environmental Quality

A report from the WHO confirmed that approximately one-quarter of the global disease burden, and more than one-third of the burden among children, stems from modifiable environmental factors (Pruss-Ustun & Corvalan, 2006). The environment also plays a major role in quality of life, years of healthy life lived, and health disparities. Poor air quality is linked to premature death, cancer, and long-term damage to the respiratory and cardiovascular systems (Healthy People, 2010b). For instance, cross-sectional and longitudinal studies suggest an association between traffic-related pollution and increased asthma morbidity and cardiopulmonary mortality. There is also evidence that pollutants such as ozone and traffic exhausts are linked to new cases of asthma (Wong, Lai, & Chris, 2004).

In order to improve health and the quality of the environment, environmental standards and regulations need to be implemented and enforced, pollution levels and human exposure need to be monitored, and the risks of pollution need to be considered in decision-making processes (America's Environmental Health Gap, 2000).

Mental Health

The burden of mental illness is among the highest of all diseases in the United States. Approximately one in four adults in the United States reported having a mental health disorder in the past year, and one in seventeen reported having a serious mental illness. Mental health disorders affect children and adolescents at an alarming rate, with one in five having a mental health disorder in 2010, the most common of which was attention deficit hyperactivity disorder (ADHD) (Reeves et al., 2011). According to the CDC's *Morbidity Mortality Weekly Report* (MMWR), the percentage of children 14 to 17 years of age with a parent-reported ADHD diagnosis increased from 7.8 to 9.5 percent from 2003 to 2007, representing a 21.8 percent increase (Visser, Bitsko, Danielson, & Perou, 2010). Prevention of mental health disorders is a growing area of research and practice (Healthy People, 2010b).

Nutrition, Physical Activity, and Obesity

Good nutrition, physical activity, and a healthy body weight are essential components of an individual's overall health and well-being (Healthy People, 2010b). Most Americans, however, do not follow a healthy diet and are not physically active at levels necessary to maintain good health. For instance, fewer than one in three adults, and an even lower proportion of adolescents, eat the recommended portions of vegetables each day (CDC, 2009b). In addition, 81.6 percent of adults and 81.8 percent of adolescents do not get the recommended amount of physical activity (US Department of Health and Human Services, 2008). As a result of these lifestyle choices, obesity rates have increased dramatically, with approximately one in three adults and one in six children and adolescents considered obese. Obesity-related conditions, including heart disease, stroke, and type 2 diabetes, are among some of the leading causes of death. Furthermore, costs associated with obesity pose a significant burden on the US medical care delivery system (Healthy People, 2010b).

Oral Health

Oral diseases cause pain and disability for millions of Americans (Healthy People, 2010b). According to the CDC (2011c), tooth decay affects children in the United States more than any other chronic infectious disease. The National Health and Nutrition Examination Survey, 2005–2008, found that the prevalence of untreated dental caries varied significantly by poverty level for all age groups (see table 3.1). In addition, 52 percent of Mexican Americans have retained their permanent teeth compared to 51 percent of non-Hispanic whites and 38 percent of African Americans (Dye, Li, & Beltrán-Aguilar, 2012).

Table 3.1 Prevalence of Untreated Dental Caries and Existing Dental Restorations in Teeth, by Sex, Race and Ethnicity, and Poverty Level: United States, 2005–2008

	Untreated Dental Caries				Dental Restoration			
Characteristic	**Total**	**Ages 5–19**	**Ages 20–64**	**Ages 65 and Over**	**Total**	**Ages 5–19**	**Ages 20–64**	**Ages 65 and over**
Total	21.5	16.6	23.7	19.9	75.5	45.9	84.3	88.5
Race and ethnicity								
Non-Hispanic white[a]	17.8	13.3	19.3	17.8	80.1	46.2	88.8	91.6
Non-Hispanic black	34.2**	22.6**	39.7**	35.8**	62.6**	40.4**	73.1**	63.7**
Mexican American	31.1**	22.4**	35.2**	36.4**	61.8**	50.1	67.4**	69.3**
Poverty level								
Below 100 percent	35.8**	25.4**	41.9	41.3**	62.7**	48.6	71.5**	63.3**
100 percent to less than 200 percent	30.5**	19.3**	37.7**	22.5**	8.8**	46.3	75.1**	85.6**
200 percent or higher[a]	15.5	12.1	16.6	15.3	80.2	44.5	89.0	92.6
Sex								
Male	24.6***	17.6	27.2**	25.1**	72.1**	44.8	80.5**	86.3**
Female[a]	18.6	15.5	20.2	15.6	78.7	47.0	88.0	90.4

Source: Dye, Li, and Beltrán-Aguilar (2012).

[a] Reference group.

** $p < 0.05$.

A growing body of research also suggests a link between oral health, specifically periodontal disease, and several chronic diseases, including diabetes, heart disease, and stroke (American Dental Association, 2009). Although these conditions can be prevented with regular visits to the dentist, only 44.5 percent of individuals 2 years of age and older had a dental visit in the past twelve months. Disparities in access to oral health also exist, with non-Hispanic whites, those with higher incomes, and those with higher education levels being more likely to report visiting a dentist in the past twelve months compared to other groups (Healthy People, 2010b).

Tobacco

Tobacco use is the single most preventable cause of disease, disability, and death in the United States and is responsible for an estimated 443,000 premature deaths each year (CDC, 2011d). Tobacco is also one of the most costly public health challenges, with cigarette smoking costing more than $193 million in medical care costs, and secondhand smoke costing an additional $10 million (CDC, 2008). Disparities in tobacco use also exist, with the lowest rates of tobacco use reported among the Asian population (9.7 percent) compared to non-Hispanic whites (22.6 percent) and Native Hawaiian or other Pacific Islanders (22.6 percent). In 2008, the prevalence of smoking was lower among those with higher education and family income levels compared to those with lower levels of education and income.

A range of social, environmental, psychological, and genetic factors are associated with tobacco use, including gender, race, ethnicity, age, income level, educational attainment, and geographic location (Healthy People, 2010b). Smoke-free protections such as bans on smoking in public places, tobacco prices and taxes, and the implementation of effective tobacco prevention programs all influence tobacco use (American Lung Association, 2012).

Race/Ethnicity, Gender, Age, and Disability

Health disparities refers to differences in the incidence and prevalence of health conditions and health status between groups based on race/ethnicity, socioeconomic status, gender, disability status, or a combination of these factors. In this section, we explore health disparities from a variety of angles, including race/ethnicity, gender, age, and disability. Eliminating disparities will require new knowledge regarding the determinants of disease, causes of health disparities, and effective interventions for prevention and treatment.

Focus Areas of Disparities

The US Department of Health and Human Services has selected six areas in which racial and ethnic minority groups experience significant disparities in health access and outcome: infant mortality, cancer screening and management, cardiovascular disease, diabetes, HIV infections and AIDS, and immunizations (CDC, 2009c).

Infant Mortality

The infant mortality rate, which is the rate at which babies less than 1 year of age die, is used to compare the health and well-being of populations across and within countries (CDC, 2009c). The infant mortality rate in the United States has continued to decline over the past several decades from 26.0 per 1,000 live births in 1960 to 6.06 per 1,000 in 2011 (Kaiser Family Foundation, 2010). Despite this decline, the United States is still ranked thirty-fourth in the world in terms of infant mortality, which is largely due to the disparities that continue to exist among various racial and ethnic groups, specifically among the African American population. For instance, compared to non-Hispanic whites, African Americans have a 2.5 times higher infant mortality rate. African American infants are also four times more likely than non-Hispanic white infants to die due to complications associated with low birth weight. This disparity between white and African American infants has persisted over the past two decades (CDC, 2009d).

Cancer Screening and Management

Cancer is the second leading cause of death in the United States, and it is expected that 577,190 Americans will die from cancer in 2012 (American Cancer Society, 2012). Cancer risk can be addressed through lifestyle modifications, including changes in diet and nutrition, exercise, and tobacco use. Since health educators are trained in theories of behavior change, they are in a unique position to begin to address some of these disparities.

In terms of breast and cervical cancers, African American women continue to have higher mortality rates compared to other racial/ethnic groups, which may be due to not receiving regular mammograms or Pap screenings and follow-up treatment (American Cancer Society, 2008). In addition, compared to all other ethnic groups, Vietnamese American women have higher cervical cancer incidence rates (CDC, 2010). Low rates of screening and treatment for women of other ethnic groups, including Hispanics or Latinas, American Indians or Alaska Natives, Asian Americans, and Pacific Islanders, are largely due to limited access to health care services, language barriers, cultural barriers, or a combination of these factors (CDC, 2009e).

Cardiovascular Disease

Heart disease and stroke are the leading causes of death for all racial and ethnic groups in the United States; however, minority and low-income populations experience a disproportionate burden of death and disability from cardiovascular disease (CVD). For instance, in 2008, African Americans were 30 percent more likely than whites to die from heart disease and 1.6 times more likely than whites to have high blood pressure (CDC, 2011e).

Numerous studies are being conducted to investigate CVD in these populations. For instance, the Multi-Ethnic Study of Atherosclerosis is designed to detect CVD noninvasively before it has produced clinical signs and symptoms in a cohort of whites, African Americans, Hispanic Americans, and Asian Americans. In addition, the Jackson Heart Study is examining the physiological, environmental, social, and genetic factors related to CVD, including the high rates of complications from hypertension in the African American population. Additional studies include the Strong Heart Study of American Indians and the Genetics of Coronary Artery Disease in Alaska Natives (NIMHD, n.d.).

Diabetes

Diabetes was the seventh leading cause of death in the United States, affecting 25.8 million individuals in 2010. Compared to whites, African Americans and Hispanics are more than twice as likely to have diabetes, and American Indians under the age of 20 have the highest prevalence of type 2 diabetes (CDC, 2011f). Early screening and treatment are the most promising strategies to reverse these trends.

The Agency for Healthcare Research and Quality (AHRQ) sponsors research that focuses on how patients and providers can work together to better manage diabetes to improve quality of life and reduce diabetes-related complications. This research has confirmed the importance of controlling blood sugar levels to prevent blindness and the importance of routine monitoring and treatment of severe foot infections to prevent amputations (Agency for Healthcare Research and Quality, 2011).

HIV Infection and AIDS

HIV infection is the leading cause of death for individuals 25 to 44 years of age in the United States and the leading cause of death for African American men ages 35 to 44. Racial and ethnic populations are disproportionately affected by the HIV/AIDS epidemic in the United States. Although African American and Hispanic individuals represent about one-quarter of the country's population, more than half of new AIDS cases reported to CDC are among these populations (CDC, 2011g). The goal of Healthy People 2020 is to eliminate these disparities by improving access to prevention and health care services for all Americans and increasing the proportion of HIV-diagnosed African Americans and Latinos with undetectable viral load by 20 percent (Healthy People, 2010b).

Immunizations

The gap between immunization rates among many racial/ethnic and white populations has narrowed; however, disparities still exist among many underserved populations, especially among adults (CDC, 2011h). For instance, in 2009, 70 percent of older non-Hispanic whites received the influenza vaccine compared to only 51 percent of older African Americans and Hispanics. Similarly, in 2010, 64 percent of non-Hispanic whites received the pneumococcal vaccine compared to 46 percent of African Americans and 39 percent of Hispanics (US Department of Health and Human Services, 2011a). Children living below the poverty level have lower immunization coverage rates as well (CDC, 2007).

In 2011, in an effort to address these issues, the US Department of Health and Human Services developed the New National Vaccine Plan, a strategic approach designed to prevent infectious diseases and reduce adverse reactions to vaccines (US DHHS, 2011a).

Gender

Data from the National Health Interview Study (NHIS) provide evidence of gender disparities in health and health outcomes at a national level. Kaplan, Anderson, and Ake (2001) used data from the NHIS to estimate life expectancy rates adjusted for quality of life for men and women in the United States and found that women lived longer than men but experienced higher morbidity during their later years. Another study examining health disparities between men and women, also conducted in Ohio, found significant differences between groups on the basis of socioeconomic status, health care system experience, health behaviors, and health outcomes. They also indicated that women were more likely than men to live at or below 200 percent of poverty and to have ever been diagnosed with cancer, while men were more likely than women to be uninsured and to have high blood pressure and heart disease and to have had a heart attack. These results can be used to encourage dialogue with policymakers and decision makers on *health equity* and equality (Frazier, 2009).

health equity
According to Healthy People 2020, the attainment of the highest level of health for all people. In order to achieve health equity, societal efforts must focus on addressing avoidable inequalities, historical and contemporary injustices, and the elimination of health-related disparities.

Age

According to the Profile of Older Americans, there were 40.4 million individuals 65 years of age or older in 2010, an increase of 5.4 million, or

15.3 percent, since 2000, and it makes individuals aged 65 and older one of the fastest-growing population segments in the United States. In terms of race and ethnicity, 20.0 percent of individuals 65 and older were of minority status in 2010. Individuals of Hispanic origin represented 6.9 percent, African Americans represented 8.4 percent, Asian or Pacific Islanders represented 5.5 percent, American Indian or Native Alaskan represented less than 1 percent, and the remaining percentage represented two or more races (US DHHS, 2011b).

Ageism
Discrimination against those who are in the later period of adulthood. For example, media articles, cartoons, and greeting cards illustrate some aspects of ageism focusing on negative aspects of the aging process.

Ageism is a term that refers to negative stereotypes and discrimination based on age (Butler, 1969). Ageism often results in the attitude that older people are unproductive, sickly, depressing, and cognitively impaired (Osgood, 1996; Palmore, 1999). Outcomes of ageism can include isolation from the community, unnecessary institutionalization, untreated medical and physical illnesses, and suicide (Palmore, 1999). Age can also be a factor in health disparities. For instance, many older Americans have fixed incomes, which can make paying for health care expenses difficult. In addition, barriers including impaired mobility or a lack of transportation can make accessing health care services a challenge for the elderly population. Furthermore, older Americans may not have the opportunity to access health information using the Internet since less than 15 percent of Americans over the age of 65 have Internet access. This may put older individuals at a disadvantage in terms of accessing information about their health and understanding the ways in which to protect their health (Brodie et al., 2000).

Disability

According to the US Census, 36 million individuals in the United States have a disability. More specifically, 10.2 million have hearing impairment and 6.5 million have vision impairment. In addition, 13.5 million individuals 5 years of age or older experience difficulty concentrating, remembering, or making decisions (US Department of Commerce, 2011). The likelihood of having a disability increases with age (less than 10 percent for those 15 years of age or younger to almost 75 percent for those 80 years of age or older). A number of disabilities can be delayed or prevented with a healthy lifestyle and access to health care.

A review of the literature suggests that disparities exist between the health of those with a disability and the general population. According to *Closing the Gap: A National Blueprint to Improve the Health of Persons with Mental Retardation* (NIMHHD, n.d.), individuals with mental retardation are more likely to receive inappropriate and inadequate treatment or be denied health care. Although this report was specific to mental retardation, it was mentioned that most, if not all, of the content of the publication could be applied to any population with a disability (Johnson & Woll, 2003).

Social Determinants of Health

The 1978 International Conference on Primary Health Care (Alma Ata Conference) called for an urgent and effective national and international action to develop and implement primary health care throughout the world, and particularly in developing countries, in a spirit of technical cooperation and in keeping with a new international economic order. The conference acknowledged disparities and urged member states to explore ways to address disparities in social determinants of health (Tejada de Rivero, 2003).

Research and subsequent international health promotion conferences have helped us better understand the social determinants of health. In fact, McGinnis, Williams-Russo, and Knickman (2002) concluded that "our genetic predispositions affect the health care we need, and our social circumstances affect the health we receive" (p. 83). These conclusions were emphasized by the WHO Commission on Social Determinants of Health, which in 2008 concluded that "health is not simply about individual behaviour or exposure to risk, but how the socially and economically structured way of life of a population shapes its health" (para. 1).

The social determinants of health include social, economic, and environmental conditions, which are shaped by the distribution of money, power, and resources at the global, national, and local levels (WHO, 2008). The research literature suggests that social determinants (see figure 3.1) predict the greatest proportion of health status variance among individuals worldwide.

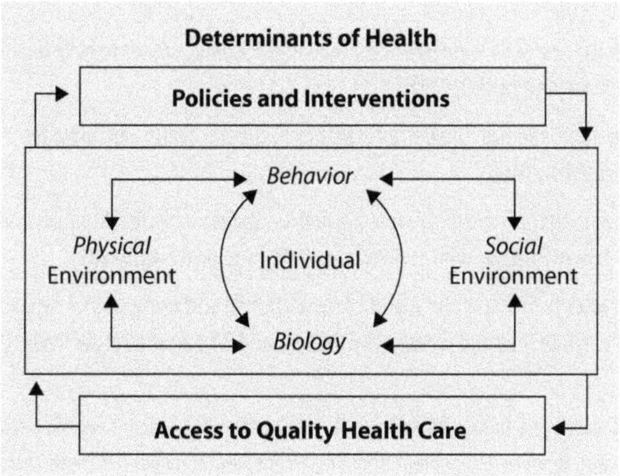

Figure 3.1 Determinants of Health
Source: Healthy People 2020 (2012).

Most health disparities affect groups marginalized because of socioeconomic status, race/ethnicity, sexual orientation, gender, disability status, geographic location, or some combination of these factors. In general, individuals from these groups have poorer health and less access to the social determinants or conditions that support health, including healthy food, good housing, good education, safe neighborhoods, and freedom from racism and other forms of discrimination (Whitehead & Dahlgren, 2007). More specifically, in terms of sexual orientation, over thirty thousand individuals from the gay, lesbian, bisexual, and transgender group die each year because of tobacco-related disease (American Cancer Society, 2005). In addition, African American gay, bisexual, and other men who have sex with men (MSM) represented an estimated 72 percent (10,600) of new infections among all African American men and 36 percent of an estimated 29,800 new HIV infections among all MSM (CDC, 2013). Statistics on selected social determinants are presented in table 3.2.

Table 3.2 Social Determinants of Health

Access to care	In 2006, adults with less than a high school diploma were 50 percent less likely to have visited a doctor in the past twelve months compared to those with at least a bachelor's degree (Pleis & Lethbridge-Çejku, 2007).
	In 2006, compared to white adults (79 percent), Asian Americans and Hispanic adults (75 percent and 68 percent, respectively) were less likely to have visited a doctor or other health professional in the past year (Pleis & Lethbridge-Çejku, 2007).
	One in four American children is born into poverty. Children living in poverty suffer twice as much tooth decay as their more affluent peers, and their disease is more likely to go untreated (CDC, 2010).
	Older adults (75 years of age or older), African Americans, poor individuals, and individuals with Medicaid coverage were more likely to have at least one emergency department visit in a twelve-month period compared to those in other age, race, income, and insurance groups (Garcia, Bernstein, & Bush, 2010).
Insurance coverage	In 2008, Asians under the age of 65 were more likely than whites to have health insurance (86.1 percent compared to 83.3 percent) (AHRQ, 2011).
	In 2008, Hispanics under the age of 65 were less likely than non-Hispanic whites to have health insurance (66.7 percent compared to 87.5 percent) (AHRQ, 2011).
	More than one in four Hispanic adults in the United States lacks a usual health care provider (Association of Hispanic Healthcare Executives, 2010).
	In 2010, insurance rates among the nonelderly were 2.6 and 1.8 times higher for Hispanics and African Americans, respectively, compared to non-Hispanic whites (DeNavas-Walt, Proctor, & Smith, 2011).
Employment	In 2010, unemployment rates were higher for African American men and women (18.4 percent and 13.8 percent, respectively) compared to white men and women (9.6 percent and 7.7 percent, respectively) (US Department of Labor, 2011).
	In 2010, unemployment rates were higher for Asian men and women (7.8 percent and 7.1 percent, respectively) compared to white men and women (9.6 percent and 7.7 percent, respectively) (US Department of Labor, 2011).
	In 2010, the jobless rates for Hispanic men and women were 12.7 percent and 12.3 percent, respectively (US Department of Labor, 2011).

Education	While the reading performance of most racial/ethnic groups has improved over the past fifteen years, minority children from low-income families are significantly more likely to have less than a basic reading level (US Department of Education, 2007). In 2007, the high school dropout rate was higher among Hispanics (21 percent) than among African Americans (8 percent), Asians/Pacific Islanders (6 percent), and whites (5 percent) (Aud, Fox, & Ramani, 2010). On the 2007 National Assessment of Educational Progress reading assessment, higher percentages of Asian/Pacific Islander and white fourth graders and eighth graders scored at or above "Proficient" than did American Indian/Alaska Native, African American, and Hispanic students at the same grade levels (Aud et al., 2010).
Access to resources	Lower-income and minority communities are less likely to have access to grocery stores with a wide variety of fruits and vegetables (Baker, Schootman, Barridge, & Kelly, 2006; Marland, Wing, Diez Roux, & Poole, 2002). Predominantly African American postal codes have about half as many chain supermarkets as predominantly white postal codes, and predominantly Latino areas have only one-third as many (Powell, Slater, Mirtcheva, Bao, & Chaloupka, 2007).
Income	Low socioeconomic status is associated with an increased risk for many diseases, including cardiovascular disease, arthritis, diabetes, chronic respiratory diseases, cervical cancer, and mental distress (Pleis & Lethbridge-Çejku, 2006). In 2010, based on median annual earnings for full-time, year-round workers, women earned 77.4 percent of men's earnings (US Department of Labor, 2010). In 2010, for full-time wage and salary workers, the earning difference between women and men varied with age, with younger women more closely approaching pay equity than older women (US Bureau of Labor Statistics, 2011).
Housing	Among all sheltered individuals over the course of one year (October 2009-September 2010), 41.6 percent were white, 9.7 percent were Hispanic, 37 percent were African American, 4.5 percent were other single races, and 7.2 percent were multiple races (Substance Abuse and Mental Health Services Administration, 2011). Among all sheltered individuals over the course of one year (October 2009-September 2010), 62 percent were male and 38 percent were female (Substance Abuse and Mental Health Services Administration, 2011).
Transportation	Rural residents must travel greater distances than urban residents to reach health care delivery sites (Agency for Healthcare Research and Quality, 2005). Compared to low-income whites, low-income minorities spend more time traveling to work and other daily destinations because they have fewer private vehicles and use public transit and car pools more frequently (Brownson & Boehmer, n.d.).

Healthy People 2020 addresses the social determinants of health through its goal of creating social and physical environments that promote good health for all (Healthy People, 2010c). In order to accomplish this goal, advances and collaboration are needed in fields such as education, child care, housing, business, law, media, community planning, transportation, and agriculture. In addition, a deeper understanding of how population groups experience their environments or *place* and the impact of place on health is needed (Institute of Medicine, 2002a). The Joint Center for Political and Economic Studies and California State University, Fresno's Central Valley Health Policy Institute examined the impact of place on health in the San

place
The relationship between the physical, social, and emotional environment that contributes to health disparities by affecting social determinants of health

Joaquin Valley. According to this report, place played a significant role in health, specifically on life expectancy rates, which varied as much as twenty-one years for some postal codes. Rates of premature death also varied, with rates in the lowest-income postal code areas nearly twice that of those in the highest-income postal code areas. Recommendations from this report include an "equity in all policies" approach, which involves considering the impact of zoning and contracting decisions on all postal codes (Daniel, 2012).

Racism and Discrimination and Their Impact on Health Education

There is no question that racism, real and perceived, plays a role in access to health care services. Several studies have reviewed the link between health outcomes and racism, but most of them have failed to point out the complex relationship between racism and health. Racism can take many forms and can be experienced from the provider to the patient as well as from the patient to the provider. Unmet expectations may be misinterpreted as racism, and subtle forms have replaced more overt forms of discrimination.

Real and perceived racism and discrimination may also play a role in the relationship between patient and health educator, although little in the research literature addresses this issue. We have already described racial and ethnic disparities in health and potential causes for these disparities, specifically those relating to social determinants of health. In addition to these causes, variations in patients' health beliefs, values, preferences, and behaviors must be considered. Some examples of these factors include variations in patient recognition of symptoms, thresholds for seeking care, ability to communicate symptoms to a provider who understands their meaning, ability to understand the prescribed management strategy, and adherence to preventive measures and medications (Gornick, 2000; Williams & Rucker, 2000). These factors can contribute to health disparities by influencing the patient-physician decision-making process and the interaction between patients and the health care delivery system (van Ryn & Burke, 2000). For these reasons, the field of cultural competence has emerged.

Racism can be addressed through the facilitation of cultural competence, which refers to "a set of congruent behaviors, attitudes, and policies that come together in a system, agency, or among professionals that enables effective work in cross-cultural situations" (CDC, 2011i). In terms of health education, health educators must learn how to develop and implement culturally appropriate health education programs, which requires a clear understanding of the relationship between culture and health. In addition, becoming culturally competent can be achieved through increasing cultural awareness, knowledge, skills, and desire; using sensitivity in communication; and applying the National Standards for Culturally and Linguistically Appropriate Services, which provides the foundation for building culturally competent health care organizations and workers (Luquis & Pérez, 2003). This movement toward cultural competence has gained national recognition and is now considered a method by which to eliminate racial and ethnic health disparities in health and health care by health policymakers, managed care administrators, academicians, providers, and consumers (Denboba, Bragdon, Epstein, Garthright, & McCann Goldman, 1998).

Primary Prevention, Health Education, and Health Disparities

Our nation spends nearly $1 trillion a year on diagnosing and treating disease, yet hundreds of thousands of deaths are due to preventable causes each year, including 400,000 due to smoking, 300,000 due to poor diet and inactivity, and 100,000 as a result of alcohol misuse (McGinnis & Foege, 1993). These deaths and other associated health problems occur disproportionately among the poor and minority populations (Snyder, 1998).

Primary prevention, or taking action before a health condition arises, is considered vital to reducing disparities in health (Mikkelsen et al., 2002). Primary prevention focuses its efforts on avoiding the onset of illness and infirmity before the development of chronic and behaviorally related diseases. In the United States, disparities exist in routine care and prevention among all racial, ethnic, and low-income groups (Health Reform, 2012). Individuals who do not have access to a usual source of primary prevention health care are more likely to turn to the hospital emergency room as their primary source of care. For instance, African Americans use the emergency department at a rate that is twice as high as that of whites. In terms of preventive care, compared to whites (57 percent), only 37 percent of Hispanics and 49 percent of African Americans received a colorectal cancer screening in 2007 (Agency for Healthcare Research and Quality, 2008). Similar patterns of limited preventive care among these groups are also observed for other chronic conditions, including obesity, HIV/AIDS, and diabetes. The Patient Protection and Affordability Care Act should address some of these concerns since it emphasizes primary prevention and increased access to health care (Wallace, 2012).

Suggestions for Working with Diverse Groups

Cultural competence has been defined as "a developmental process defined as a set of values, principles, behaviors, attitudes, and policies that enable health professionals to work effectively across racial, ethnic, linguistically diverse populations" (Joint Committee on Health Education and Promotion Terminology, 2012, p. 11). Cultural competence or proficiency does not require a health educator to adopt others' racial or ethnic cultural practices or require him or her to become an expert in every possible cultural group. It does, however, require that health educators use their abilities in four areas—awareness, knowledge, experience, and skills—and be willing to make a commitment to a lifelong process of change.

The following general recommendations, based on the professional literature and our own personal experience, are designed to give health educators practical suggestions for dealing with different cultural groups:

- *Differentiate among culture, race, and ethnicity.* Although these terms are often used as synonyms for convenience, they are not the same. Erroneous classifications may lead us to make erroneous assumptions about people. For instance, we might think a person to be of a given race given his or her skin color, but this person's cultural identity or ethnicity may not correspond to that color.
- *Avoid stereotypes.* Many publications, including this book, highlight some cultural health values documented in the professional literature. But not every member of a particular group will ascribe to those generally accepted standards. Keep in mind, for example, that not everyone over the age of 65 uses a walker and that many people over 65 enjoy a satisfying social life that includes dancing and sexual activity.
- *Ascertain acculturation levels.* Acculturation has been defined as the degree to which an immigrant adopts the culture and behaviors of the host country. Income, education, and language preference are all proxies for acculturation, but they do not represent a complete picture. A highly educated, English-proficient, first-generation immigrant may practice alternative medicine while proficiently navigating the US health care system.
- *Be cognizant of language preference.* Generally first-generation immigrants require translation of written materials and spoken words into their native language; less obvious is the need to provide materials in languages other than English to a number of those who are the second and subsequent generations in the United States. Meeting individuals' language preference is a key factor in delivering culturally appropriate health education programs because it allows people to communicate their needs and wants in an appropriate way. Being cognizant of language preference also refers to selecting and using the terminology employed by the target population rather than the technical language of health educators. Finally, it also refers to having qualified personnel,

regardless of cultural or ethnic background, who are proficient in the language needed.

- *Be cognizant of what you do not know.* People may provide the answers they think you want to hear. Avoid the trap of not pushing further to better understand the sociocultural world of others.
- *Be clear about your objectives.* One of the easiest ways to lose an educational opportunity is to be insufficiently organized. Your goals and objectives need to be clear, well articulated, and developed in conjunction with the target population. This is part of the empowerment process (Anspaugh, Dignan, & Anspaugh, 2000).
- *Remember family dynamics.* US-trained health educators tend to focus on individuals rather than on the social networks these individuals share. This process, although expedient, goes against the basic cultural values of some groups. Family members are a powerful and strong source of support to many cultural and ethnic groups in the United States. This may be a residual of having once lived in communities less affluent than their current home—communities where, as Casken (1999) points out, "the ties to the family ensure that no one goes hungry or homeless" (p. 408). Furthermore, Casken continues, "although the family's or individual's economic situation in the natal territory might have been no better than that in the immigrant territory, the lack of viable economic resources more than compensated for the invisible social commitments that support communities in their home territories" (p. 414).
- *Create strong coalitions.* Successful programs incorporate a group's strengths and explore ways to make weaknesses into opportunities. This can be accomplished only when members of the target group are deeply involved in the planning and implementation process. The creation of strong coalitions not only increases the chances for a successful program, but almost guarantees that the program will become institutionalized.
- *Develop trust.* Target population members may show deference and respect given a health educator's title and institutional affiliation, but that does not mean they trust the health educator. The health educator needs to become familiar with the target population, participate in community events, and be accepted into the everyday life of the community before trust can be achieved. He or she needs to become a familiar face in the community and participate in activities other than his or her own programs.
- *Select communication methods carefully.* Many entry-level health educators feel comfortable with developing written materials and

distributing them among the target population, yet they may have little, if any, regard for people's language preference and literacy level. Although written materials are well accepted in the majority culture, not everyone can read or likes to get printed materials, an approach that may be perceived to be too clinical. This issue is compounded when the materials are poorly developed and show, among other problems, spelling errors.

- *Incorporate cultural assessments.* One of the first things that we need to do as health educators is to include a cultural assessment into all program needs assessments.
- *Incorporate cultural values, beliefs, and practices into programs.* Health education interventions that have no relevance to the target community will not succeed. Along with information gathered from Western-style medicine, we need to include information that is relevant to the community. Whenever possible provide a contrast between the Western and non-Western approaches to health and illness, beliefs, and practices (Kim, McLeod, & Shantzis, 1992). Be careful not to show reverence for one and disdain for the other.
- *Involve members of the target group in the planning and decision-making process.* The participants may include healers, informal leaders, and community organizers.
- *Accommodate different learning styles.* As health educators, we cannot afford to forget that not everyone learns in the same manner. Some people like to read, others to explore on their own, and others to be shown. Be sure to incorporate activities that address the different learning styles that are likely to be found in your target group.
- *Make a commitment to multiculturalism.* No one can ask you to change your beliefs any more than you can ask someone else to change his or hers. In working with diverse groups, however, it is important to have a good understanding of one's own culture, stereotypes, and, in some cases, prejudices. Only when we can be honest with ourselves can we reach members of other ethnic groups or, in some cases, members of our own ethnic group who may not fit our socioeconomic profile (Airhihenbuwa, 1995).
- *Work within existing social networks.* Needs assessment data should yield information about existing groups and support in the community. Involving as many of them as possible makes it easier to work with the community rather than on the community.
- *Bring information back to the target audience.* One of the greatest, and accurate, criticisms of university-based health educators is that

they use people—in other words, they collect data and publish their results, but do little for the people who contributed to the data collection process, and then they retreat to their ivory tower. Although it is important to share the knowledge gained through our interventions with the scientific community, it is just as important to share the findings with the target community. These findings must be presented in a way that is useful to the community and furthers the empowerment process.

- *Understand traditional health beliefs*. Each of us, regardless of cultural heritage, holds numerous health beliefs. In North America, we tend to recommend that people who have flu-type symptoms eat chicken soup and get plenty of rest. Members of the Hmong culture believe that epilepsy is caused by ancestral spirits that have entered the body. Members of the Greek culture believe in the *Mati* or the evil eye—the belief that individual misfortune is caused by the envy of another. Greeks refer to envious people as having the ability to cast the evil eye on a person with good fortune (one of wealth, beauty, or good health, for example). The curse of the evil eye is broken by reciting a secret prayer, which is received from an older relative of the opposite sex, or performing the sign of the cross and spitting in the air three times. Understanding and respecting those beliefs will make the practice of health education in a multicultural setting much easier.
- *Respect religious beliefs*. The kahuna lapa'au in Hawaiian traditions helps people heal with the aid of a helping spirit known as the Akau (Mokuau & Tauili'ili, 1992). Similarly, Confucian ideology, Buddhism, and Taoism influence some Asian cultures (Hoylord, 2002). Although most of us in the United States value a separation of church and state, several groups do not make that distinction. We must be careful not to offend or contradict the religious beliefs that the target population holds.
- *Make it easy for the target audience to participate*. This applies the principle of the golden rule, which requires health educators to make their programs as user friendly as possible. Bring the program to the residences of the target audience, employ bilingual experts, or hold the program after work hours. Each of these steps shows respect and will increase your ability to reach the target audience.

Conclusion

Rapid demographic changes have contributed to the development of health disparities among some segments of the population. Issues related to access, language, and history may play a role in people's ability to avail themselves of health education programs. This chapter presents information related to the six priority areas the CDC has identified as requiring immediate attention to decrease health disparities. The information presented in this chapter can be used as the basis for not only supporting the goals denoted in Healthy People 2020, but also for developing health education and prevention programs designed to reach diverse groups while contributing to the elimination of health disparities.

Points to Remember

- Optimal health is not only the absence of disease or infirmity but also the result of a person's cultural background, race and ethnicity, educational level, and access to health care.
- Despite medical advances in health care and medical treatments, not everyone has access to the same services.
- Healthy People 2020 makes addressing health disparities a national priority for the next decade.
- Knowing yourself is an important skill to have in order to deliver health education to diverse groups.

Case Study

A Vietnamese person who survived the war has come to the United States and during the past five years has become a struggling family business owner. Recently he experienced chest problems but has not gone to the doctor because he does not have health insurance, and at 162 percent of the federal poverty line, he does not quality for government assistance. After several months of dealing with the issue with traditional remedies, his partner has finally convinced him to seek help, so he comes to you, a health educator.

1. When a person is hesitant in bringing up health issues, what is the first step you should take as a health educator to assist him or her?
2. What are some of the issues you must deal with?
3. How prepared are you to deal with those issues?
4. Do you need more information? If so, what additional information do you need? Be specific.
5. Knowing what you know, outline how you could best help this person. Provide a rationale for your response.

KEY TERMS

Ageism

Health disparity

Health equity

Place

References

Agency for Healthcare Research and Quality. (2005). *Health care disparities in rural areas: Selected findings from the 2004 national healthcare disparities report.* Retrieved from http://www.ahrq.gov/research/ruraldis/ruraldispar.htm

Agency for Healthcare Research and Quality. (2008). *National healthcare disparities report.* Retrieved from http://www.ahrq.gov/qual/qrdr08.htm

Agency for Healthcare Research and Quality. (2011). *Disparities in health care quality among racial and ethnic minority groups: Selected findings from the 2010 national healthcare quality and disparities report.* Retrieved from http://www.ahrq.gov/qual/nhqdr10/nhqrdrminority.10.pdf

Airhihenbuwa, C. O. (1995). *Health and culture: Beyond the Western paradigm.* Thousand Oaks, CA: Sage.

America's Environmental Health Gap. (2000). *Why the country needs a nationwide health tracking network.* Retrieved from http://www.healthyamericans.org/reports/files/healthgap.pdf

American Cancer Society. (2005). *Smoking and the LGBT community.* Retrieved from http://www.lgbthealth.org/doc/lbgttobacco.pdf

American Cancer Society. (2008). *Cancer facts and figures 2008.* Retrieved from http://www.cancer.org/cancerfactsandfigures/cancer-facts-figures-2008

American Cancer Society. (2012). *Cancer facts and figures—2012—American cancer society.* Retrieved from http://www.cancer.org/research/cancerfactsfigures/acspc-031941

American Dental Association. (2009). *Lifestyle behaviors that promote oral health also decrease risks for chronic disease.* Retrieved from http://www.ada.org/3127.aspx

American Lung Association. (2012). *Tobacco policy statement.* Retrieved from http://www.lung.org/associations/charters/plains-gulf/advocacy/tobacco-policy-statement.html

Anspaugh, D., Dignan, M., & Anspaugh, S. (2000). *Developing health promotion programs.* Long Grove, IL: Waveland Press.

Association of Hispanic Healthcare Executives. (2010). *Quarter of Latinos get no health information from medical professionals, new survey finds.* Retrieved from http://www.jobs.ahhe.org/?p=68

Aud, S., Fox, M. A., & Ramani, A. K. (2010). *Status and trends in the education of racial and ethnic groups.* Washington, DC: US Department of Education. Institute of Education Sciences. Retrieved from http://www.air.org/files/AIR-NCEracial_stats_trends1.pdf

Baker, E., Schootman, M., Barridge, E., & Kelly, C. (2006). Access to foods that enable individuals to adhere to dietary guidelines: The role of race and poverty. *Preventing Chronic Disease, 3*(3), 1–11.

Brodie, M., Flournoy, R. E., Altman, D. E., Blendon, R. J., Benson, J. M., & Rosenbaum, M. D. (2000). Health information, the Internet, and the digital divide. *Health Affairs, 19*(6), 255–265.

Brownson, R. C., & Boehmer, T. K. (n.d.). *Patterns and trends in physical activity, occupation, transportation, land use, and sedentary behaviors. TRB Special Report 282. Does the built environment influence physical activity? Examining the evidence.* Retrieved from http://www.trb.org/downloads/sr282papers/sr282Brownson.pdf

Butler, R. N. (1969). Age-ism: Another form of bigotry. *Gerontologist, 9,* 243–246.

Casken, J. (1999). Pacific Islander health and disease: An overview. In R. M. Huff & M. V. Kline (Eds.), *Promoting health in multicultural populations: A handbook for practitioners* (pp. 397–417). Thousand Oaks: Sage.

Centers for Disease Control and Prevention. (2000).

Centers for Disease Control and Prevention. (2007). *Eliminate disparities in adult and child immunization rates.* Retrieved from http://www.cdc.gov/omhd/amh/factsheet/immunization.htm

Centers for Disease Control and Prevention. (2008). Annual smoking—attributable mortality, years of potential life lost, and productivity losses—United States, 2000–2004. *Morbidity and Mortality Weekly Report, 57*(45), 1226–1228.

Centers for Disease Control and Prevention. (2009a). *Health disparities.* Retrieved from http://www.cdc.gov/omhd/topic/healthdisparities.html

Centers for Disease Control and Prevention. (2009b). *State indicator report on fruits and vegetables.* Retrieved from http://www.fruitsandvegetablesmatter.gov/health_proffessionals/statereport.html

Centers for Disease Control and Prevention. (2009c). *Eliminating racial and ethnic health disparities.* Retrieved from http://www.cdc.gov/omhd/about/disparities.htm

Centers for Disease Control and Prevention. (2009d). *Surveys and data collection systems.* Retrieved from http://www.cdc.gov/nchs/surveys.htm

Centers for Disease Control and Prevention. (2009e). *Eliminate disparities in cancer screening and management.* Retrieved from http://www.cdc.gov/omhd/AMH/factsheets/cancer.htm#4

Centers for Disease Control and Prevention. (2011a). *Health disparities among racial/ethnic populations.* Retrieved from http://www.cdc.gov/nccdphp/dach/chhep/disparities.htm

Centers for Disease Control and Prevention. (2011b). *CDC health disparities and inequities report—United States, 2011.* Retrieved from http://www.cdc.gov/mmwr/pdf/other/su6001.pdf

Centers for Disease Control and Prevention. (2011c). *Children's oral health.* Retrieved from http://www.cdc.gov/oralhealth/topics/child.htm

Centers for Disease Control and Prevention. (2011d). *Smoking and tobacco use.* Retrieved from http://www.cdc.gov/tobacco/data_statistics/fact_sheets/health_effects/tobacco_related_mortality/

Centers for Disease Control and Prevention. (2011e). *National vital statistics report.* Retrieved from http://www.cdc.gov/nchs/data/nvsr/nvsr59/10.pdf

Centers for Disease Control and Prevention. (2011f). *Eliminate health disparities in cardiovascular disease (CVD).* Retrieved from http://www.cdc.gov/omhd/AMH/factsheets/cardio.htm

Centers for Disease Control and Prevention. (2011g). *Basic statistics.* Retrieved from http://www.cdc.gov/hiv/topics/surveillance/basic.htm

Centers for Disease Control and Prevention. (2011h). *Immunization.* Retrieved from http://www.cdc.gov/nchs/fastats/immunize.htm

Centers for Disease Control and Prevention. (2011i). *Social determinants of health.* Retrieved from http://www.cdc.gov/socialdeterminants/Definitions.html

Centers for Disease Control and Prevention. (2013). *HIV in the United States: At a glance.* Retrieved from http://www.cdc.gov/hig/resources

Centers for Disease Control and Prevention. (2010). *Children's oral health.* Retrieved from: http://www.cdc.gov/oralhealth/publications/factsheets/index.htm

Daniel, A. (2012). *Report shows health disparities in valley zip codes.* Retrieved from http://www.californiahealthline.org/features/2012

DeNavas-Walt, C., Proctor, B. D., & Smith, J. C. (2011). *Income, poverty, and health insurance coverage in the United States: 2010.* Retrieved from http://www.census.gov/prod/2011pubs/p60–239.pdf

Denboba, D. L., Bragdon, J. L., Epstein, L. G., Garthright, K., & McCann Goldman, T. (1998). Reducing health disparities through cultural competence. *American Journal of Health Education, 29,* S47-S53.

Dye, B. A., Li, X., & Beltrán-Aguilar, E. D. (2012, May). *Selected oral health indicators in the United States, 2005–2008.* Hyattsville, MD: US Department of Health and Human Services.

Frazier, L. A. (2009). *Unhealthy differences: Health disparities between men and women in Ohio.* Columbus: Health Policy Institute of Ohio.

Garcia, T. C., Bernstein, A. B., & Bush, M. A. (2010). *Emergency department visitors and visits: Who used the emergency room in 2007? NCHS Data Brief,* 38, 1–8.

Gornick, M. F. (2000). Disparities in Medicare services: Potential causes, plausible explanations, and recommendations. *Health Care Financing Review, 21,* 23–43.

Health Reform. (2012). *Health disparities: A case for closing the gap.* Retrieved from http://www.healthreform.gov/reports/healthdisparities/

Healthy People 2020. (2010a). *Disparities.* Retrieved from http://www.healthypeople.gov/2020/about/disparitiesAbout.asp

Healthy People 2020. (2010b). *Leading health indicators.* Retrieved from http://www.healthypeople.gov/2020/LHI

Healthy People 2020. (2010c). *Social determinants of health.* Retrieved from http://www.healthypeople.gov/2020/topicsobjectives2020/overview.aspx

House, J. S., & Williams, D. R. (2000). Understanding and reducing socioeconomic and racial/ethnic disparities in health. In B. D. Smedley & S. L. Syme (Eds.), *Promoting health: Intervention strategies from social and behavioral research* (pp. 81–124). Washington, DC: National Academies Press.

Hoylord, E. (2002). Health-seeking behaviors and social change: The experience of the Hong Kong Chinese elderly. *Qualitative Health Research, 12*(6), 731–750.

Institute of Medicine (2002a). *Disparities in health care: Methods for studying the effects of race, ethnicity, and SES on access, use, and quality of health care.* Retrieved from http:///www.iom.edu/media/Files/Activitypercent20Files/Quality/NHDRGuidelines/DisparitiesGornick.pdf

Institute of Medicine. (2002b). *Unequal treatment: Confronting racial and ethnic disparities in health care.* Washington, DC: National Academy Press.

Joint Committee on Health Education Terminology. (2012). Report of the 2011 Joint Committee on Health Education and Promotion Terminology. *American Journal of Health Education, 43*(2), 1–19.

Johnson, J. L., & Woll, J. (2003). A national disgrace: Health disparities encountered by persons with disabilities. *Disability Studies Quarterly, 23*(1), 61–74.

Kaiser Family Foundation. (2010). *Infant mortality rate (deaths per 1,000 live births), linked files, 2005–2007.* Retrieved from http://www.statehealthfacts.org/comparemaptable.jsp

Kaplan, R., Anderson, J., & Ake, C. (2001). Gender differences in quality-adjusted life expectancy: Results from the national health interview survey. *Clinical Journal of Women's Health, 1*(1), 191–198.

Kim, S., McLeod, J., & Shantzis, C. (1992). *Cultural competence for evaluators working with Asian American Communities: Some practical considerations.* In M. A. Orlandi, R. Weston, & L. G. Epstein (Eds.), *Cultural competence for evaluators.* Rockville, MD: Office of Substance Abuse and Prevention.

Luquis, R., & Pérez, M. (2003). Achieving cultural competence: The challenges for health educators. *American Journal of Health Education, 34*(3), 131–138.

Marland, K., Wing, S., Diez Roux, A., & Poole, C. (2002). Neighborhood characteristics associated with the location of food stores and food service places. *American Journal of Preventive Medicine, 22*(1), 23–29.

McGinnis, J. M., & Foege, W. H. (1993). Actual causes of death in the United States. *Journal of the American Medical Association, 270,* 2207–2213.

McGinnis, J. M., William-Russo, P., & Knickman, J. R. (2002). The case for more active policy attention to health promotion. *Health Affairs, 21,* 78–93.

Mikkelsen, L., Cohen, L., Bhattacharyya, K., Valenzuela, I., Davis, R., & Gantz, T. (2002). *Eliminating health disparities: The role of primary prevention.* Oakland, CA: Prevention Institute.

Mokuau, N., & Tauli'ili, P. (1992). Families with Native Hawaiian and Pacific Islander roots. In E. W. Lynch & M. J. Hanson (Eds.), *Developing cross-cultural competence: A guide for working with young children and their families.* Baltimore, MD: Paul H. Brookes.

National Institute on Minority Health and Health Disparities. (2009). *American recovery and reinvestment act of 2009.* Retrieved from http://www.nimhd.nih.gov/recovery/godissemination.asp

National Institute on Minority Health and Health Disparities. (n.d.). *Health disparities—closing the gap.* Retrieved from http://www.nimhd.nig.gov/hdfactsheet_gap.asp

National Institutes of Health. (2010). *Health disparities defined.* Retrieved from http//crchd.cancer.gov/disparities/defined

Osgood, N. J. (1996). *Society does not respect the elderly.* In C. P. Cozic (Ed.), *An aging population: Opposing viewpoints.* San Diego, CA. Greenhaven Press.

Palmore, E. B. (1999). *Ageism: Negative and positive* (2nd ed.). New York: Springer.

Pettit, M. L., & Nienhaus, A. R. (2010). The current scope of health disparities in the US: A review of the literature. *Health Educator, 42* (2), 47–55.

Pleis, J. R., & Lethbridge-Çejku, M. (2007). *Summary health statistics for US adults: national health interview survey, 2006.* Retrieved from http://www.cdc.gov/nchs/nhis.htm

Powell, L. M., Slater, S., Mirtcheva, D., Boa, Y., & Chaloupka, F. J. (2007). Food store availability and neighborhood characteristics in the United States. *Preventive Medicine, 44*(3), 189–195.

Price, J. H., McKinney, M. A., & Braun, R. E. (2011). Social determinants of racial/ethnic health disparities in children and adolescents. *Health Educator, 43*(1), 2–12.

Pruss-Ustun, A., & Corvalan, C. (2006). *Preventing disease through healthy environments.* Geneva, Switzerland: World Health Organization. Retrieved from http://www.who.int/quantifying_ehimpacts/publications/preventingdisease.pdf

Reeves, W. C., Strine, T. W., Pratt, L. A., Thompson, W., Ahluwalia, I., Dhingra, S. S., . . . Safran, M. A. (2011). Mental illness surveillance among adults in the United States. *Morbidity and Mortality Weekly Report, 60*(3), 1–32.

Robert Wood Johnson Foundation. (2009). *Education matters for health.* Retrieved from http://www.commissionhealth.org

Snyder, L. (1998). Eliminating racial and ethnic disparities in health. *Public Health Reports, 13,* 372–375.

Substance Abuse and Mental Health Services Administration. (2011). *Individuals experiencing homelessness.* Retrieved from http://www.homeless.samhsa.gov/Resource/View.aspx?id=48800

Sudano, J. J., & Baker, D. W. (2006). Explaining U.S. racial/ethnic disparities in health declines and mortality in late and middle age: The roles of socioeconomic status, health behaviors, and health insurance. *Social Science and Medicine, 62*(4), 909–922.

Tejada de Rivero, D. A. (2003). Alma-Alta revisited. *Perspectives in Health Magazine.* Retrieved from http://www.paho.org/english/dd/pin/Number17_article1_4.htm

US Bureau of Labor Statistics. (2011). *Table 1. Median usual weekly earnings of full-time wage and salary workers, by selected characteristics, 2010 annual averages, "highlights of women's earnings in 2010.* Retrieved from http://www.catalyst.org/publication/217/womens-earnings-and-income

US Census Bureau. (2012). *Population estimates.* Retrieved from http://www.census.gov/popest/

US Department of Commerce. (2011). *Profile America facts for features.* Retrieved from http://www.census.gov/newsroom/releases/archieves/facts_for_features_special_edition

US Department of Education. (2007). *National assessment of educational progress: 2007. Reading assessments.* Retrieved from http://www.nationreportcard.gov/reading_2007/data.asp

US Department of Health and Human Services. (2008). *Physical activity guidelines for Americans.* Retrieved from http://www.health.gov/PAGuidelines

US Department of Health and Human Services. (2011a). *News release.* Retrieved from http://www.hhs.gov/news/press/2011pres/02/20110216b.htm

US Department of Health and Human Services. (2011b). *A profile of older Americans: 2010.* Retrieved from http://www.aoa.gov/aoaroot/aging/Profile2010

US Department of Labor. (2010). *Table PINC-05. Work experience in 2010-people 15 years old and over by total money earnings in 2010, age, race, Hispanic origin, and sex.* Retrieved from http://www.bls.gov/cps/cpsaat39.htm

US Department of Labor. (2011). *Employment situation summary.* Retrieved from http://www.bls.gov/news.release/empsit.nr0.htm

van Ryn, M., & Burke, J. (2000). The effect of patient race and socio-economic status on physician's perceptions of patients. *Social Science and Medicine, 50,* 813–828.

Visser, S. N., Bitsko, R. H., Danielson, M. L., & Perou, R. (2010). Increasing prevalence of parent-reported attention-deficit/hyperactivity disorder among children—United States, 2003 and 2007. *Morbidity and Mortality Weekly Report, 59*(44), 1439–1443.

Wallace, G. (2012). *"Obamacare": The word that defined the health care debate.* Retrieved from http://www.articles.cnn.com/2012–06–25/politics/politics_obamacare-word-debate_1_health-reform-law-health-care-affordable-care-act_s=PM:POLITICS

Whitehead, M., & Dahlgren, G. (2007). *Concepts and principles for tackling social inequities in health: Levelling up part I.* Retrieved from http://www.euro.who.int/document/e89383.pdf

Williams, D. R., & Rucker, T. D. (2000). Understanding and addressing racial disparities in health care. *Health Care Financing Review, 21,* 75–90.

Wong, G. W., Lai, K., & Chris, K. W. (2004). Outdoor air pollution and asthma. *Pulmonary Medicine, 10*(1), 62–66.

World Health Organization. (2008). *Social determinants of health.* Retrieved from http://www.who.int/social_determinants/en/

CHAPTER 4

COMPLEMENTARY AND ALTERNATIVE MEDICINE IN CULTURALLY COMPETENT HEALTH EDUCATION

Helda Pinzon-Perez

With the emergence of such health-related fields as complementary and alternative medicine (CAM), a new body of knowledge is expanding the horizons of health educators' practice. Culturally competent health educators need to understand the value of scientific and cultural constructs related to alternative forms of healing.

Health educators are being called on to explore their role in educating the public at large about complementary and alternative medicine, *holistic health*, and *integrative medicine or healing* (Johnson & Johnson, 2004). This chapter provides an overview of the principles involved in the practice of complementary healing, alternative medicine, and holistic health, as well as a description of the use of these modalities in the United States and worldwide. It includes a description of common CAM modalities in racial and ethnic groups in the United States and presents an analysis of the applications and future challenges for health education posed by these emerging fields.

Use of CAM

The 2007 statistics on the use of CAM, gathered through the National Health Interview Survey (NHIS), indicate that 38.3 percent of the adult population and 12 percent

LEARNING OBJECTIVES

After completing this chapter, you will be able to

- Recognize the similarities and differences among complementary healing, alternative medicine, and holistic health.
- Learn statistical data regarding the use of CAM in the United States.
- Identify complementary and alternative medicine practices in racial and ethnic groups.
- Discuss the impact of complementary healing, alternative medicine, and holistic health on the practice of culturally competent health education.
- Identify the potential challenges and future applications of complementary healing, alternative medicine, and holistic health for health educators.

holistic health
Practices oriented toward an integration of the body, the mind, the spirit, and the environment

integrative medicine or healing
A multidisciplinary process that has resulted in benefits such as improved clinical outcomes, reduction in hospital days, decreased hospitalizations, decreased pharmacological costs, and fewer outpatient surgeries

of children in the United States use CAM therapies. These statistics were published in December 2008 by the National Center for Complementary and Alternative Medicine (NCCAM) and the National Center for Health Statistics from the Centers for Disease Control and Prevention. The 2007 NHIS collected information from 23,393 people aged 18 years or older and 9,417 children and adolescents younger than 18. The results indicated an increase of 2.3 percent in the use of CAM by adults as compared to the 2000 results (NCCAM, 2008a). Selected results of this study are presented in box 4.1.

BOX 4.1 USE OF COMPLEMENTARY AND ALTERNATIVE MEDICINE

Following are selected results of the 2007 National Health Interview Survey: Complementary and Alternative Medicine Use in the Past Twelve Months among Adults in the United States.

In Adults

- CAM use in the adult population is higher for women and people with high levels of education.
- The most commonly used CAM practices by adults are nonvitamin and nonmineral natural products.
- An increased use of deep breathing exercises, therapy, and yoga was documented in the 2007 survey.
- The use of CAM therapies for head or chest colds decreased since 2002.
- By gender, 33.5 percent of male respondents and 48.2 percent of female respondents indicated their use of CAM therapies.
- By education, 20.8 percent of CAM users had less than a complete high school education; 31.0 percent were high school graduates or GED recipients; 45.0 percent had some college studies; 47.2 percent had an associate of arts degree; 49.6 percent had a bachelor of arts or science degree; and 55.4 percent had a master's, doctorate, or professional degree.
- By age, the highest use of CAM was in the age group 50 to 59 years old (44.1 percent), followed by the 60 to 69 group (41 percent), 40 to 49 group (40.1 percent), 30 to 39 group (39.6 percent), 18 to 29 group (36.3 percent), 70 to 84 group (32.1 percent), and 85 years and over (24.2 percent).
- By poverty status, 28.9 percent of respondents who used CAM were in the "poor" group, 30.9 percent in the "near-poor" group, and 43.3 percent in the "not poor" group.
- By marital status, 36.0 percent of CAM users were never married, 37.6 percent were married, and 38.1 percent were cohabitating,, 38.5 percent were divorced or separated, and 26.1 percent were widowed.
- By health insurance coverage, among those who were under 65 years, 42.7 percent had private insurance, 30.6 percent had public insurance, and 31.5 percent were uninsured. Among

those who were 65 and over, 37.1 percent had private insurance, 29.1 percent had public insurance, and 11.1 percent were uninsured.

- The most common CAM therapies that adults reported using in the 2007 survey are natural products (17.7 percent), deep breathing (12.7 percent), meditation (9.4 percent), chiropractic/osteopathic (8.6 percent), massage (8.3 percent), yoga (6.1 percent), diet-based therapies (3.6 percent), progressive relaxation (2.9 percent), guided imagery (2.2 percent), and homeopathic treatment (1.8 percent).
- The therapies that showed a significant increase in the 2007 survey as compared to the 2002 survey were deep breathing (11.6 percent in 2002, 12.7 percent in 2007), meditation (7.6 percent in 2002, 9.4 percent in 2007), massage (5 percent in 2002, 8.3 percent in 2007), and yoga (5.1 percent, 6.1 percent).
- The most commonly used natural products reported in the 2007 survey were fish oil/omega 3 (37.4 percent), glucosamine (19.9 percent), echinacea (19.8 percent), flaxseed oil/pills (15.9 percent), and ginseng (14.1 percent).
- Among adults, the diseases and conditions for which CAM is used for are back pain (17.1 percent), neck pain (5.9 percent), joint pain (5.2 percent), arthritis (3.5 percent), anxiety (2.8 percent), and cholesterol (2.1 percent).
- An estimated 83 million adults spent $ 33.9 billion out-of-pocket for alternative therapies.

In Children

- The use of CAM therapies is greater for children whose parents have used CAM (23.9 percent), for children whose parents have more than a high school diploma (14.7 percent), and whose families delayed conventional care because of a concern with cost (16.9 percent).
- Most use of CAM therapies is by adolescents ages 12 to 17 (16.4 percent) as compared to younger children.
- The most common CAM therapies used by children are natural products (3.9 percent), chiropractic and osteopathic (2.8 percent), deep breathing (2.2 percent), yoga (2.1 percent), homeopathic treatments (1.3 percent), and traditional healers (1.1 percent).
- The most common natural products used by children are echinacea (37.2 percent), fish oil/omega 3 (30.5 percent), combination herb pills (17.9 percent), and flaxseed oil/pills (16.7 percent).
- The diseases and conditions for which CAM is used in children include back or neck pain (6.7 percent), head or chest cold (6.6 percent), anxiety/stress (4.8 percent), other musculoskeletal condition (4.2 percent), attention deficit hyperactivity disorder (2.5 percent), and insomnia (1.8 percent).
- The use of CAM therapies by ethnicity is: white children (12.8 percent), Hispanic children (7.9 percent), and black children (5.9 percent).

Sources: National Center for Complementary and Alternative Medicine (2008a); Barnes, Bloom, and Nahin (2008).

Pearson, Johnson, and Nahin (2006) stated that over 1.6 million Americans use CAM practices for insomnia or sleeping disorders. Of those, 65 percent use herbal products, and 39 percent use mind-body therapies. Barnes, Powell-Griner, McFann, and Nahin (2004) found that CAM has most commonly been used to treat low-back pain, neck-related problems, joint pain, and depression. Other uses they mentioned are the treatment of sinusitis (1.2 percent), cholesterol problems (1.1 percent), asthma (1.1 percent), hypertension (1.0 percent), and menopause (0.8 percent).

According to the 2007 NHIS, 11.2 percent of the total out-of-pocket health care expenses is associated with CAM use. In addition, 354 million visits were done to consult CAM providers, and 835 million purchases were associated with CAM products and services, as well as $33.9 billion spent out-of-pocket by US adults on CAM visits (National Center for Complementary and Alternative Medicine, 2008b). In contrast, the 2002 NHIS revealed that 19 percent of US adults used herbal medicine, functional foods such as garlic, and animal-based supplements such as glucosamine during the twelve months preceding the survey. Among the natural products most often used by respondents were echinacea (40.3 percent), ginseng (24.1 percent), ginkgo biloba (21.1 percent), and garlic supplements (19.9 percent) (Barnes et al., 2004).

Definitions of Concepts in Nontraditional Healing

Health educators need to have a clear understanding of each of the terms used in nontraditional healing, including *complementary* and *alternative medicine, conventional medicine, integrative medicine* or *healing, holistic health*, and *folk and traditional medicine.* Understanding what each of these areas encompasses is important for health educators because they are educational agents with whom consumers of nontraditional healing will consult for clarification.

folk and traditional medicine
The treatment of illnesses through remedies and therapies that are based on experience and knowledge transmitted throughout generations in an apprenticeship model

CAM is defined by the National Center for Complementary and Alternative Medicine (NCCAM, 2011a) as the medical and health care practices, systems, and products that are not included yet in the conventional, Western, allopathic medicine delivery system and are now in the process of being studied under rigorous scientific inquiry.

Conventional medicine, also known as *allopathic care* or *biomedicine,* has been defined as the body of scientific knowledge practiced by doctors of medicine, doctors of osteopathic medicine, and allied health professionals such as psychologists, physical therapists, and registered nurses, among others (NCCAM, 2011a). Health educators have been active educational agents in the field of conventional medicine. They now need to increase their presence in CAM areas.

Complementary medicine and *alternative medicine* are terms with distinct meanings. *Complementary medicine* describes practices used simultaneously with conventional medicine (NCCAM, 2011a), for example, the use of aromatherapy following surgery to alleviate discomfort. In contrast, *alternative medicine* is used instead of *conventional medicine,* as in the case of using a specific diet for the therapeutic treatment of cancer instead of using chemotherapy (NCCAM, 2011a). Health educators with multiple interests may initially find less resistance to becoming professionally involved in complementary medicine. They may find that health care professionals have less initial resistance to becoming involved in complementary medicine because it acknowledges the value of both conventional and traditional healing.

complementary medicine
Practices used simultaneously with conventional medicine

alternative medicine
Practices used instead of conventional medicine, as in the case of a specific diet for the therapeutic treatment of cancer instead of using chemotherapy

Traditional medicine is defined by the World Health Organization (WHO, 2008) as the group of practices that incorporates knowledge and skills that are culturally rooted in the theories, beliefs, and experiences of indigenous groups aimed toward promotion of health, prevention of disease, and treatment of physical and mental illnesses. Traditional medicine employs indigenous health traditions and cultural healing constructs involving the use of plants, animal remedies, mineral-based medicines, and spiritual means. According to WHO (2008), traditional medicine practices employed by groups outside the indigenous cultures are often defined as alternative or complementary medicine.

Folk medicine is defined as the treatment of illnesses through remedies and therapies that are based on experience and knowledge transmitted throughout generations in an apprenticeship model (WebMD, 2012). Traditional and folk medicine have gained recognition among health educators because of their interest in culturally competent health care. Conducting further studies on these forms of medicine is important for the growth of the health education profession.

The NCCAM (2006a) also uses the term *integrative medicine,* which it defines as a combination of conventional medical practices and CAM therapies. Integrative medicine systems promote the equal importance and scientific value of mainstream and alternative healing mechanisms—for example, the simultaneous use of massage therapy and conventional medications to alleviate low-back pain (NCCAM, 2006a).

Lemley (2012) defines integrative medicine as a healing-oriented medicine that looks at the individual in a holistic manner and integrates elements of the body, the mind, and the spirit into the development of healthy lifestyles. According to Lemley, integrative medicine is based on six principles: (1) it involves a partnership between the patient and the practitioner, (2) it involves conventional and alternative therapies based on the needs of the client, (3) it facilitates the body's natural healing, (4) it looks at conventional and alternative medicine in a critical manner, (5) it acknowledges the value of science for both conventional and CAM practices, and (6) it is offered by practitioners who are themselves committed to self-development.

The Consortium of Academic Health Centers for Integrative Medicine (2011) states that integrative medicine is guided by evidence and provides patients with multiple therapeutic approaches to obtain optimal healing and maximum well-being. This consortium calls for a comprehensive and compassionate health care system that offers integrative services at the individual and community levels. The American Association of Integrative Medicine (2006) adds that patients are the most important members of the medical team. No current data exist on the number of practitioners and customers of integrative medicine. According to the American Association of Integrative Medicine (2012), additional research in this area is greatly needed.

The various terms used to denote CAM were differentiated in 2002 by the National Center for Complementary and Alternative Medicine. The clarification in the definition of terms such as *holistic health, folk medicine,* and *CAM* was an effort to provide a clear basis for understanding CAM and other modalities among health practitioners. Health educators ought to contribute toward the understanding of this new field by becoming actively involved in research exploring the number of people using this modality, their reasons for such use, and their experiences with it.

Pinzon-Perez (2005) has advocated for a broader understanding of these concepts and the use of more inclusive terms such as *holistic, complementary, alternative,* and *integrative healing.* Currently, the focus on medical practices denoted in terms such as *complementary, alternative,* and *integrative medicine* narrows the scope of these practices and limits their applications to the field of medicine. There is a need to expand the focus of these terms to embrace healing and thus to make them more applicable in fields such as health education and allied health professions. Health education publications on holistic and integrative healing are needed.

Patterson and Graf (2000) have described the relevance of integrating complementary and alternative medicine into the health education curriculum. Chng, Neill, and Fogle (2003) have advocated for conducting research on CAM and integrative medicine among college student populations and for exploring the application of these terms in the field of health education.

Holistic health describes practices oriented toward an integration of the body, the mind, the spirit, and the environment (NCCAM, 2011a). Holistic health should be an important domain in the field of health education because this discipline ought to view health in a comprehensive manner.

Integrative medicine or *healing* refers to a multidisciplinary process that has resulted in benefits such as improved clinical outcomes, reduction in hospital days, decreased hospitalizations, decreased pharmacological costs, and fewer outpatient surgeries (Sarnat & Winterstein, 2004). Integrative healing is comprehensive and multisectorial.

Health educators need to conduct more studies to expand the understanding of these conceptual definitions and their applications to health education. It is important that health educators create a body of knowledge unique to the domains and needs of the health education practice. Some recommendations for health educators in this regard are conducting research on holistic health and integrative healing; expanding the competencies and responsibilities of health educators to address newly emerging fields such as CAM, integrative healing, and holistic health; and designing culturally appropriate strategies to educate individuals and communities on these new forms of healing.

Modalities of CAM

The NCCAM (2011a) groups CAM practices into four categories:

- *Natural products,* which include herbal medicines, also known as botanicals, vitamins, minerals, and probiotics. Many of these natural products are commercialized as dietary supplements.
- *Mind and body medicine,* which focuses "on the interactions among the brain, body, and behavior, with the intent to use the mind to affect physical functioning and promote health" (NCCAM, 2011a). This category includes practices such as meditation, yoga, acupuncture, deep-breathing exercises, guided imagery, hypnotherapy, progressive relaxation, qi gong, and tai chi.
- *Manipulative and body-based practices,* which "focus primarily on the structures and systems of the body, including the bones and joints, soft tissues, and circulatory and lymphatic systems" (NCCAM, 2011a)—for example, spinal manipulation, osteopathic manipulation, and massage therapy.
- *Other CAM practices,* which includes various subcategories—for example:
  - Movement therapies such as the Feldenkrais method, Alexander technique, pilates, Rolfing structural integration, and Trager psychophysical integration.
  - Practices embraced by traditional healers.
  - Manipulation of energy fields such as in magnet therapy, light therapy, Reiki, and healing touch.
  - Whole medical systems such as ayurveda, homeopathy, traditional Chinese medicine, and naturopathy (NCCAM, 2011a).

In the past, the National Center for Complementary and Alternative Medicine divided CAM therapies into five major categories, set out in box 4.2, based on mechanisms of action and modalities of treatment.

BOX 4.2 CATEGORIES OF CAM PREVIOUSLY USED BY NCCAM

Whole Medical Systems

Whole medical systems are built on complete systems of theory and practice. Often these systems have evolved apart from and earlier than the conventional medical approach used in the United States. Examples of whole medical systems that have been developed in Western cultures include homeopathic medicine and naturopathic medicine. Examples of systems that have been developed in non-Western cultures include traditional Chinese medicine and Ayurveda.

Mind-Body Medicine

Mind-body medicine uses a variety of techniques designed to enhance the mind's capacity to affect bodily function and symptoms. Some techniques that were considered CAM in the past have become mainstream (e.g., patient support groups and cognitive-behavioral therapy). Other mind-body techniques are still considered CAM, including meditation, prayer, mental healing, and therapies that use creative outlets such as art, music, or dance.

Biologically Based Practices

Biologically based practices in CAM use substances found in nature, such as herbs, foods, and vitamins. Some examples are dietary supplements, herbal products, and the use of other so-called natural but as yet scientifically unproven therapies (e.g., using shark cartilage to treat cancer).

Manipulative and Body-Based Practices

Manipulative and body-based practices in CAM are based on manipulation or movement of one or more parts of the body–for example, chiropractic or osteopathic manipulation, and massage.

Energy Medicine

Energy therapies involve the use of energy fields. They are of two types:

- Biofield therapies, intended to affect energy fields that purportedly surround and penetrate the human body. The existence of such fields has not yet been scientifically proven. Some forms of energy therapy manipulate biofields by applying pressure or manipulating the body by placing the hands in, or through, these fields. Examples include qi gong, Reiki, and therapeutic touch.
- Bioelectromagnetic-based therapies, which involve the unconventional use of electromagnetic fields, such as pulsed fields, magnetic fields, or alternating-current or direct-current fields.

Source: NCCAM (2007a).

CAM modalities studied in the 2007 NHIS were related to (1) biologically based therapies, which included chelation therapy; nonvitamin, nonmineral natural products; and diet-based therapies; (2) mind-body therapies, which included biofeedback, meditation, guided imagery, progressive relaxation, deep breathing exercises, hypnosis, yoga, tai chi, and qi gong; (3) alternative medical systems, which included acupuncture, Ayurveda, homeopathic treatment, naturopathy, and traditional healers; and (4) manipulative and body-based therapies, which included chiropractic or osteopathic manipulation, massage, and movement therapies (Barnes et al., 2008).

Barnes et al. (2008) presented the definitions of CAM modalities used for the 2007 NHIS conducted by the Centers for Disease Control and Prevention's (CDC) National Center for Health Statistics (NCHS). These definitions are presented in box 4.3. Box 4.4 displays the definitions of traditional and folk modalities of CAM used in the 2007 NHIS.

BOX 4.3 SELECTED MODALITIES OF CAM AS DEFINED FOR THE 2007 NHIS

Acupuncture: A family of procedures involving stimulation of anatomical points on the body by a variety of techniques. American practices of acupuncture incorporate medical traditions from China, Japan, Korea, and other countries. The acupuncture technique that has been most studied scientifically is penetrating the skin with thin, solid, metallic needles that are manipulated by the hands or by electrical stimulation.

Alexander technique: A movement therapy that uses guidance and education on ways to improve posture and movement. The intent is to teach a person how to use muscles more efficiently in order to improve the overall functioning of the body. Examples of the Alexander technique as CAM are using it to treat low-back pain and the symptoms of Parkinson's disease.

Atkins diet: A diet that emphasizes a drastic reduction in the daily intake of carbohydrates (40 grams or less), countered by an increase in protein and fat.

Ayurveda: A system of medicine that originated in India several thousand years ago. A chief aim of ayurvedic practices is to cleanse the body of substances that can cause disease and thereby help reestablish harmony and balance. In the United States, Ayurveda is considered a type of CAM and a whole medical system.

Biofeedback: Uses simple electronic devices to teach clients how to consciously regulate bodily functions, such as breathing, heart rate, and blood pressure, in order to improve overall health. Biofeedback is used to reduce stress, eliminate headaches, recondition injured muscles, control asthmatic attacks, and relieve pain.

Chelation therapy: A chemical process in which a substance is used to bind molecules, such as metals or minerals, and hold them tightly so that they can be removed from a system such as the body.

Chiropractic care: This care involves the adjustment of the spine and joints to influence the body's nervous system and natural defense mechanisms to alleviate pain and improve general health. It is primarily used to treat back problems, headaches, nerve inflammation, muscle spasms, and other injuries and traumas.

Deep breathing: Slow and deep inhalation through the nose, usually to a count of 10, followed by slow and complete exhalation for a similar count. The process may be repeated five to ten times several times a day.

Energy healing therapy: The channeling of healing energy through the hands of a practitioner into the client's body to restore a normal energy balance and therefore health. It has been used to treat a wide variety of ailments and health problems and is often used in conjunction with other alternative and conventional medical treatments.

Guided imagery: A series of relaxation techniques followed by the visualization of detailed images, usually calm and peaceful in nature. If used for treatment, individuals will visualize their body free of the specific problem or condition. Sessions are typically twenty to thirty minutes in length and may be practiced several times a week.

Homeopathy: A system of medical practices based on the theory that any substance that can produce symptoms of disease or illness in a healthy person can cure those symptoms in a sick person. For example, someone suffering from insomnia may be given a homeopathic dose of coffee. Administered in diluted form, homeopathic remedies are derived from many natural sources, including plants, metals, and minerals.

Hypnosis: An altered state of consciousness characterized by increased responsiveness to suggestion. The hypnotic state is attained by first relaxing the body and then shifting attention toward a narrow range of objects or ideas suggested by the hypnotist or hypnotherapist.

Macrobiotic diet: A diet low in fat that emphasizes whole grains and vegetables and restricts the intake of fluids. Of particular importance is the consumption of fresh, unprocessed foods.

Massage: A manipulation of muscle and connective tissue to improve the function of those tissues and promote relaxation and well-being.

Meditation: A group of techniques, most of which started in Eastern religious or spiritual traditions, whereby a person learns to focus attention and suspend the stream of thoughts that normally occupy the mind.

Naturopathy: An alternative medical system proposing that there is a healing power in the body that establishes, maintains, and restores health. Practitioners work with the patient with a goal of supporting this power through treatments such as nutrition and lifestyle counseling, dietary supplements, medicinal plants, exercise, homeopathy, and treatments from traditional Chinese medicine.

Nonvitamin, nonmineral, natural products: Products taken by mouth that contain a dietary ingredient intended to supplement the diet other than vitamins and minerals. Examples include herbs or herbal medicine (as single herbs or mixtures), other botanical products such as soy or flax products, and dietary substances such as enzymes and glandulars.

Osteopathic manipulation: A full-body system of hands-on techniques to alleviate pain, restore function, and promote health and well-being.

Qi gong: An ancient Chinese discipline combining the use of gentle physical movements, mental focus, and deep breathing directed toward specific parts of the body. The exercises are normally performed two or more times a week for thirty minutes at a time.

Reiki: An energy medicine practice that originated in Japan. The practitioner places his or her hands on or near the person receiving treatment, with the intent to transmit ki, believed to be life force energy.

Tai chi: A mind-body practice that originated in China as a martial art. A person doing tai chi moves his or her body slowly and gently while breathing deeply and meditating (tai chi is sometimes called moving meditation).

Yoga: Combines breathing exercises, physical postures, and meditation to calm the nervous system and balance body, mind, and spirit. Usually performed in classes, with sessions conducted once a week or more and roughly lasting forty-five minutes each.

Source: Barnes et al. (2008).

Boxes 4.2, 4.3, and 4.4 provide important theoretical definitions for health educators that will enhance their ability to deliver health education

BOX 4.4 TRADITIONAL AND FOLK MODALITIES OF CAM USED IN THE 2007 NHIS.

Botanica: A traditional healer who supplies healing products, sometimes associated with spiritual interventions.

Curandero: A type of traditional folk healer. Originally found in Latin America, they specialize in treating illness through the use of supernatural forces, herbal remedies, and other natural medicines.

Espiritista: A traditional healer who assesses a patient's condition and recommends herbs or religious amulets in order to improve this person's physical or mental health or to help him or her overcome a personal problem.

Hierbero or *Yerbera:* A traditional healer or practitioner with knowledge of the medicinal qualities of plants.

Native American healer or medicine man: A traditional healer who uses information from the spirit world in order to benefit the community. People see Native American healers for a variety of reasons, but especially to find relief or a cure from illness or to find spiritual guidance.

Shaman: A traditional healer who is said to act as a medium between the invisible spiritual world and the physical world. Most shamans gain knowledge through contact with the spiritual world and use the information to perform tasks such as divination, influencing natural events, and healing the sick or injured.

Sobador: A traditional healer who uses massage and rub techniques in order to treat patients.

Traditional healer: Someone who employs any one of a number of ancient medical practices that are based on indigenous theories, beliefs, and experiences handed down from generation to generation.

Yerbera: See *Hierbero.*

Source: Barnes et al. (2008).

about CAM effectively. The responsibilities and competencies delineated by the National Commission for Health Education Credentialing (2008b) are directly linked to health educators' knowledge of concepts and theories. Responsibilities such as acting as a resource person in health education and communicating health and health education needs, concerns, and resources related to CAM require health educators to have a solid understanding of these operational and theoretical definitions.

The Competencies Update Project (CUP), undertaken between 1998 and 2004 by the American Association for Health Education, the National Commission for Health Education Credentialing, and the Society for Public Health Education, delineated the role of the health educator as a three-tiered hierarchical model. This new framework defined the responsibilities and competencies of health educators based on their level of practice (National Commission for Health Education Credentialing, 2007).

Entry-level health educators, defined as those with a bachelor's or master's degree and fewer than five years of experience, need to expand their body of knowledge on the types and modalities of CAM. Advanced level 1 health educators, those with a bachelor's or master's degree and five years or more of experience, ought to engage in the design, implementation, and evaluation of educational programs related to CAM. Advanced level 2 health educators, defined as those with a doctoral degree and five or more years of experience, ought to engage in research projects and scientific discovery related to CAM.

CAM in Racial and Ethnic Groups

The use of CAM varies by cultural group. A study on breast cancer conducted by Lee (cited by Jones, 2001) revealed that half of the women in the study used at least one type of alternative medicine and one-third used two types. The types of CAM used by participating females varied among cultural groups: African-American women used spiritual healing methods (36 percent), Hispanic/Latino women used nutritional therapies (30 percent) and spiritual healing (26 percent), Chinese women used herbal remedies (22 percent), and white women used dietary therapies (35 percent) and massage and acupuncture (21 percent) (Jones, 2001).

The results of the 2007 NHIS indicated that by ethnicity, the highest use of CAM therapies was in American Indian/Alaska Natives (50.3 percent), followed by Native Hawaiian and other Pacific Islanders (43.2 percent), non-Hispanic whites (43.1 percent), Asians (39.9 percent), blacks or African Americans (25.5 percent), and Hispanics (23.7 percent) (Barnes et al., 2008). Additional information on the use of CAM therapies by racial and ethnic groups is described below.

African Americans

Of the blacks/African Americans responding to the 2007 NHIS, 25.5 percent indicated they used CAM therapies: 12.3 percent used biologically based therapies, 14.8 percent used mind-body therapies, 1.4 percent used alternative medical systems, 0.2 percent used energy healing therapies, and 6.5 percent used manipulative and body-based therapies (Barnes et al., 2008). According to Spector (2009), examples of CAM remedies used by black populations include the use of asafetida worn around the neck to prevent infectious diseases, the use of copper and silver bracelets worn on the wrist of baby girls to prevent illness until young childhood, and the use of sassafras tea for the treatment of respiratory illnesses.

Latinos/Hispanics

In the 2007 NHIS, 3.7 percent of Hispanic respondents revealed their use of CAM: 11.8 percent used biologically based therapies, 10.6 percent used mind-body therapies, 3.0 percent used alternative medical systems, 0.1 percent used energy healing therapies, and 6.7 percent used manipulative and body-based therapies (Barnes et al., 2008). According to Spector (2009), CAM practices among Hispanic/Latino populations are highly influenced by religious beliefs and theories such as the hot and cold origin of ailments. In this theory, disease is the result of an imbalance of the body's main humors: hot and cold. For Latinos/Hispanics, cold diseases such as asthma should be treated with hot remedies such as herbal products and massage. Hot diseases such as diabetes and hypertension should be treated with cold remedies such as nopal and aloe vera juice (Spector, 2009). Examples of CAM practices in this group include visiting shrines, offering prayers, consultation with holistic healers, use of *parteras* (midwives), treatment by *sobanderos* (massage healers) and *hueseros* (bone settlers) and use of camomile, spearmint, orange leaves, and sweet basil teas and infusions (Spector, 2009).

Within the Hispanic or Latino origin group in the 2007 NHIS, 29.7 percent of the adult Puerto Ricans respondents used CAM therapies, followed by Dominicans (28.2 percent), Mexican Americans (27.4 percent), Central or South Americans (23.4 percent), Cuban or Cuban Americans (22.9 percent), and Mexicans (18.2 percent). In addition, the 2007 survey revealed that Puerto Ricans and Mexican Americans were more likely than Mexican adults to use biologically based CAM therapies or manipulative and body-based therapies (Barnes et al., 2008).

Among Puerto Ricans who used CAM, 14.2 percent used biologically based therapies, 16.8 percent used mind-body therapies, 2.4 percent used alternative medical systems, and 7.6 percent used manipulative and body-based therapies (Barnes et al., 2008). Flores-Pena and Evanchuck (1994) mentioned that *Santeria* and the use of *botanicas* are common among Puerto Rican populations. *Santeros* use storytelling and prayers to saints as a mechanism to restore health. *Botanicas* are small stores where people can purchase herbs, ointments, and incense prescribed by *santeros* or spiritual healers (Spector, 2009).

Among Mexicans who used CAM, 8.9 percent used biologically based therapies, 6.9 percent used mind-body therapies, 3.9 percent used alternative medical systems, and 4.1 percent used manipulative and body-based therapies (Barnes et al., 2008). Among Mexican Americans who used CAM, 14.0 percent used biologically based therapies, 11.6 percent used mind-body therapies, 2.1 percent used alternative medical systems, and 7.9 percent used manipulative and body-based therapies (Barnes et al., 2008). According to Tafur, Crowe, and Torres (2009) Mexicans and Mexican Americans use traditional healing practices associated with *curanderismo* for folk illnesses such as *mal de ojo* (evil eye or bad eye), *caida de la mollera* (fallen anterior fontanelle), and *envidia* (envy).

Among Cuban or Cuban Americans who used CAM, 11.2 percent used biologically based therapies, 14.1 percent used mind-body therapies, and 8.5 percent used manipulative and body-based therapies (Barnes et al., 2008).

Appelbaum et al. (2006) stated that Cubans are worldwide leaders in the use of natural and traditional medicine. According to these authors, practices that Cubans use and are taught in medical schools include herbal therapies, acupuncture, moxibustion, massage, mind-body modalities, and hypnosis.

Among Dominicans who use CAM, 12.3 percent used biologically based therapies, 18.5 percent used mind-body therapies, and 5.3 percent used manipulative and body-based therapies (Barnes, 2008). In writing on medicinal plants used in the east region of the Dominican Republic, Portorreal Liriano (2011) noted that Dominicans primarily use herbal medicine for the treatment of ailments. Some of the plants that this group use include albahaca morada (known in English as opal basil) for gastrointestinal concerns, pana (breadfruit) tree for low back pain, artemesia for menstrual disorders, anamu for the prevention of infection and to heal wounds, and apasote (epizote) for parasitic diseases and as an antibacterial.

Among Central or South Americans who use CAM, 18.2 percent used biologically based therapies, 10.0 percent used mind-body therapies, 3.5 percent used alternative medical systems, and 7.4 percent used manipulative and body-based therapies (Barnes et al., 2008). According to Fontaine (2011), Central and South Americans use a variety of CAM therapies, such as consultation with holistic healers, the use of herbs and nutritional supplements, as well as prayer, meditation, and massage.

Whites

In the 2007 NHIS, 43.1 percent of white respondents said they used CAMs: 22.7 percent used biologically based therapies, 21.4 percent used mind-body therapies, 3.7 percent used alternative medical systems, 0.7 percent used energy healing therapies, and 18.7 percent used manipulative and body-based therapies (Barnes et al., 2008). According to Spector (2009), this group includes healing traditions from people with German, Irish, English, Italian, Polish, French, and Scottish ancestries. Examples of CAM practices used by this group include naturopathy, diet-based therapies, biofeedback, chiropractic, meditation, and home remedies such as peppermint and cinnamon teas, castor oil, onion poultices, and honey.

Asians and Pacific Islanders

This group is divided into two major categories in the 2007 NHIS. The first group is composed of non-Hispanic Asians. In the 2007 NHIS, 39.9 percent of Asian respondents stated their use of CAM: 19.6 percent used biologically based therapies, 23.4 percent used mind-body therapies, 5.4 percent used alternative medical systems, 0.3 percent used energy healing therapies, and 11.1 percent used manipulative and body-based therapies. The second group is composed of Native Hawaiians and other Pacific Islanders: 43.2 percent of respondents indicated their use of CAM. Within this group, 26.1 percent used biologically based therapies, and 24.5 percent used mind-body therapies (Barnes et al., 2008). Fontaine (2011) and Spector (2009) explained the importance of understanding the yin (representing the female, negative energy) and yang (representing the male, positive energy) in the genesis and management of disease. The group of Asian and Pacific Islanders uses CAM practices such as Tai Chi, Ayurveda, massage, acupuncture, moxibustion, cupping, coining, and traditional Chinese medicine. Tai chi, Ayurveda, massage, and acupuncture are defined in Box 4.3. Moxibustion involves the application of heat coming from a dried plant; cupping refers to applying a hot cup to the skin to create suction; and coining refers to rubbing the edge of a coin in the skin to produce therapeutic heat (Spector, 2009; Fontaine, 2011).

American Indian and Alaska Natives

In the 2007 NHIS, 50.3 percent of American Indian and Alaska Native respondents used CAM: 23.7 percent used biologically based therapies, 23.3 percent used mind-body therapies, 13.2 percent used alternative medical systems, and 13.4 percent used manipulative and body-based therapies (Barnes et al., 2008). According to Fontaine (2011), spirituality and natural medicine are core concepts of CAM use among American Indian and Alaska Natives. Examples of CAM practices in this group include smudging, sweat lodges, drumming and chanting, dancing, acupressure, use of herbs, and consultations with medicine women and medicine men.

Summary

Although there are some differences in CAM use by cultural groups, the 2007 NHIS statistics on the use of CAM revealed that the most commonly used therapies across cultural groups in the United States are nonvitamin, nonmineral natural products (17.7 percent) and deep breathing exercises (12.7 percent) (Barnes et al., 2008). Therapies such as acupuncture for back pain, insomnia, and smoking cessation; massage for musculoskeletal problems; and meditation for depression and anxiety are commonly used by all groups regardless of race or ethnicity (NCCAM, 2008a).

At the international level, a review of the use of traditional, complementary, and alternative medicine among 123 member states of the WHO revealed that CAM and traditional medicine are widely used around the world. In Africa, over 80 percent of Ethiopians use traditional medicine. In the Americas, a 1999 study revealed that 70 percent of Canadians have used one or more natural health products. In the Eastern Mediterranean region, 70 percent of the Pakistani rural population has used CAM and traditional medicine. In Europe, one-eighth of the British population has tried complementary or alternative medicine, and 90 percent of them are ready to use it again. In Southeast Asia, 70 percent of rural Indonesians have used CAM practices. In the Western Pacific region, 95 percent of Chinese hospitals have units for traditional medicine (WHO, 2001).

According to WHO (2001), the most commonly cited reasons for the use of these healing practices around the world are that they are more affordable, more closely related to the patient's ideology, and less paternalistic than biomedicine. CAM and traditional medicine constitute important sources of medical care in various nations around the globe.

Chan (2008), in an address to the WHO congress on traditional medicine, indicated that 60 percent of children in some African regions are treated at home with herbal remedies. Robinson and Zhang (2011) stated that 70 to 95 percent of the population in developing countries use traditional medicine for primary care. For instance, it is estimated that 90 percent of the population in Ethiopia, 75 percent in Mali, 70 percent in Rwanda, and 60 percent in Tanzania and Uganda use traditional medicine. In developed nations, 80 percent of the population in Germany, 70 percent in Canada, 49 percent in France, and 48 percent in Australia use CAM (Robinson & Zhang, 2011).

National Center for Complementary and Alternative Medicine

The NCCAM, created in 1998, is the lead federal entity supporting scientific research initiatives in CAM areas. Studies on the applications of holistic health and alternative medicine in areas of scientific discovery, such as health education, medicine, social work, and nursing, have been supported by NCCAM. A precursor agency, the Office for Alternative Medicine, existed from 1992 to 1998 (NCCAM, 2007b).

As one of the twenty-seven institutes and centers of the NIH, this agency promotes rigorous scientific inquiries on healing practices, educates CAM researchers, and informs the public on the latest findings related to CAM practices. The role and priorities of the NCCAM are presented in box 4.5.

The information in box 4.5 is particularly relevant for health educators within the framework of the new responsibilities and competencies delineated by the Competencies Update Project. Responsibility VII states that health educators should communicate and advocate for health and health education (Gilmore, Olsen, Taub, & Connell, 2005). The NCCAM focus areas reveal a need for health educators to take an active and leading role in advocating for the advancement of scientific research on CAM,

BOX 4.5 NCCAM ROLE AND PRIORITIES

NCCAM's mission is to define, through rigorous scientific investigation, the usefulness and safety of complementary and alternative medicine interventions and their roles in improving health and health care. NCCAM achieves its mission through basic, translational ("bench-to-bedside"), and clinical research; research capacity building and training; and education and outreach programs.

The NCCAM priorities are:

- Advancing scientific research in the United States and around the world.
- Supporting training opportunities for new researchers and encouraging experienced researchers to study CAM.
- Providing timely and accurate information about CAM research through a website, a national information clearinghouse, fact sheets, a lecture series, continuing medical education models, and publications.
- Supporting rigorous and scientifically designed clinical trials to ensure the safety and effectiveness of CAM therapies.
- Building a scientific evidence base about CAM therapies, whether they are safe, and whether they work for the conditions for which people use them and, if so, how they work.

Source: Adapted from NCCAM (2011a).

sharing news and information on emerging CAM practices, and supporting the integration of proven CAM therapies.

NCCAM provides funding for research centers intended to advance scientific knowledge on CAM. The budget for this entity has continued to increase since it was established in 1996.

NCCAM now sponsors centers of excellence for research on CAM, developmental centers for research on CAM, centers for dietary supplements research, and international centers for research on CAM. These centers conduct basic and translational research, as well as observational studies and clinical investigations on topics such as herbs, dietary supplements, antioxidants, polyphenols, Chinese herbal medicine, and osteopathic manipulative treatment. The 2012 funding priorities of NCCAM include research on the impact of CAM modalities in alleviating chronic pain syndromes, reducing inflammatory processes, maximizing health and wellness, and improving quality of life (NCCAM, 2011b). In 2006, the CAM research priorities were approaches to anxiety and depression; secondary prevention and management of hypertension, atherosclerosis, and congestive heart failure; ethnomedicine; immune modulation and enhancement; inflammatory bowel syndrome and irritable bowel syndrome; insomnia; liver diseases; obesity and metabolic syndrome; infectious respiratory diseases; gender health; and health disparities (NCCAM, 2006b).

NCCAM also offers funding for training and educational programs at the undergraduate, graduate, and postdoctoral levels. The focus of these training opportunities is the development of culturally competent research and delivery systems for CAM. The health education profession needs to extend its body of knowledge to new domains such as CAM. Health educators can find CAM research and training opportunities at the NCCAM.

CAM and Health Education

Health educators have embraced the concepts promoted by holistic health and integrative healing (Chng et al., 2003). According to Pinzon-Perez (2005), the practice of health education is based on a holistic understanding of human life and the multidimensional nature of health. Terms such as *holistic health* and *integrative medicine* or *healing* are often found in the health education vocabulary and have become integral to this practice.

Health educators are defined as practitioners who have scientific training in the design, development, and evaluation of activities that help to improve the health of all people (NCHEC, 2008a). The NCHEC defines certified health education specialists (CHES) as professionals who have met eligibility requirements and have passed a competency-based examination on the seven areas of responsibility of health educators (NCHEC, 2008a). A new designation, master certified health education specialist (MCHES), is used for health educators who have had multiple courses on health education, have fulfilled experience requirements, and have an ongoing commitment to the advancement of health education as a professional field (NCHEC, 2008b). The emerging fields of CAM, holistic health, and integrative healing pose new challenges for CHES and MCHES in the areas of advocacy, needs assessment, program planning, and program evaluation. Multiple strategies for educating the public on CAM, in settings such as schools, communities, health care facilities, businesses, colleges, and government agencies, need to be developed.

NCCAM has made a call to health professionals to educate the public on how to select a CAM provider. Responsibility VI of the Responsibilities and Competencies of health educators says that these professionals should act as resource persons in health education (NCHEC, 2008b). Health educators should be knowledgeable about CAM so they can educate others. An important goal in this educational process is to educate consumers on how to select CAM practitioners. Selecting the appropriate CAM provider will protect consumers and increase the likelihood of success in treatment. The NCCAM guidelines for selecting a CAM practitioner may need to be transmitted by health educators to their clients. These guidelines are presented in box 4.6.

BOX 4.6 NCCAM GUIDELINES FOR SELECTING A CAM PRACTITIONER

- If you are seeking a CAM practitioner, speak with your primary health care provider(s) or someone you believe to be knowledgeable about CAM regarding the therapy in which you are interested. Ask if he or she has a recommendation for the type of CAM practitioner you are seeking.
- Inquire about education, training, licenses, and certifications of the CAM provider. Compare the practitioner's qualifications with the training and licensing standards for that profession.
- Make a list of CAM practitioners, and gather information about each one before making your first visit. Ask basic questions about their credentials and practice. Where did they receive their training? What licenses or certifications do they have? How much will the treatment cost?
- Check with your insurer to see if the cost of therapy will be covered.
- After you select a practitioner, make a list of questions to ask at your first visit. You may want to bring a friend or family member who can help you ask questions and note answers.
- Come to the first visit prepared to answer questions about your health history, including injuries, surgeries, and major illnesses, as well as prescription medicines, vitamins, and other supplements you may take.
- Assess your first visit and decide if the practitioner is right for you. Did you feel comfortable with the practitioner? Could the practitioner answer your questions? Did he or she respond to you in a way that satisfied you? Does the treatment plan seem reasonable and acceptable to you?
- Ask if it is possible to have a brief consultation in person or by phone with the practitioner. This will give you a chance to speak with the practitioner directly. This consultation may or may not involve a charge.
- Ask if there are diseases or health conditions in which the practitioner specializes and how frequently he or she treats patients with problems similar to yours.
- Ask if the practitioner believes the therapy can effectively address your complaint and if any scientific research supports the treatment's use for your condition.
- Ask about the number of patients the practitioner typically sees in a day and the average time spent with each patient.

- Ask about charges and payment options. How much do treatments cost? If you have insurance, does the practitioner accept your insurance or participate in your insurer's network? Even with insurance, you may be responsible for a percentage of the cost.
- Ask about the hours appointments are offered. How long is the wait for an appointment? Consider whether this will be convenient for your schedule.
- Ask about office location. If you are concerned, ask about public transportation and parking. If you need a building with an elevator or a wheelchair ramp, ask about them.
- Ask what will be involved in the first visit or assessment.
- Observe how comfortable you feel during these first interactions.

Source: Adapted from (NCCAM, 2004, 2011c).

Currently the body of knowledge on the application of CAM in the field of health education is limited. Patterson and Graf (2000), Chng et al. (2003), Johnson and Johnson (2004), Pinzon-Perez (2005), Synovitz, Gillan, Wood, Martin-Nordness, and Kelly (2006), Pérez and Luquis (2008), Stanczak and Heuberger (2009), Johnson, Priestley, Porter, and Petrillo (2010), Geiger Thomas, Bojana, and Devlin (2011), and Synovitz and Larson (2013) have published valuable articles and books or presented papers at national conferences on the importance of CAM in health education. For example, Synovitz and Larson (2013), in their book on complementary and alternative medicine for health professionals, discussed CAM therapies from a consumer's health perspective. They presented an analysis of health insurance coverage of CAM and a discussion on CAM and the Patient Protection and Affordable Care Act.

Geiger et al. (2011) wrote on the role of health educators in supporting global health. In this article, they called on health educators to be actively involved in the achievement of the United Nations Millennium Development Goals. They proposed a strategy to achieve such goals by determining the value of CAM therapies for the poor and vulnerable throughout the world.

Johnson et al. (2010) conducted a national study to examine US health educators' attitudes toward CAM and their use of common CAM therapies. The results of this study indicated that health educators have positive attitudes toward CAM. This study revealed that approximately 90 percent of health educators have used at least one CAM therapy in the past twelve months, with female health educators reporting more positive attitudes toward the use of CAM.

Stanczak and Heuberger (2009), who conducted a study on the use of probiotics among participants, called for health educators to become resource people and educate consumers on CAM.

Synovitz et al. (2006) conducted research on college students' CAM use in relation to health locus of control and spirituality level. Their findings indicated that internal locus of control was positively associated with use of CAM therapies and with spirituality level. Internal locus of control was defined in this study as the person's belief that she or he has control over their health status.

These and other studies have major implications for health education since they have established a founding body of knowledge of CAM for this profession. Additional studies are needed to increase the understanding of the applications of CAM for health educators.

In box 4.7, I discuss the applications of the studies conducted by Patterson and Graf, Chng et al., and Johnson and Johnson. I also provide valuable insights on the applications and challenges for health education posed by the emergence of CAM.

BOX 4.7 CAM, HOLISTIC HEALTH, AND INTEGRATIVE HEALING: APPLICATIONS AND CHALLENGES FOR HEALTH EDUCATION

- The increasing pattern of use of CAM, holistic health, and integrative healing practices has motivated health educators and other practitioners in the behavioral and medical fields to conduct and publish research in this area.
- In the field of health education, professional development organizations such as AAHE, SOPHE, and others have started to provide grants, under the umbrella of *cultural competence*, to find out the applications of CAM, holistic health, and integrative healing in this field. Although this is a promising start, more funding is needed to motivate health education practitioners to conduct research in these areas.
- CAM, holistic health, and integrative healing are now being addressed in professional development agendas for health educators.
- According to Johnson and Johnson (2004), health educators need to be aware of the current status of CAM use in the U.S., become familiar with different forms of CAM therapy, discuss commonly used CAM therapies with clients, assist clients in their selection of appropriate CAM therapies to promote health and prevent disease, encourage clients to communicate the use of CAM therapies to their health care providers, have continuing education opportunities in CAM from professional organizations, and offer CAM courses in professional health education preparation programs.
- In health education . . . no national standards have been developed yet to unify the curriculum for the training of health educators on CAM, holistic health and integrative healing.

Most efforts to teach health educators about these issues have been developed as part of curriculums that address cultural competence and *cultural proficiency.*

- Patterson and Graf (2000) wrote a cornerstone article in defense of requiring complementary and alternative medicine training in the curriculum for health educators. These authors presented a well-founded rationale to support their premise that CAM should be taught as a separate course, or in the absence of enough resources, be integrated into existing health education courses.
- Section 3 of Article VI of the Code of Ethics for the Health Education Profession, "Responsibility in Professional Preparation," indicates that health educators should be involved in professional preparation and professional development programs that provide them with materials that are accurate, up-to-date and timely.
- It is essential that entry-level health educators become knowledgeable of the scientific and cultural basis of the various forms of CAM, holistic health practices, and integrative healing therapies. This knowledge will provide health educators with the professional skills to become accurate health resources.
- Academic training on CAM, holistic health and integrative healing should be included at the undergraduate and graduate levels.
- Creating standards related to CAM, holistic health and integrative healing for the professional preparation of health educators implies a revision of the requirements for Certified Health Education Specialists (CHES). Although CHES certification addresses issues related to cultural competence and proficiency, it needs to be extended to assess health educators' knowledge and scientific understanding of basic forms of CAM, holistic health and integrative healing... This indicates that health educators with CHES designation should be professionals with scientific and socio-cultural knowledge on alternative and complementary healing practices.
- An additional challenge for health educators is to generate knowledge on the applications of integrative healing to the practice of health education... Theses, doctoral dissertations and professional research on this issue should be encouraged at all levels of professional preparation.

Source: Pinzon-Perez (2005). Reprinted with permission.

cultural competence
A developmental process defined as a set of values, principles, behaviors, attitudes, and policies that enable health professionals to work effectively across racial, ethnic, and linguistically diverse groups

cultural proficiency
The end point of cultural competence, in which the individual develops the ability to respond appropriately to groups of diverse ethnic and cultural backgrounds

The nursing profession could serve as a valuable example to health educators on the importance of establishing formal education programs and standards of practice on CAM, traditional medicine, and holistic health. The American Holistic Nurses Association (AHNA), an organization founded in 1981, has served as a bridge between the biomedical perspective in nursing and the alternative and complementary healing paradigm (AHNA, 2004). This organization has developed philosophical principles that can be adopted by health educators interested in CAM, traditional medicine, and holistic health.

Some of the philosophical principles that health educators could adhere to include the understanding that nurses, as well as health educators, (1) can have a professional practice that promotes wholeness; (2) can motivate individuals to become responsible health consumers; (3) should provide services to individuals, families, and communities in ways that integrate the body, the mind, and the spirit; and (4) should advocate for the understanding that illness is an opportunity for individuals to regain their wholeness (AHNA, 2004). According AHNA, nurses should begin by developing lifestyles congruent with a philosophy of wholeness. Health educators too should consider embracing this concept and developing for themselves lifestyles oriented toward inner self-enhancement and holistic health—lifestyles that will ultimately enable them to provide a better quality of health education services.

A possible strategy for enhancing the understanding of CAM in health education would be to create ad hoc and standing committees in professional organizations, such as the American Association for Health Education and the Society for Public Health Education, to stimulate scientific inquiry and develop a specific body of knowledge on the integration of CAM into health education. Patterson and Graf (2000) have made a call to health educators to incorporate CAM into the health education curriculum. Of particular relevance in the development of a specific body of knowledge on CAM for health education is the study of culturally competent health education programs in relation to CAN, holistic health, and integrative healing.

Culturally competent health education programs should include constant dialogue and further research on how to incorporate training, publications, and professional development in CAM, traditional medicine, and holistic health into the delivery of health education services. Examples of culturally competent health education programs on CAM should be published and made known to the professional health education body. Funding for research and publications on this area ought to be a priority for professional health education organizations and individual members.

There is also a need to add classes at the undergraduate and graduate levels in which future health educators can learn about and discuss the implications of CAM for their professional practice. Synovitz et al. (2006) have supported this need, finding it relevant in light of the results of their study on college students' use of CAM therapies. There is also a need to consider the development of academic certificate programs and international research cooperative agreements on CAM.

Potential challenges in future applications of complementary healing, alternative medicine, and holistic health for the health education profession include defining health educators' competencies and responsibilities associated with CAM practices, enhancing the body of knowledge relating to CAM in health education professional practice, and stimulating dialogues in the health education professional community on alternative, complementary, and holistic healing practices and on their use within a context of cultural respect and rigorous scientific inquiry. CHES and MCHES ought to be involved in the challenge of promoting research on CAM and health education, as well as to educate consumers based upon evidence-based results.

Suggestions for Working with Diverse Groups

Smith and Wilbur (2008) stated that cultural competence is an essential skill when working with diverse groups. They ask for health education specialists to make a strong pledge for current and future health education specialists to develop strategies to work effectively with diverse populations. Smith and Wilbur used the Swahili word *harambe*, which means being united physically, in spirit, and in mind, to illustrate the true nature of health educators working with diverse groups. Health educators need to acknowledge and embrace the cultural and spiritual beliefs that influence the use of CAM therapies among diverse populations.

Working with diverse groups implies looking at new paradigms in the use of health services. One of these new paradigms is the use of CAM therapies as regular sources of health and well-being. According to Chan (2008), the use of traditional medicine is widely spread around the world, and for that reason, traditional and Western medicine need to blend within the context of primary health care. World Health Assembly resolution 62.13, passed in May 2009 by the WHO member states, called for governments to acknowledge the value of these traditional practices while regulating them to ensure safety and effective use (Robinson & Zhang, 2011).

Xue (2008), from the WHO Collaborating Centre for Traditional Medicine, has urged global governments to respect and preserve traditional medicine, especially for those whose major, and maybe the only, source of health care comes from holistic health practices. Xue emphasized that education is the critical element in ensuring a safe and effective utilization of traditional, complementary, and alternative medicine. In this context, health educators play a pivotal role since education is the core of the health educator's job. Educational initiatives related to CAM use should be based on such concepts as cultural competence and cultural humility.

Effective work with diverse groups involves the development of national policies on the use of CAM and its inclusion into national health systems. World Health Assembly resolution 62.13 urged member states to share knowledge and resources to strengthen the communication between conventional and traditional practitioners and to promote research on effective and culturally sensitive mechanisms when working with diverse populations (Robinson & Zhang, 2011). The need for health care providers to understand traditional forms of medicine used among various populations around the world has been described by Fadiman (1997) in her book *The Spirit Catches You and You Fall Down*, which describes how coining treatments used by the Hmong population have sometimes been misinterpreted by health care providers as child endangerment. Fadiman called for better intercultural communication among patients, families, and health care providers.

The National Commission for Health Education Credentialing, the Society for Public Health Education, and the American Association for Health Education delineated in the Competencies Update Project 7 responsibilities, 35 competencies, and 163 subcompetencies, emphasizing the need for health educators to conduct a self-assessment of their progress toward achieving cultural competency in their professional practice (Johnson Vaughn, 2008). A relevant suggestion for health educators working with diverse groups is to maintain a critical attitude toward themselves and a vigilant introspection of their cultural competency levels. Cultural competency in health education involves an advocacy role toward the value, respect, and acknowledgment of various health practices of traditional and holistic nature among diverse populations.

It is important that health educators maintain a critical view of CAM based on research and evidence-based practice. Health educators should be aware of the benefits and risks associated with the use of CAM and need to keep themselves updated on the latest research data. For instance, benefits of CAM have been documented in a journal database of the National Library of Medicine, which includes forty systematic reviews of alternative medicine practices documenting the usefulness of acupuncture for osteoarthritis, knee pain, back pain, insomnia, and nausea, as well as the benefits of massage for back pain (Barnes et al., 2008). Among risks described by the NCCAM (2012) are the possibility of medication interactions, for example in the case of Saint John's wort, which interacts with antidepressants, as well as the possibility of product contamination such in the case of dietary supplements that contain active ingredients found in prescription drugs. In addition, cost considerations should be taken into account when selecting a CAM therapy. The NCCAM (2012) has made a call to health professionals, including health educators, to help users become informed consumers, participate in adverse-event reporting systems, and check their website for alerts and advisories on emerging products.

Conclusion

Complementary and alternative medicine practices are amply used in the United States. The 2007 National Health Interview Survey documented that 38.3 percent of the adult population and 12 percent of children in the United States use CAM therapies. By ethnicity, the NHIS revealed that the highest use of CAM therapies was in American Indian/Alaska Natives (50.3 percent), followed by Native Hawaiian and other Pacific Islanders (43.2 percent), non-Hispanic whites (43.1 percent), Asians (39.9 percent), blacks or African Americans (25.5 percent), and Hispanics (23.7 percent).

NCCAM is the lead federal entity supporting scientific research initiatives related to CAM. It groups CAM practices into four categories: natural products, mind and body medicine, manipulative and body-based practices, and other CAM practices. The clarification of terms such as *complementary and alternative medicine, conventional medicine, folk* or *traditional medicine, integrative medicine* or *healing,* and *holistic health* is of special relevance for the health education practice.

Points to Remember

- Health educators face a new body of knowledge related to the emergence of fields such as complementary and alternative medicine. There are new challenges for health educators regarding their role in complementary and alternative healing practices.
- It is vital that health educators create a body of knowledge on CAM unique to the domain and needs of the health education practice. Further research in this area is needed.
- Of particular relevance in the development of a specific body of knowledge on CAM for health education is the study of culturally competent

health education programs related to complementary and alternative medicine, holistic health, and integrative healing.

- When working with diverse groups, health educators ought to be critical and vigilant of their own cultural-competence skills and maintain an attitude of humility and self-improvement.
- The National Center for Complementary and Alternative Medicine is a reliable source of information on CAM, integrative healing, and holistic health for health educators and clients.

Case Study

A significant number of clients in a health care facility have reported using CAM and traditional healing practices. As a member of the health care team, you, the health educator, have been commissioned to provide culturally competent health education on CAM, traditional medicine, and holistic health to these clients.

1. What steps would you follow to assess the health education needs of this group?
2. What topics would you suggest including in the educational plan for this group?
3. What resources (websites, articles, organizations) would you use in designing the health education program for this group?
4. What elements would you take into account when designing a culturally competent health education program for this group?

KEY TERMS

Alternative medicine
Complementary medicine
Cultural competence
Cultural proficiency
Folk and traditional medicine
Holistic health
Integrative medicine or healing

References

American Association of Integrative Medicine. (2006). *Member testimonials.* Retrieved from http://aaimedicine.com/about_testimonials.php

American Association of Integrative Medicine. (2012). *About.* Retrieved from http://www.aaimedicine.com/about/

American Holistic Nurses Association. (2004). *About AHNA*. Retrieved from http://www.ahna.org/about/about.html

Appelbaum, D., Kligler, B., Barrett, B., Frenkel, M., Guerrera, M., Kondwani., Tattelman, E. (2006). *Natural and traditional medicine in Cuba: Lessons for US medical schools*. Retrieved from http://www.medicc.org/mediccreview/articles/mr_50.pdf

Barnes, P., Powell-Griner, E., McFann, K., & Nahin, R. (2004). *Complementary and alternative medicine use among adults: United States, 2002* (CDC advance data from Vital and Health Statistics, Report 343). Hyattsville, MD: National Center for Health Statistics. Retrieved from nccam.nih.gov/news/camstats.htm

Barnes, P. M., Bloom, B., & Nahin, R. L. (2008). *Complementary and alternative medicine use among adults and children: United States, 2007.* Hyattsville, MD: National Center for Health Statistics. 2008. Retrieved from http://nccam.nih.gov/sites/nccam.nih.gov/files/news/nhsr12.pdf

Chan, M. (2008). *Address at the WHO Congress on Traditional Medicine*. from http://www.who.int/dg/speeches/2008/20081107/en/index.html

Chng, C. L., Neill, K., & Fogle, P. (2003). Predictors of college students' use of complementary and alternative medicine. *American Journal of Health Education, 34*(5), 267–271.

Consortium of Academic Health Centers for Integrative Medicine. (2011). *About us*. Retrieved from http://www.imconsortium.org/about/home.html

Fadiman, A. (1997). *The spirit catches you and you fall down*. New York, NY: Farrar, Straus, and Giroux.

Flores-Pena, Y., & Evanchuck, R. (1994). *Santeria garments and altars*. Jackson: University of Mississippi Press.

Fontaine, K. (2011). *Complementary and alternative therapies for nursing practice*(3rd ed.). Upper Saddle River, NJ: Pearson Education.

Geiger, B., Thomas, D., Bojana, B., & Devlin, M. (2011). The role of health education specialists in supporting global health and the Millennium Development Goals. *International Electronic Journal of Health Education, 14*, 37–45. Retrieved on March 29, 2012, from http://www.aahperd.org/aahe/publications/iejhe/upload/11_B-Geiger.pdf

Gilmore, G. D., Olsen, L. K., Taub, A., & Connell, D. (2005). Overview of the National Health Educator Competencies Update Project, 1998–2004. *American Journal of Health Education, 32* (6), 363–370.

Johnson, P., & Johnson, R. (2004). *Current status of complementary and alternative health practices in the US: Implications for health education professionals*. Paper presented at the 2004 AAHPERD national convention, New Orleans, LA.

Johnson, P., Priestley. J., Porter, K. & Petrillo, J. (2010 May/June). Complementary and alternative medicine: attitudes and use among health educators in the United States. *American Journal of Health Education, 41*, 167–177. Retrieved from http://www.aahperd.org/aahe/publications/ajhe/upload/MayJune-2010–2.pdf

Johnson Vaughn, E. (2008). *Cultural competence in health education and health promotion*. San Francisco, CA: Jossey-Bass.

Jones, M. (2001). Ethnnicity may affect alternative, complementary therapy choices. *Journal of the National Cancer Institute, 93*(20), 1522–1523.

Lemley, B. (2012). *What is integrative medicine?* Retrieved from http://www.drweil.com/drw/u/ART02054/Andrew-Weil-Integrative-Medicine.html

National Center for Complementary and Alternative Medicine. (2004). *Selecting a CAM practitioner.* Retrieved from http://nccam.nih.gov/health/practitioner/index.htm

National Center for Complementary and Alternative Medicine. (2006a). *NCCAM facts-at-a-glance*. Retrieved from http://nccam.nih.gov/about/ataglance

National Center for Complementary and Alternative Medicine. (2006b). *Research funding priorities*. Retrieved from http://nccam.nih.gov/research/priorities/index.htm#5

National Center for Complementary and Alternative Medicine. (2007a). *What is CAM?* Retrieved from http://nccam.nih.gov/health/whatiscam

National Center for Complementary and Alternative Medicine. (2007b). *CAM basics*. Retrieved from http://nccam.nih.gov/health/whatiscam/pdf/D347.pdf

National Center for Complementary and Alternative Medicine. (2008a). *The use of complementary and alternative medicine in the United States*. Retrieved from http://nccam.nih.gov/news/camstats/2007/camsurvey_fs1.htm

National Center for Complementary and Alternative Medicine. (2008b). *CAM costs overall*. Retrieved from http://nccam.nih.gov/news/camstats/costs/costdatafs.htm#overall

National Center for Complementary and Alternative Medicine. (2011a). *What is complementary and alternative medicine?* Retrieved from http://nccam.nih.gov/health/whatiscam#informed

National Center for Complementary and Alternative Medicine. (2011b). *Research funding priorities*. Retrieved from http://nccam.nih.gov/grants/priorities

National Center for Complementary and Alternative Medicine. (2011c). *Selecting a complementary and alternative medicine practitioner.* Retrieved from http://nccam.nih.gov/health/decisions/practitioner.htm

National Center for Complementary and Alternative Medicine. (2012). *Safe use of complementary health products and practices*. Retrieved from http://nccam.nih.gov/health/safety

National Commission for Health Education Credentialing. (2007). *Competencies Update Project*. Retrieved from http://www.nchec.org/aboutnchec/cup/cup.htm

National Commission for Health Education Credentialing. (2008a). *What is a certified health education specialist (CHES)?* Retrieved from http://www.nchec.org/aboutnchec/faq/

National Commission for Health Education Credentialing. (2008b). *Responsibilities and competencies for health education specialists*. Retrieved from http://www.nchec.org/credentialing/responsibilities/

Patterson, S., & Graf, H. (2000). Integrating complementary and alternative medicine into the health education curriculum. *Journal of Health Education, 31*, 346–351.

Pearson, N. J., Johnson, L. L., & Nahin, R. L. (2006). Insomnia, trouble sleeping, and complementary and alternative medicine: Analysis of the 2002 National Health Interview Survey data. *Archives of Internal Medicine, 166*, 1775–1782.

Pérez, M., & Luquis, R. (2008). *Cultural competence in health education and health promotion*. San Francisco, CA: Jossey-Bass.

Pinzon-Perez, H. (2005). Complementary and alternative medicine, holistic health, and integrative healing: Applications in health education. *American Journal of Health Education, 36*(3), 174–178.

Portorreal Liriano, F. (2011). *Plantas Medicinales en el Este Dominicano* [Medicinal Plants in the East Region of the Dominican Republic]. San Pedro de Macorís, RD: Instituto de Investigaciones Científicas. Universidad Central del Este.

Robinson, M., & Zhang, X. (2011). *The world medicines situation 2011: Traditional medicines: Global situation, issues, and challenges* (3rd ed.). Geneva: World Health Organization. Retrieved March 28, 2012, from http://www.who.int/medicines/areas/policy/world_medicines_situation/WMS_ch18_wTraditionalMed.pdf

Sarnat, R. L., & Winterstein, J. (2004). Clinical and cost outcomes of an integrative medicine IPA. *Journal of Manipulative Physiological Therapies, 27*(5), 336–347.

Smith, B., & Wilbur, K. (2008). Foreword. In M. A. Pérez & R. R. Luquis (Eds.), *Cultural competence in health education and health promotion*. San Francisco, CA: Jossey-Bass,

Spector, R. (2009). *Cultural diversity in health and illness* (7th ed.). Upper Saddle River, NJ: Pearson Education.

Stanczak, M., & Heuberger, R. (2009). Assessment of the knowledge and beliefs regarding probiotic use. *American Journal of Health Education, 40*(4), 207–211.

Synovitz, L., Gillan, W., Wood, R., Martin-Nordness, M., & Kelly, J. (2006). An exploration of college students' complementary and alternative medicine use: Relationship to health locus of control and spirituality level. *American Journal of Health Education, 37*(2), 87–96.

Synovitz, L., & Larson, K. (2013). *Complementary and alternative medicine for health professionals: A holistic approach to consumer health*. Burlington, MA: Jones & Bartlett Learning.

Tafur, M., Crowe, T., & Torres, E. (2009). A review of curanderismo and healing practices among Mexicans and Mexican Americans. *Occupational Therapy International, 16*(1), 82–88.

WebMD. (2012). *Folk medicine.* Retrieved from http://dictionary.webmd.com/terms/folk-medicine

World Health Organization. (2001). *Legal status of traditional medicine and complementary/alternative medicine: A worldwide review.* Retrieved from http://whqlibdoc.who.int/hq/2001/WHO_EDM_TRM_2001.2.pdf

World Health Organization. (2008). *Traditional medicine.* Retrieved from http://www.who.int/mediacentre/factsheets/fs134/en/

Xue, C. (2008). *Traditional, complementary, and alternative medicine: Policy and public health perspectives. Bulletin of the World Health Organization.* Retrieved from http://www.who.int/bulletin/volumes/86/1/07–046458/en/index.html

CHAPTER 5

SPIRITUALITY AND CULTURAL DIVERSITY

Vickie D. Krenz

Voluminous studies from the psychological and sociological fields have investigated the association of regular church attendance and practices with health outcomes. The plethora of research has demonstrated that *religion* and spiritual beliefs can contribute to improved health, life expectancy, mental health, social support, and quality of life. This chapter provides an overview of the role of religion and *spirituality*, the emotional or experiential expression of "feelings or experiences of awe, wonder, harmony, peace, or connectedness with the universe or a higher power" (Johnstone et al., 2009, p. 147), on health behaviors and cultural diversity in the broader context. To address the concept of spirituality from the standpoint of a comparison between religious theologies would exhaust the limits of a chapter.

The topic of religion and spirituality on health outcomes has been clouded by the subjective perceptions of these terms, which have been used interchangeably to reflect the interrelatedness of the religious and spiritual dimensions. However, there is a need to differentiate these concepts. Johnstone, Yoon, Franklin, Schopp, and Hinkebein (2009) proposed that religion is a reflection of the behavioral aspects of religious practices, including the "frequency of participation in culturally based activities/practices (e.g., prayer/meditation, attendance at services, reading religious texts, performance of rituals, etc.)" (p. 147). However, Driskell and Lyon (2011) point out that it

LEARNING OBJECTIVES

After completing this chapter, you will be able to

- Discuss the religious and spiritual trends in the United States.
- Discuss the importance of worldview on spiritual and religious beliefs.
- Understand and explain the role of religion and spirituality on health behaviors and cultural diversity.

religion
The practice or participation in culturally based activities, including prayer and meditation, attendance at services, reading religious texts, and performance or rituals (Johnstone, Yoon, Franklin, Schopp, & Hinkebein, 2009)

spirituality
The emotional or experiential expression of "feelings or experiences of awe, wonder, harmony, peace, or connectedness with the universe or a higher power" (Johnstone et al., 2009, p. 147)

atheist
The disbelief in or denial of the existence of a God or supreme being.

agnostic
The belief that the existence or nature of God or the ultimate origin of the universe is known or knowable

is not sufficient to use religious behaviors and self-identified denomination as the measure of religiosity; religious beliefs, they say, are a stronger indicator for understanding the role of religion.

Spirituality is a subjective expression of beliefs with individual experiences and interpretations about the universe. Increased attention to spirituality in the research literature has shown the complexity of definitions from different disciplines and perspectives. Most often the concept of spirituality is described as character, well-being, or a sense of meaning and purpose (Miller & Thoresen, 2003; Murray & Zenter, 1989; Heelas, 2005). Other definitions of *spirituality* have focused on the connectedness of an individual with self, community, or a greater power (Reed, 1992; Gomez & Fisher, 2003; Rowold, 2011). As Meezenbroek and colleagues (2012) noted, the concept of spirituality has many meanings that reflect the breadth of individual religious and secular experiences.

Religious and Spiritual Trends in the United States

Religion remains very important in the American landscape. Findings from the U.S. Census Bureau (2012) and the American Religious Identification Survey (ARIS) (Kosmin & Keysar, 2006, 2009) indicated that 82.5 percent of Americans reported some form of religious identity. In the United States, Christianity remains the most commonly cited religious affiliation. Overall, the religious profile of Americans consisted of 52.5 percent Protestant/other Christian, 23.6 percent Catholic, 1.9 percent Mormon, 1.6 percent Jewish, 0.5 percent Muslim, 2.4 percent other non-Christian religion. Nevertheless, as table 5.1 shows, there is a growing segment of American's religious affiliation in the Non/*Atheist*/*Agnostic* category, with 15.0 percent of the population now self-reporting as believing in no God, no religion, humanistic, ethical culture, and secular (Kosmin & Keysar, 2009). Similar findings have been reported by the Pew Forum (Pew Forum on Religion and Public Life, 2009), with 16.1 percent of Americans self-identifying as unaffiliated (e.g., atheist, agnostic, nothing in particular). Furthermore, findings from the ARIS (Kosmin & Keysar, 2009) revealed that the percentage of Americans who self-identified as Christian declined from 86.2 percent in 1990 to an estimated 76.0 percent in 2008.

Overall, there has not been a shift to other world religions or new religious movements but a steady rejection of organized religions. The Gallup Poll findings reflect the changes in Americans' self-reported church, synagogue, or mosque attendance. Based on more than 800,000 randomized telephone interviews, 43.1 percent of the respondents reported weekly or almost weekly attendance (Newport, 2010). In contrast, 45 percent of the respondents reported

Table 5.1 U.S. Religious Traditions, 2008

Religious Tradition	Percent of Responses
Evangelical Protestant churches[a]	26.3
Mainline Protestant churches[b]	18.1
Historically black churches[c]	6.9
Catholic	23.9
Unaffiliated[d]	16.1
Jewish[e]	1.7
Mormon[f]	1.7
Other faiths[g]	1.2
Buddhist[h]	0.7
Jehovah's Witness	0.7
Orthodox[i]	0.6
Muslim[j]	0.6
Hindu[k]	0.4
Other Christian[l]	0.3
Other world religions	<0.3

Source: Pew Forum on Religion and Public Life. (2010). U.S. Religious Landscape Survey, http://religions.pewforum.org/

[a]Includes evangelical denominations of Baptist, Methodist, nondenominational, Lutheran, Presbyterian, Pentecostal, Anglican/Episcopalian, Restorationist, Congregationalist, Holiness, Reformed, Adventist, Anabaptist, Pietist, other Evangelical, Protestant nonspecific.

[b]Includes mainline denominations of Baptist, Methodist, nondenominational, Lutheran, Presbyterian, Anglican/Episcopalian, Restorationist, Congregationalist, Reformed, Anabaptist, Friends, other/Protestant nonspecific.

[c]Includes historically black denominations Baptist, Methodist, nondenominational, Pentecostal, Holiness, Protestant nonspecific.

[d]Includes atheist, agnostic, nothing in particular.

[e]Includes Reform, Conservative, Orthodox, other Jewish groups, Jewish nonspecific.

[f]Includes Church of Jesus Christ of Latter-Day Saints, Community of Christ, Mormon nonspecific.

[g]Includes Unitarians and other liberal faiths, new age, Native American religions.

[h]Includes Theravada (Vipassana), Mahayana (Zen), Vajrayana (Tibetan), other Buddhist groups, Buddhist nonspecific.

[i]Includes Greek Orthodox, Russian Orthodox, other Orthodox church, Orthodox nonspecific.

[j]Includes Sunni, Shia, other Muslim groups, Muslim nonspecific.

[k]Includes Vaishnava, Shaivite, other Hindu groups, Hindu nonspecific.

[l]Includes metaphysical, other.

that they seldom or never attend church, synagogue, or mosque. Respondents who reported more frequent church attendance included non-Hispanic blacks (55 percent), those over 65 years of age (53 percent), black Hispanics (52 percent), those who are married (48 percent), females (47 percent), and white Hispanics (46 percent). In contrast, respondents who reported less frequent church attendance were males (39 percent), not married (36 percent), 18 to 29 years old (35 percent), and Asian (31 percent).

Most recently, Saad (2012b) reported that confidence in organized religion is at an all-time low since the 1970s. Only 44 percent of Americans surveyed reported that they have a great deal or quite a lot of confidence in the church or organized religion. The Pew Forum (2009) identified other reasons that American have become unaffiliated with churches: hypocrisy among religious people, an overemphasis on rules and not enough emphasis on spirituality, and too much focus on money and power among religious leaders. Nevertheless, Americans have maintained strong spiritual beliefs in spite of a growing dissatisfaction with religious institutions.

There has been a steady decline in mainline church attendance among Americans, with an upward shift to a nondenominational identity. Kosmin, Keysar, Cragun, and Navarro-Rivera (2009) reported an increase in the number of Americans who reject all forms of organized religion. In 2008, 20 percent of Americans did not indicate a religious identity and these "nones" (no stated religious preference, atheist, or agnostic) grew from 8.1 percent in 1990 to 15.0 percent in 2008. Young adults (18 to 29 years) were more likely than other age groups to self-identify as nones. Of particular interest, Latinos have increasingly self-reported as none, from 4 percent to 12 percent (1990 and 2008, respectively). Nones tend to be more educated compared to the general US adult population. Furthermore, 19 percent of males self-identify as none compared to 12 percent of females. These findings are consistent with the Pew Forum (2009) study on religion and public life for American adults who self-identify as unaffiliated with any particular religious group.

While Americans have demonstrated dissatisfaction with organized religion, there remains an interest in spirituality. ARIS (Kosmin & Keysar, 2009) findings indicated that 70 percent of Americans continue to believe in a personal God. In comparison, an estimated 12 percent of Americans are atheists (no God) or agnostic (unknowable or unsure), and 12 percent are deistic (they believe in a higher power but no personal God).

Immigration has had a small but significant impact on religious groups in the United States. According to Kosmin and Keysar (2009), Catholics have increased to over 173 million members due to immigration, primarily from Latin American countries. However, the percentage of Catholics declined from 26.2 percent to 25.1 percent between 1990 and 2008. Among Hispanics, immigration has been shown to have an impact on self-identified religious affiliation. Spanish speakers were more likely to self-identify as Catholic as compared to English speakers, who were more likely to self-identify as Baptist or mainline religious denominations. Similarly, the Pew Forum (2008) reported that 46 percent of immigrants self-reported as Catholic, with 72 percent among Mexican immigrants and 51 percent among other Latin American immigrants.

These changing trends in religious self-identification have also been noted among racial groups. According to Kosmin and Keysar (2009), blacks (non-Hispanic) are more likely to attend church, with 55 percent doing so on a weekly or almost weekly basis. Among Hispanics, 52 percent of black Hispanics reported regular church attendance as compared to 46 percent white Hispanics. Only 41 percent of non-Hispanic whites reported regular church attendance. Asians have the lowest self-reported church attendance, with only 31 percent attending church weekly or almost weekly.

Shifts in religious affiliation have been documented over the past three decades. ARIS findings (Kosmin & Keysar, 2009) revealed that white (non-Hispanic) Catholics declined from 27 percent in 1990 to 21 percent in 2008, with an increase in ex-Catholic respondents who now self-identify as none. This trend was also evident in the decline of white mainline Christians during the same time frame. Blacks demonstrated a similar trend from 1990 to 2001, moving from former Baptists to none. Since 2001, blacks have tended to self-identify as generic Christian and conservative Protestant (e.g., African Methodist).

Similarly, Asian Americans have demonstrated changes in religious self-identification over time. There has been an observable decline among Asians in self-identity as Catholics, with 27 percent in 1990, 20 percent in 2001, and 17 percent in 2008. Asian immigration has resulted in an increase of self-identified adherents in Eastern religions, from 8 percent in 1990 to 21 percent in 2008. There remains a trend among Asians to self-identify as none (Kosmin & Keysar, 2009).

Self-identification with an organized religion has been associated with educational attainment. Since 1990, organized religious traditions have increased the percentage of college graduates (25 years and older) among their adherents. As noted in table 5.2, Jewish and Eastern religions' educational attainment exceeded other religious traditions in 2008. Muslim and non-Christian traditions demonstrated a decline in educational attainment (Kosmin & Keysar, 2009).

Geographical location is important in Americans' church attendance. Church attendance is highest in the South (51 percent) compared to the Midwest (44 percent), East (38 percent), and West (37 percent). However, a striking phenomenon has been the dramatic increase in the nones across all geographical regions in the United States. Regions that have been predominantly Catholic (50 percent in New England and 43 percent in the middle Atlantic regions) have demonstrated significant shifts into the none category (Kosmin and Keysar, 2009).

Interestingly, Kosmin and colleagues (2009) described the nones as a diverse group of people who do not identify with more formalized American

Table 5.2 Percentage of College Graduates in the Population Age 25 and Over by Religious Tradition, 1990–2008

	1990	2008
US national population		
Protestant	21	27
Baptist	11	16
Christian generic	22	26
Mainline Christian	26	35
Pentecostal/Charismatic	9	13
Protestant denominations	13	21
Historically black churches	—	16
Catholic	22	27
Jewish	50	57
Mormon	22	31
Muslim	41	35
Eastern religions	44	59
New religions movements and other religions	35	33
None/unaffiliated	28	31
Don't know/refused	29	31

Sources: Kosmin, and Keysar (2009). Pew Forum on Religion and Public Life. (2010). U.S. Religious Landscape Survey, http://religions.pewforum.org/

religions, including irreligious, unreligious antireligious, and anticlerical. The majority of nones (73 percent) grew up in religious homes, with 55 percent having parents with the same religion. Interestingly, 55 percent of nones reported that they have had some form of a religious initiation ceremony (e.g., baptism, Christening, circumcision, bar mitzvah, or naming ceremony). As noted in table 5.3, the nones represent a highly educated group that includes 17 percent with less than a high school diploma, 25 percent high school graduate, 24 percent some college, 20 percent college graduate, 11 percent postgraduate, and 3 percent other or refused to answer. Furthermore, 33 percent of nones accept human evolution as compared to only 15 percent of the general U.S. population. It is clear that the nones are a growing and significant religious group that is as culturally diverse as other religious affiliations.

Since the majority of Americans self-identify as Christian, the influence of the Bible is a key issue in American religious practice. Brown (1980) reported that reading the Bible was the most influential factor contributing to moral behavior. More recently, Jones (2011) reported that only three in ten Americans interpret the Bible as the literal word of God. In contrast,

Table 5.3 Characteristics of Those with a Religious Self-Identification of None

Religious Self-Identity	Percentage of Responses
Atheist	7
Rational skeptics	
Hard agnostic (there is no way to know)	19
Soft agnostic (I'm not sure)	16
Deist (there is a higher power but no personal God)	25
Theist (there is definitely a personal God)	27
Gender	
Male	60
Female	40
Race/ethnicity	
White	72
Irish	33
British	20
Italian	9
Jewish	4
Black	8
Hispanic/Latino	12
Asian	3
Other	5
Educational level	
Less than high school	17
High school graduate	25
Some college	24
College graduates	20
Postgraduate	11
Other/refused to answer	3

Source: Kosmin and colleagues (2009).

49 percent of Americans consider the Bible inspired by God but not to be taken literally, and 17 percent view the Bible as an ancient book of fables or legends. Those who were very religious, with lower education and lower income, were more likely to believe that the Bible is the actual word of God. In comparison, those who attend church nearly weekly or monthly, with middle or higher incomes and higher education (college graduate/postgraduate), were more likely to believe that the Bible is the inspired word of God. Only 46 percent of Protestants (self-identified Christians, not including

Catholics or Mormons) and 66 percent of Catholics believe that the Bible is the inspired word of God.

It is evident that Americans have shifted their religious self-identification away from organized religious denominations. Church attendance has dropped significantly across most racial, gender, and traditional denominations. Immigration has expanded the breadth of religions represented in the United States to include Islam, Hindu, Buddhist, and Sikh. A comparative religion approach can provide descriptive information on the theological basis of organized religions. As Kosmin and Keysar (2009) and the Pew Forum on Religion and Public Life (2009) noted, there remains considerable diversity both between and within traditional religious groups. For example, Baptist denominations consist of numerous subcategories, including Southern, American, Free-Will, Missionary, Conservative, and African American. Similarly, Catholic classifications include Roman Catholic, Greek Orthodox, and Eastern Rites. Jewish traditions include Reformed, Conservative, and Orthodox Judaism. Buddhism consists of three major groups: Zen, Theravada, and Tibetan Buddhism.

Furthermore, the beliefs of individuals are not a homogeneous reflection of broader religious beliefs and practices of organized religious denominations. For example, Saad (2012a) reported that 38 percent of Catholics and 33 percent of Protestants considered themselves to be pro-choice. Newport (2012a, 2012b) reported that 82 percent of Catholics and 90 percent of non-Catholics perceived birth control as morally acceptable and that 38 percent of Protestants, 51 percent of Catholics, and 88 percent of those who reported no religious identity supported legal same-sex marriage.

Worldview and Spiritual Beliefs

In a discussion of spirituality, it is fitting to understand how individuals conceptualize reality and their perceptions of the universe. Scientific empiricism in the twentieth century challenged the basic tenets of Protestant Christianity. The term *worldview* (*Weltanschauung*) is a philosophical and theological concept that focuses on individual inner subjectivity in relation to an external world. It strives to identify the meaning and value of the universe and of human life. From a Protestant Evangelical theological perspective, the individual worldview is centered on the issue of the divine revelation of God to human existence. A key concept is the validity of the biblical doctrines of Jesus as the incarnated Son of God. Existential philosophers challenged this belief with objective rationality to the external world and history. The external reality is defined by a scientific empirico-mathematical approach that quantifies time and the sequence of events. People experience

worldview
The broader reflection of an individual's subjective perceptions of the world, including individual experiences, well-being, and meaning or purpose of life

this external reality through a mathematical sequence of predictable events (Barth, 1962; Bultmann, 1961; Kant, 1878; Moltmann, 1967).

Philosophers and theologians have debated the authenticity of the historical events that form the basis for Christian religious faith (e.g., the Immaculate Conception; the personification of God in Jesus Christ; the Trinity of Father, Son, and Holy Spirit; the Resurrection). Evangelical Christianity holds the events of the New Testament as the divine personal communication of God to man. Furthermore, God centers this disclosure in personal relationships with humans. Existential scholars (Kierkegaard, 1936; Marsh, 1952; Ott, 1965) have argued the sequence of time and the nonobjective experience of God. There can be no act of God as a historic event, and religion must be interpreted with inner subjective experience.

Within the context of spirituality and the worldview is how individuals perceive the universe (i.e., the cosmos) in relation to their individual experience with God (or supreme being). The concept of cosmological dualism contrasts the universe as an open or closed continuum. In an open continuum, God interacts in human experiences (Torrance, 1969, 1971). In contrast, in a closed continuum, God is spatially separated from the universe and cannot interact in human experiences (Newton, 1953). Based on subjective perceptions, individuals may believe that God is continuously involved in their personal experiences. In contrast, individuals may perceive that God (or the absence of a God) is removed from active involvement in the human experience.

As with the shift in ideologies, there has emerged a broader conceptual framework for religious and spiritual expression. The self-identification of religious identity remains subjective but can be viewed on a continuum that encompasses ideologies that include *monotheism* (belief in one god), *polytheism* (belief in more than one god), and *pantheism* (belief that god is everywhere and in everything, but is not an individual being), deism (a higher power but no personal god), agnostic (unknown or unsure), or atheism (belief in no god) (Rosten, 1975). Religious perceptions can acknowledge individual expression in the name or names that may be attributed to a specific spiritual entity or entities, including *God, Yahweh, El Shaddai, Elohim, Ayllah, Great Spirit,* or *science* (Henry, 1976).

monotheism
Belief in one God

polytheism
Belief in more than one God

pantheism
The belief that there is no God, but rather a sense of awe or reverence for nature or the universe

More recently, the research literature has identified the concept of spirituality as a factor in health outcomes. The existential concept of the worldview has evolved to encompass a broader reflection of individual psychological experiences and well-being. Numerous authors (Cole, Hopkins, Tisak, Steel, & Carr, 2008; Meezenbroek et al., 2012; Rippentrop, Altmaier, & Burns, 2006) have recognized that spirituality does not necessitate religiosity but reflects the psychological experiences of religiosity and spirituality.

Koenig and Larsen (2001) characterized spirituality as including life satisfaction, feelings of the meaning and purpose of life, and worldview. Cook (2004) proposed that spirituality includes the connectedness of oneself to someone or something beyond the human experience, including the universality, a transcendent reality, or higher power (i.e., God). Greenfield, Vaillant, and Marks (2009) expanded this concept to include experiences that are related to the "sense of connection with a transcendent, integration of self, feelings of awe, gratitude, compassion, and forgiveness" (p. 2).

Spirituality is a subjective expression of beliefs with individual experiences and interpretations about the universe. For some individuals, the belief that a higher deity, "God," is actively involved in human events allows for the potential to attribute circumstances or situations to something that God has given them. The "blessings," "punishments," or "tests" can explain circumstances that are beyond individual control. Therefore, faith in a divine plan or intervention cushions the uncontrollable events that may defy an individual's ability to cope (e.g., the loss of a loved one, changes in health status, financial loss). Spirituality, then, becomes a source of comfort and well-being (i.e., God allowed the event to happen).

Impact of Religiosity and Spirituality on Health and Well-Being

The impact of religiosity and spirituality on health and well-being has been well established. Hill and associates (2000) and McSherry and Cash (2004) noted the difficulties in operational definitions for these concepts, including such terms as *religion, religiosity, spirituality,* and *well-being.* Although these terms represent interrelated constructs, there remains a need for clear definitions and precise measurement. Most often, self-reported religious affiliation or self-perceived level of religion or spirituality (e.g., "How religious/spiritual do you consider yourself to be?") has been used to categorize religious practice (Pearce, Little, & Perez, 2003; Zinnbauer & Pargament, 2005). In addition, Sloan and Bagiella (2002) noted that there remains little empirical evidence that supports the beneficial health outcomes of religious involvement.

Health Practices

Research has pointed to the impact of religion on health outcomes. Newport, Sangeeta, and Witters (2010a) reported that very religious and moderately religious Americans were more likely to practice healthy behaviors compared to nonreligious Americans. Their findings revealed that that 14.9 percent of very religious and 26.6 percent of moderately religious respondents were nonsmokers (as compared to 27.6 percent of nonreligious).

Interestingly, 68.1 percent of very religious and 58.1 percent of moderately religious respondents reported having had five or more servings of fruits and vegetables at least four times in the past week as compared to 55.1 percent of nonreligious. In addition, 53.3 percent of very religious and 49.3 percent of moderately religious respondents indicated that they had exercised at least thirty minutes at least three days in the last week (as compared to 47.9 percent of nonreligious).

Many religious faiths consider the human body to be sacred and subscribe to practices to ensure physical well-being. These prescriptions often include prohibition of harmful substances (e.g., tobacco, alcohol, illicit drugs), dietary practices, or exercise guidelines. Krause (2003) reported that religious affiliation with a fundamentalist church was protective for alcohol use. In comparison, people who had liberal religious beliefs were healthier but less happy. Frequent religious involvement and affiliation in early adolescence (age 14) has been shown to delay timing for first intercourse (Jones, Darroch, & Singh, 2005).

Harrigan (2011) analyzed data from the National Health Interview Survey to examine the impact of prayer on health habits. The results demonstrated that 13,179 (59 percent) of the participants who prayed for their health reported that they engaged in positive health habits, including frequent vigorous exercise, increased use of relaxation techniques, support groups, meditation, and use of traditional and complementary and alternative medicine therapies. Of these, 76.5 percent were white, 16.0 percent were black, 5.5 percent were Asian, and 2.0 percent were other. Females (51.9 percent) were slightly more likely to pray for their health as compared to males (48.1 percent). However, there were no statistically significant differences between participants by race/ethnicity, age, income, gender, or place of birth.

Research findings consistently document the impact of religious practices and spirituality on positive health outcomes. For example, as part of their theological doctrines, Seventh-Day Adventists follow a vegetarian diet and refrain from negative health habits such as smoking and alcohol consumption. Montgomery and associates (2007) demonstrated that an Adventist lifestyle among black adherents contributed to better health outcomes as compared to blacks nationally. Fraser and Shavlik (2001) documented that California Seventh-Day Adventists had higher life expectancies than other white Californians due to their diet, exercise, and lack of smoking.

Similar positive health outcomes have been observed in Mormons residing in Utah. Lyon, Gardner, and West (1980) demonstrated that Mormons showed a lower incidence of smoking-related cancers as compared to non-Mormons. As the authors noted, Mormon teaching prohibits alcohol and tobacco use, as well as conservative sexual activity. Similar studies (Daniels, Merrill, Lyon, Stanford, & White, 2004) have supported that Mormon religious practices are associated with lower rates of breast cancer.

Mental Health

The mental health field has produced a vast array of data on the impact of religiosity and spirituality on well-being outcomes. Religious participation was associated with more purpose in life and personal growth among older adults. "Very religious" individuals are less likely to report having been diagnosed with depression over the course of their lifetime. Newport, Sangeeta, and Witters (2010b) reported that lifetime clinical diagnosis of depression was 15.6 percent among the very religious, 20.4 percent among the moderately religious, and 18.7 percent among the nonreligious. Similarly, Green and Elliott (2010) noted that individuals who identified as religious tended to report greater happiness and optimism for coping with difficult situations. Furthermore, very religious Americans are also less likely to report experiencing the daily negative emotions of worry, stress, sadness, and anger than are their moderately religious and nonreligious counterparts. Wong, Rew, and Slaikeu (2006) investigated adolescent mental health outcomes using a meta-analysis of twenty articles between 1998 and 2004. The findings demonstrated that higher levels of religiosity and spirituality were positively associated with better mental health outcomes among adolescents.

Adherence to religious beliefs has also been shown to be a source of negative mental health outcomes. Yorulmaz, Gencoz, and Woody (2009) and Inozu, Karanchi, and Clark (2012) reported that highly religious Christians and Muslim students tended to have greater levels of obsessionality related to personal guilt and personal responsibility for controlling unwanted intrusive thoughts. Williams, Lau, and Grisham (2013) demonstrated a relationship between religiosity and obsessive-compulsive symptoms among university students with moderate religiosity levels. However, the authors suggested that obsessional thinking was attributed to the teaching of certain underlying religious doctrines (e.g., wishing harm on a hated individual).

Catastrophic Illnesses

The role of religiosity and spirituality on catastrophic illness such as cancer has received considerable attention. Numerous studies (Koffman, Morgan, Edmonds, Speck, & Higginson, 2008; Stewart & Yuen, 2011) have demonstrated that religiosity and spirituality can be a positive coping strategy for dealing with physical illnesses. A number of studies (Levine, Aviv, Yoo, Ewing, & Au, 2009; Wilkinson, Saper, Rosen, Welles, & Culpepper, 2008) have reported the beneficial effect of prayer as a means to cope with disease. Peterman, Fitchett, Brady, Hernandez, and Cella (2002) noted the need for measures to address spiritual well-being among cancer and other chronic illness patients. Similarly, Cotton, McGrady, and Rosenthal (2010) noted that there remains the need for a developmentally relevant religious/spirituality scale to reliably measure adolescent well-being outcomes. Thus, there is a need to assess spiritual well-being in the development of health education interventions for age-specific populations.

Nelson and colleagues (2009) developed a theoretical framework addressing the relationship among religiosity, spirituality, and depression with male prostate cancer. The sense of meaning and peace was the main component in reducing depression with activities and interventions that were not exclusive to religious involvement. Similarly, Maliski, Connor, Williams, and Litwin (2010) found that faith in God was a motivator among African American men diagnosed with prostate cancer to cope with their perceptions and achieve purposeful acceptance or resignation.

The role of spirituality has been shown to have a stronger role on quality-of-life measures among cancer patients. Schnoll, Harlow, and Brower (2000) found that spirituality was a significant factor in psychological adjustment among women with breast cancer. Rippentrop et al. (2006) investigated emotional well-being, functional well-being, interpersonal/social well-being, and treatment satisfaction in sixty-one cancer patients. Their results demonstrated that spirituality has a stronger relation with quality of life than religiosity measures. Tanyi and Werner (2007) reported consistent findings with African American women on hemodialysis for end-stage renal disease.

Braam, Klinkenber, Galenkamp, and Deeg (2012) compared previous depressive symptoms and religiousness with proxy respondents of Longitudinal Aging Study Amsterdam patients for moods in the last week of life. Interviews with after-death proxy respondents of the deceased sample members revealed that previous depressive symptoms, church membership, church attendance, and religious beliefs were associated with an increased likelihood of depression in the last week of life. However, patients without previous depressive symptoms were more likely to have a sense of peace.

Individuals may attribute their illnesses to God's will as some form of test. Zaldivar and Smolowitz (1994) reported that 78 percent of non–Mexican American Hispanic adults with diabetes believed that their disease was "God's will." Similar findings have been reported for Arab

American women and their breast cancer (Obeidat, Lally, & Dickerson, 2012). Ismail, Wright, Rhodes, and Small (2005) reported that South Asians (e.g., Muslims, Sikhs, and Hindus) believed their epilepsy was the result of fate, the will of God, or punishment for past life sins. In contrast, Vuckovic, Williams, Schneider, Ramirez, and Gullion (2012) found that shamanic practitioners believe that illness is the result of being "dispirited" (a separation of the soul from the body).

Of particular interest, Morita, Tsunoda, Inoue, and Chihara (2000) focused on the existential concerns of terminally ill Japanese cancer patients. The existential distress these cancer patients experienced included loss of autonomy, lowered self-esteem, and hopelessness. Furthermore, terminally ill Japanese cancer patients are more likely to request hastened death, with 21 percent expressing the desire to die and 10 percent to hasten death. In comparison, Ando, Morita, Lee, and Okamoto (2008) reported that Japanese terminally ill cancer patients who faced their illness with positive meaning and acceptance demonstrated spiritual well-being. Breitbart and colleagues (2000) reported that the strongest predictors for the request were depression and helplessness. Ando, Morita, Ahn, Marquez-Wong, and Ide (2009) demonstrated that cultural differences may contribute to the concerns of terminally ill cancer patients. In addition, greater attention to spiritual well-being of terminally ill patients is needed by health care professionals.

Spiritually Based Interventions

Several interventions have been developed to address the spiritual beliefs and religious practices among patients with chronic illnesses. McCauley, Haaz, Tarpley, Koenig, and Barlett (2011) evaluated the effectiveness of a spiritual intervention (a video and workbook) to encourage patients' spiritual coping. The results did not demonstrate statistically significant improvements between the intervention and control groups in pain, mood, health perceptions, illness intrusiveness, and self-efficacy. However, the program was associated with increased energy and required no additional clinician time. Kemppainen and colleagues (2012) used a mantram (a sacred word or phrase) spiritually based intervention with patients with HIV disease to improve coping and manage physical symptoms. Ando and colleagues (2008, 2009) conducted short-term life review interviews to address the primary concerns of terminally ill cancer patients. The focus of the intervention was to improve spiritual well-being with attention to the culturally specific primary concerns of patients.

Spiritually based interventions have also been used for educational and early screening programs. Holt and colleagues (2011) and Katz and associates (2004) tailored culturally focused colorectal cancer education programs for African Americans. Church-based approaches have been used to address health-related issues. Ma, Gao, Tan, Chae, and Rhee (2012) addressed screening and vaccination for hepatitis B virus among Korean Americans using Korean church leaders. Numerous researchers (Dodani, Kramer, Williams, Crawford, & Kriska, 2009; Whitt-Glover, Goldmon, Karanja, Heil, & Gizlice, 2012) have implemented a diabetes prevention program with community-based churches using physical activity for African Americans. Similarly, diabetes prevention interventions targeted for the Latino community have been implemented through Catholic churches. Bopp, Fallon, and Marquez (2011) implemented a culturally and spiritually relevant physical activity intervention for Latinos in three Catholic churches. Baig and colleagues (2012) developed a peer-based self-management program for Latinos with diabetes. It is apparent that faith-based approaches can be used to tailor health messages to specific spiritual communities.

Religiosity/Spirituality and Cultural Diversity

Religious beliefs and practices in the United States are as diverse as its cultures and people. The breadth of formal religious practices ranges from a belief in a personal God to the belief in no God. However, Christianity has remained the predominant religion in the United States, with 78 percent of all adults identifying with a Christian faith and 92 percent saying they believe in God (Kosmin & Keysar, 2009). While Americans have become dissatisfied with organized religions, there remains a strong interest in the spirituality that is not tied to racial, gender, educational, or income categories.

Age

Epner and Baile (2012) pointed out that cultural processes frequently differ within the same ethnic or social group. These processes are reflected by the variation within groups by age, gender, political association, class, religion, and ethnicity. The Pew Forum (2008) reported variations in religious affiliation by age. As shown in table 5.4, younger Americans were less likely to report a Protestant religious affiliation as compared to older Americans. As noted previously, younger Americans were more likely to report Eastern religions, Muslim, and unaffiliated religious traditions. In comparison, older Americans were more likely to report Protestant or Catholic religious traditions.

Table 5.4 Percentage of Age Composition by Religious Traditions, 2008

	Ages 18–29	Ages 30–49	Ages 50–69	Ages 70 and Over	Total Percentage
US national population	22%	38%	28%	12	100%
Catholic	21	38	28	13	100
Baptist	11	31	37	21	100
Mainline Christian	18	35	33	14	100
Christian generic	25	41	25	9	100
Pentecostal/Charismatic	16	34	36	14	100
Protestant denominations	22	36	28	14	100
Mormon/Church of the Latter Day Saints	22	40	28	10	100
Jewish	21	28	33	18	100
Eastern religions	37	40	20	3	100
Muslim	42	45	12	1	100
New religious movements and other religions	24	40	27	9	100
None	29	41	23	7	100

Source: Kosmin and Keysar, (2009).

Race and Ethnicity

Racial and ethnic groups have demonstrated shifts in religious traditions from 1990 to 2008. Table 5.5 displays the self-reported religious traditions by racial/ethnic composition. White Americans represent predominantly Protestant and Catholic religious traditions. Blacks, in comparison, are more likely to self-report as Baptist and Christian generic. Hispanics continue to self-report as Catholics, with a growing number of individuals shifting to Christian generic. Asians and other races are more likely to self-report as Eastern religions and none. As noted previously, there continues to be a dramatic shift among all racial and ethnic groups from formal Christian groups to the "none" religious tradition.

Gender

Gender differences are evident in organized religious participation and church attendance. ARIS findings (Kosmin & Keysar, 2009) revealed that females were more likely to report participation in formal Christian groups, including Pentecostals (58 percent), Baptists (57 percent), and mainline Christians (56 percent). In comparison, males were more likely to

Table 5.5 Composition of Racial/Ethnic Groups by Religious Tradition 1990, 2001, 2008

	White Non-Hispanic			Black Non-Hispanic			Hispanic			Asian and Other Races		
	1990	2001	2008	1990	2001	2008	1990	2001	2008	1990	2001	2008
Catholic	27%	23%	21%	9%	7%	6%	66%	57%	59%	27%	20%	17%
Baptist	15	15	15	50	46	45	7	5	3	9	4	3
Mainline Christian	21	22	17	12	10	7	4	3	1	11	6	6
Christian generic	17	11	15	9	10	15	8	11	11	13	11	10
Pentecostal/charismatic	3	3	3	6	7	7	3	4	3	2	1	0
Protestant denominations	2	3	3	4	4	6	2	3	4	2	1	2
Mormon/ Church of the Latter Day Saints	2	2	2	0	0	0	1	1	0	2	0	0
Jewish	2	2	2	0	0	0	1	1	0	1	0	0
Eastern religions	0	0	0	0	0	0	0	0	0	8	22	21
Muslim	0	0	0	1	1	1	0	0	0	3	8	8
New religious movements and other religions	1	1	1	1	1	1	1	1	1	1	1	1
None	8	15	16	6	11	11	6	13	12	16	22	27
Don't know or refused to answer	2	4	4	1	2	2	1	3	5	4	5	5

Source: Kosmin and Keysar (2009).

self-identify as none (60 percent), Eastern religions (53 percent), Muslim (52 percent), and new religious movements/other religions (52 percent), such as Scientology, new age, Spiritualist, Unitarian-Universalist, and deist.

Religious Belief Systems and Faith-Based Programs

Religious beliefs and belief systems represent a subjective expression of beliefs with individual experiences and interpretations about the universe. Spirituality and religious beliefs have been shown to have an impact on health outcomes. Although formalized religious affiliation has declined among Americans, faith-based organizations have remained a central focus of many racial and ethnic communities. Wingood, Simpson-Robinson, Braxton, and Raiford (2011) noted that faith-based organizations provide stable and influential social structures for many communities, in particular, African American communities.

In recent years, there has been greater focus on the role of faith-based organizations in health education and health promotion programs. Bopp and Fallon (2013) demonstrated that faith-based organizations have strong connections to large groups and represent an access point for health promotion and wellness programming. In particular, community-based participatory models have used faith-based organizations to address health disparities as a part of the Racial and Ethnic Approaches to Health (REACH) 2010 initiatives. Collie-Akers, Schultz, Carson, Fawcett, and Ronan (2009) partnered with the Kansas City-Chronic Disease Coalition to engage neighborhoods and faith-based organizations in health promotion strategies to reduce cardiovascular disease and diabetes. Wingood et al. (2011) developed a successful community-based participatory relation between a university and a church to design and implement a faith-based HIV intervention. Similarly, Wilcox and colleagues (2007) implemented a statewide faith-based physical activity initiative with African Methodist Episcopal volunteers across South Carolina.

Conclusion

The multicultural approach to cultural competence should be receptive to diversity that exists in religious and spiritual expressions. Applying the framework of comparative religions to represent cultural norms would lead to considerable misperceptions. There continues to be a shifting in religious affiliations across the United States.

A key implication in cultural diversity is to recognize the breadth of spiritual expressions that transcend formalized religions and their practices. Contemporary religious beliefs encompass a wide range of beliefs, from monotheism to atheism. Furthermore, there is broad cultural diversity and spiritual beliefs within formalized religions. Thus, it is essential to not presuppose that all Protestants and Orthodox adherents absolutely prescribe to the official doctrines and tenets of their denomination. Rather, it is essential to recognize that spirituality is a personal experience within the concept of an individual worldview.

Furthermore, it is important to recognize the importance of faith-based organizations as a central focus in many racial and ethnic communities. These organizations represent excellent potential community-based partnerships that have strong ties to communities with health disparities. Community-based participatory models have demonstrated that faith-based organizations can provide strong connections for health and wellness promotion programming.

Points to Remember

- Religion is a complex reflection of culturally based religious practices, including church attendance, prayer, and other rituals. Spirituality is the subjective expression of individual beliefs of well-being or one's place in the universe.
- It is important to recognize the diversity in individuals' worldview and that spirituality has a wide range of expressions even within religious affiliations.
- Fewer than half of Americans report attending church, yet spirituality is important to the majority of Americans. Spirituality is a dynamic and complex perception that may change with an individual's experiences and age.

Case Study

Edgar and Sophia are Hispanic college juniors. While raised in a Catholic home, Edgar has grown away from his childhood religion and attends Mass with his mother only when he goes home occasionally. Edgar is not sure if there is a God and questions the tenets of the Catholic Church. Edgar's father identifies as Catholic but no longer believes that the church is relevant for today's world.

Sophia was raised Catholic and continues to attend Mass on a monthly basis. Her mother is a deeply religious woman who is actively involved in her church. Her father attends Mass with her mother but is not as active with church activities.

Over the past several weeks, Edgar and Sophia's relationship has grown more intense, and the couple has begun to have sexual intercourse. Edgar is not ready to have children and wants to wait until he has completed his education. Sophia does not believe in using birth control to prevent pregnancy. However, Edgar continues to pressure Sophia to use birth control pills to prevent the chance of a pregnancy at this time.

1. What would be the best description of Edgar's worldview, and how does it reflect his current religious identification?
2. How could an individual's sexual behaviors be influenced by his or her worldview?
3. How would a health educator address other aspects of sexual health, such as sexually transmitted diseases, if the couple solely focuses on the use of the pill to prevent pregnancy?
4. How would Sophia and Edgar's worldviews affect their use of other preventive behaviors, such as the use of condoms or a diaphragm?

KEY TERMS

Agnostic
Atheist
Monotheism
Pantheism
Polytheism
Religion
Spirituality
Worldview

References

Ando, M., Morita, T., Ahn, S. H., Marquez-Wong, F., & Ide, S. (2009). International comparison study of the primary concerns of terminally ill cancer patients in short-term life review interviews among Japanese, Koreans, and Americans. *Palliative Support and Care, 7,* 349–355.

Ando, M., Morita, T., Lee, V., & Okamoto, T. (2008). A pilot study of transformation, attributed meanings to the illness, and spiritual well-being for terminally ill cancer patients. *Palliative Support and Care, 6,* 335–340.

Baig, A. A., Locklin, C. A., Wilkes, A. E., Oborski, D. D., Acevedo, J. C., Gorawara-Bhat, R., . . . Chin, M. H. (2012). "One can learn from other people's experiences": Latino adults' preferences for peer-based diabetes interventions. *Diabetes Education, 38,* 733–741.

Barth, K. (1962). *Theology and church* (L. P. Smith, Trans.). Naperville, IL: Alec R. Allensen.

Bopp, M., & Fallon, E. A. (2013). Health and wellness programming in faith-based organizations: A description of a nationwide sample. *Health Promotion Practice, 14,* 122–131. doi:10.1177/1524839912446478

Bopp, M., Fallon, E. A., & Marquez, D. X. (2011). A faith-based physical activity intervention for Latinos: Outcomes and lessons. *American Journal of Health Promotion, 25,* 168–171.

Braam, A. W., Klinkenberg, M., Galenkamp, H., & Deeg, D.J.H. (2012). Late-life depressive symptoms, religiousness, and mood in the last week of life. *Depression Research and Treatment, 2012,* 1–10.

Breitbart, W., Rosenfeld, B., Pessin, H., Kaim, M., Funesti-Esch, J., Galietta, M., . . . Brescia, R. (2000). Depression, hopelessness, and desire for hastened death in terminally ill patients with cancer. *Journal of the American Medical Association, 284,* 2907–2911.

Brown, H.O.J. (1980). What's the connection between faith and works? The Gallup Poll establishes Bible reading as most discernible factor shaping moral behavior. *Christianity Today, 24,* 26–29.

Bultmann, R. (1961). Bultmann replies to his critics. In H. W. Hartsch (Ed.), *Kerygma and myth: A theological debate, vol. 2.* London: S.P.C.K.

Cole, S. C., Hopkins, C. M., Tisak, J., Steel, J. L., & Carr, B. I. (2008). Assessing spiritual growth and spiritual decline following a diagnosis of cancer: Reliability and validity of the spiritual transformation scale. *Psycho-Oncology, 17,* 112–121.

Collie-Akers, V., Schlutz, J. A., Carson, V., Fawcett, S. T., & Ronan, M. (2009). REACH 2010: Kansas City, Missouri: Evaluating mobilization strategies with neighborhood and faith organizations to reduce risk for health disparities. *Health Promotion Practice, 10,* 118S–127S.

Cook, C.C.H. (2004). Addiction and spirituality. *Addiction, 99,* 539–551.

Cotton, S., McGrady, M. E., & Rosenthal, S. L. (2010). Measurement of religiosity/spirituality in adolescent health outcomes research: Trends and recommendations. *Journal of Religion and Health, 49,* 414–444.

Daniels, M., Merrill, R. M., Lyon, J. L., Stanford, J. B., & White, G. L. (2004). Associations between breast cancer risk factors and religious practices in Utah. *Preventive Medicine, 38,* 28–38.

Dodani, S., Kramer, M. K., Williams, L., Crawford, S., & Kriska, A. (2009). Fit body and soul: A church-based behavioral lifestyle program for diabetes prevention in African Americans. *Ethnicity and Disease, 19,* 135–141.

Driskell, R. L., & Lyon, L. (2011). Assessing the role of religious beliefs on secular and spiritual behaviors. *Review of Religious Research, 52,* 386–404.

Epner, D. E., & Baile, W. F. (2012). Patient-centered care: The key to cultural competence. *Annuals in Oncology, 23,* 33–42.

Fraser, G. E., & Shavlik, D. J. (2001). Ten years of life: Is it a matter of choice? *Archives of Internal Medicine, 161,* 1645–52.

Gomez, R., & Fisher, J. W. (2003). Domains of spiritual well-being and development and validation of a spiritual well-being questionnaire. *Personality and Individual Differences, 35,* 1107–1121.

Green, M., & Elliott, M. (2010). Religion, health, and psychological well-being. *Journal of Religion and Health, 49,* 149–163.

Greenfield, E. A., Vaillant, G. E., & Marks, N. F. (2009). Do formal religious participation and spiritual perceptions have independent linkages with diverse dimensions of psychological well-being? *Journal of Health and Social Behavior, 50,* 196–212.

Harrigan, J. T. (2011). Health promoting habits of people who pray for their health. *Journal of Religion and Health, 50,* 602–607.

Heelas, P. (2005). *The spiritual revolution: Why religion is giving way to spirituality.* Malden, MA: Blackwell.

Henry, C.F.H. (1976). *God, revelation and authority, vol. 2: God who speaks and shows.* Waco, TX: Word Books.

Hill, P. C., Pargament, K. I., Wood, R. W., McCullough, M. E., Swyers, J. P., Larson, D. B., & Zinnbauer, B. J. (2000). Conceptualizing religion and spirituality: Points of commonality, points of departure. *Journal for the Theory of Social Behaviour, 30,* 51–77.

Holt, C. L., Shipp, M., Eloubedid, M., Fouad, M. N., Britt, K., & Norena, M. (2011). Your body is the temple: Impact of a spiritually based colorectal cancer educational intervention delivered through community health advisors. *Health Promotion Practice, 12,* 577–588.

Inozu, M., Karanci, A. N., & Clark, D. A. (2012). Why are religious individuals more obsessional? The role of mental control beliefs and guilt in Muslims and Christians. *Journal of Behavioral Therapy and Experimental Psychiatry, 43,* 959–966. doi:10.1016/j.jbtep.2012.02.004

Ismail, H., Wright, J., Rhodes, P., & Small, N. (2005). Religious beliefs about causes and treatment of epilepsy. *British Journal of General Practice, 55,* 26–31.

Johnstone, B., Yoon, D. P., Franklin, K. L., Schopp, L., & Hinkebein, J. (2009). Re-conceptualizing the factor structure of the Brief Multidimensional Measure of Religiousness/Spirituality. *Journal of Religion and Health, 48,* 146–163.

Jones, J. M. (2011, July 8). *In U.S., 3 in 10 say they take the Bible literally: Plurality view Bible as inspired word of God but say not everything in it should be taken literally. Gallup Poll, Princeton, NJ.* Retrieved from http://www.gallup.com/poll/148427/Say-Bible-Literally.aspx

Jones, R. K., Darroch, J. E., & Singh, S. (2005). Religious differentials in the sexual and reproductive behaviors of young women in the United States. *Journal of Adolescent Health, 36,* 279–288.

Kant, I. (1878). *Critique of pure reason* (J.M.D. Meiklejohn, Trans.). London: George Bell.

Katz, M. L., James, A. S., Piqnone, M. P., Hudson, M. A., Jackson, E., Oates, V., & Campbell, M. K. (2004). Colorectal cancer screening among African

American church members: A qualitative and quantitative study of patient-provider communication. *Bio Medical Center Public Health, 4*, 62.

Kemppainen, J., Bormann, J. E., Shively, M., Kelly, A., Becker, S., Bone, P., . . . Gifford, A. L. (2012). Living with HIV: Responses to a mantram intervention using the critical incident research method. *Journal of Alternative and Complementary Medicine, 18*(1), 76–82.

Kierkegaard, S. (1936). *Philosophical fragments*. Princeton, NJ: Princeton University Press.

Koenig, H. G., & Larson, D. B. (2001). Religion and mental health: Evidence for an association. *International Review of Psychiatry, 13*, 67–78.

Koffman, J., Morgan, M., Edmonds, P., Speck, P., Higginson, I. J. (2008). I know he controls cancer: The meanings of religions among black Caribbean and white British patients with advanced cancer. *Social Science and Medicine, 67*, 780–789.

Kosmin, B. A., & Keysar, A. (2006). *Religion in a free market: Religious and non-religious Americans, who, what, why, where*. Hartford, CT: Institute for the Study of Secularism in Society and Culture, Trinity College.

Kosmin, B. A., & Keysar, A. (2009). *American religious identification survey, 2008*. Hartford, CT: Institute for the Study of Secularism in Society and Culture, Trinity College.

Kosmin, B. A., Keysar, A., Cragun, R., & Navarro-Rivera, J. (2009). *American nones: The profile of the no religion population*. Hartford, CT: Institute for the Study of Secularism in Society and Culture, Trinity College.

Krause, N. (2003). Race, religion, and abstinence from alcohol in later life. *Journal of Aging and Health, 15*, 508–533.

Levine, E. G., Aviv, C., Yoo, G., Ewing, C., & Au, A. (2009). The benefits of prayer on mood and well-being on breast cancer survivors. *Support Care and Cancer, 17*, 295–306.

Lyon, J. L., Gardner, J. W., & West, D. W. (1980). Cancer incidence in Mormons and non-Mormons in Utah during 1967–1975. *Journal of the National Cancer Institute, 65*, 1055–1061.

Ma, G. X., Gao, W., Tan, Y., Chae, W. G., & Rhee, J. (2012). A community-based participatory approach to a hepatitis B intervention for Korean Americans. *Progress in Community Health Partnerships: Research, Education, and Action, 6*, 7–16.

Maliski, S. L., Connor, S. E., Williams, L., & Litwin, M. S. (2010). Faith among low-income, African American/black men treated for prostate cancer. *Cancer Nursing, 33*, 470–478.

Marsh, P. (1952). *The fullness of time*. New York: Harper.

McCauley, J., Haaz, S., Tarpley, M. J., Koenig, H. G., & Barlett, S. J. (2011). A randomized controlled trial to assess effectiveness of a spiritually-based intervention to help chronically ill adults. *International Journal of Psychiatry and Medicine, 41*, 91–105.

McSherry, W., & Cash, K. (2004). The language of spirituality: An emerging taxonomy. *International Journal of Nursing Studies, 41*, 151–161.

Meezenbroek, E. J., Garssen, B., van den Berg, M., van Dierendonck, D., Visser, A., & Schaufeli, W. (2012). Measuring spirituality as a universal human experience: A review of spirituality questionnaires. *Journal of Religion and Health, 51*, 336–354.

Miller, W. R., & Thoresen, C. E. (2003). Spirituality, religion, and health: An emerging research field. *American Psychologist, 58*, 24–35.

Moltmann, J. (1967). *Theology of hope.* New York: Harper.

Montgomery, S., Herring, P., Yancy, A., Beeson, L., Butler, T., Knutsen, S., . . . Fraser, G. (2007). Comparing self-reported disease outcomes, diet, and lifestyles in a national cohort of black and white Seventh-Day Adventists. *Prevention of Chronic Disease, 4*, A62.

Morita, T., Tsunoda, J., Inoue, S., & Chihara, S. (2000). An exploratory factor analysis of existential suffering in Japanese terminally ill cancer patients. *Psychooncology, 9*, 164–168.

Murray, R. B., & Zenter, J. B. (1989). *Nursing concepts for health promotion.* London: Prentice Hall.

Nelson, C., Jacobson, C. M., Weinberger, M. I., Bhaskaran, V., Rosenfeld, B., Breitbart, W., & Roth, A. J. (2009). The role of spirituality in the relationship between religiosity and depression in prostate cancer patients. *Annuals of Behavioral Medicine, 38*, 105–114.

Newport, F. (2010). *Americans' church attendance inches up in 2010.* Gallup Poll. Retrieved from http://www.gallup.com/poll/141044/Americans-Church-Attendance-Inches-2010.aspx

Newport, F. (2012a). *Americans, including Catholics, say birth control is morally OK.* Gallup Poll. Retrieved from http://www.gallup.com/poll/154799/Americans-Including-Catholics-Say-Birth-Control-Morally.aspx

Newport, F. (2012b). *Half of Americans support legal gay marriage: Democrats and independents in favor; Republicans opposed.* Gallup Poll. Retrieved from http://www.gallup.com/poll/154529/Half-Americans-Support-Legal-Gay-Marriage.aspx

Newport, F., Sangeeta, A., & Witters, D. (2010a). *Very religious Americans lead healthier lives.* Gallup Poll. Retrieved from http://www.gallup.com/poll/145379/Religious-Americans-Lead-Healthier-Lives.aspx

Newport, F., Sangeeta, A. & Witters, D. (2010b). *Very religious Americans report less depression, worry.* Gallup Poll. Retrieved from http://www.gallup.com/poll/144980/Religious-Americans-Report-Less-Depression-Worry.aspx

Newton, I. (1953). Fundamental principles of natural philosophy. In H. S. Thayer (Ed.), *Newton's philosophy of nature.* New York: Harper.

Obeidat, R. F., Lally, R. M., & Dickerson, S. S. (2012). Arab American women's lived experience with early-stage breast cancer diagnosis and surgical treatment. *Cancer Nursing, 35*, 302–311. doi:10.1097/NNC.0b013e318231db09

Ott, H. (1965). *Theology and preaching.* Philadelphia, PA: Westminster Press.

Pearce, M. J., Little, T. D., & Perez, J. E. (2003). Religious and depressive symptoms among adolescents. *Journal of Clinical Child and Adolescent Psychology, 329*, 267–276.

Peterman, A. H., Fitchett, G., Brady, M. J., Hernandez, L., & Cella, D. (2002). Measuring spiritual well-being in people with cancer: The functional assessment of chronic illness therapy—spiritual well-being scale (FACIT-Sp). *Annals of Behavioral Medicine, 24*, 49–58.

Pew Forum on Religion and Public Life. (2008, February). *US religious landscape and dynamic.* Washington, DC: Author.

Pew Forum on Religion and Public Life. (2009). *Faith in flux: Changes in religious affiliation in the U.S.* Retrieved from http://www.pewforum.org/Faith-in-Flux.aspx

Pew Forum on Religion and Public Life. (2010). U.S. Religious Landscape Survey. Retrieved from http://religions.pewforum.org/

Reed, P. G. (1992). An emerging paradigm for the investigation of spirituality in nursing. *Research in Nursing and Health, 15*, 349–357.

Rippentrop, A. E., Altmaier, E. M., & Burns, C. P. (2006). The relationship of religiosity and spirituality to quality of life among cancer patients. *Journal of Clinical Psychology in Medical Settings, 13*, 29–35.

Rosten, L. (1975). *Religions of America: Ferment and faith in an age of crisis.* New York, NY: Simon and Schuster.

Rowold, J. (2011). Effects of spiritual well-being on subsequent happiness, psychological well-being, and stress. *Journal of Religion and Health, 50*(4), 950–963.

Saad, L. (2012a, May 29). *In U.S., non-religious, postgrads are highly "pro-choice."* Gallup Poll. Retrieved from http://www.gallup.com/poll/154946/Non-Christians-Postgrads-Highly-Pro-Choice.aspx

Saad, L. (2012b, July 12). *U.S. confidence in organized religion at low point.* Gallup Poll. Retrieved from http://www.gallup.com/poll/155690/Confidence-Organized-Religion-Low-Point.aspx

Schnoll, R. A., Harlow, L. L., & Brower, L. (2000). Spirituality, demographic and disease factors, and adjustment to cancer. *Cancer Practice, 8*, 298–304.

Sloan, R. P., & Bagiella, E. (2002). Claims about religious involvement and health outcomes. *Annals of Behavioral Medicine, 24*, 14–21.

Stewart, D. E., & Yuen, T. (2011). A systematic review of resilience in the physically ill. *Psychosomatics, 52*, 199–209.

Tanyi, R. A., & Werner, J. S. (2007). Spirituality in African American and Caucasian women with end-stage renal disease on hemodialysis treatment. *Health Care for Women International, 28*, 141–154.

Torrance, T. F. (1969). *Space, time and incarnation.* New York, NY: Oxford University Press.

Torrance, T. F. (1971). *God and rationality.* New York: Oxford University Press.

U.S. Census Bureau. (2012). *Self-described religious identification of adult population, 1990, 2001, and 2008.* Retrieved from http://www.census.gov/compendia/statab/2012/tables/12s0075.pdf

Vuckovic, N. H., Williams, L. A., Schneider, J., Ramirez, M., & Gullion, C. M. (2012). Long-term outcomes of shamanic treatment for temporomandibular joint disorders. *Permanente Journal, 16,* 28–35.

Whitt-Glover, M. C., Goldmon, M. V., Karanja, N., Heil, D. P., & Gizlice, Z. (2012). Learning and developing individual exercise skills (L.A.D.I.E.S.) for a better life: A physical activity intervention for black women. *Contemporary Clinical Trials, 33,* 1159–1171.

Wilcox, S., Laken, M., Anderson, T., Bopp, M., Bryant, D., Carter, R., . . . Yancy, A. (2007). The Health-e-AME faith-based physical activity initiative: Description and baseline findings. *Health Promotion Practice, 8,* 69–78. doi:10.1177/1524839905278902

Wilkinson, J. E., Saper, R. B., Rosen, A. K., Welles, S. L., & Culpepper, L. (2008). Prayer for health and primary care: Results from the 2002 National Health Interview Survey. *Family Medicine, 40,* 638–644.

Williams, A. D., Lau, G., & Grisham, J. R. (2013). Thought-action fusion as a mediator of religiosity and obsessive-compulsive symptoms. *Journal of Behavioral Therapy and Experiential Psychiatry, 44,* 207–12. doi:10.1016/j.jbtep.2012.09.004

Wingood, G. M., Simpson-Robinson, L., Braxton, K., & Raiford, J. L. (2011). Design of a faith-based HIV intervention: Successful collaboration between a university and a church. *Health Promotion Practice, 12,* 823–831. doi:10.1177/1524839910372039

Wong, Y. J., Rew, L., & Slaikeu, K. D. (2006). A systematical review of recent research on adolescent religiosity/spirituality and mental health. *Issues in Mental Health Nursing, 27,* 161–183.

Yorulmaz, O., Gencoz, T., & Woody, S. (2009). OCD cognitions and symptoms in different religious contexts. *Journal of Anxiety Disorders, 23,* 401–406. Retrieved from http://dx.doi.org/10.1016/j.janxdis.2008.11.001

Zaldivar, A., & Smolowitz, J. (1994). Perceptions of the importance placed on religion and folk medicine by non–Mexican-American Hispanic adults with diabetes. *Diabetes Educator, 20,* 303–306.

Zinnbauer, B. J., & Pargament, K. I. (2005). Religiousness and spirituality. In R. F. Paloutzian & C. L. Park (Eds.), *Handbook of the psychology of religion and spirituality* (pp. 21–42). New York, NY: Guilford Press.

CHAPTER 6

HEALTH EDUCATION THEORETICAL MODELS AND MULTICULTURAL POPULATIONS

Raffy R. Luquis

LEARNING OBJECTIVES

After completing this chapter, you will be able to

- Explain cultural competence in terms of two theoretical models.
- Discuss the influence of culture, heritage, family, religion, and spirituality, among other factors, on health behaviors and practices.
- Apply culture-based assessment frameworks to the development of health education and promotion programs.

In the past decade, the population of the United States has reached its most racially and ethnically diverse composition yet. US Census Bureau (2008) projections of population growth indicate that the number of Hispanics, African Americans, Asians and Pacific Islanders, Native Americans and Alaska Natives, and members of other racial and ethnic groups will continue to grow in the next few decades. In fact, estimates are that by 2030, the non-white population will have increased to 45 percent of the US total (US Census Bureau, 2008). (See chapter 1 for a more complete description of the demographic changes.) Thus, the increasing diversification of the population confirms the health education field's need to incorporate the concepts of multicultural groups and cultural competence into every aspect of the planning, implementation, and evaluation processes of health education and promotion programs (Luquis & Pérez, 2003).

Cultural competence is "a developmental process defined as a set of values, principles, behaviors, attitudes, and policies that enable health professionals to work effectively across racial, ethnic, and linguistically diverse groups" (Joint Committee on Health Education and Promotion Terminology, 2012, p. 11). It is essential that health educators incorporate theoretical models so that cultural competence and related concepts can be considered in needs assessments and in the development and implementation

cultural competence
A developmental process defined as a set of values, principles, behaviors, attitudes, and policies that enable health professionals to work effectively across racial, ethnic, and linguistically diverse groups

of culturally and linguistically appropriate health education and promotion programs:

> The National Center for Cultural Competence [NCCC] (2000) defined culture as: Integrated pattern of human behavior that includes thoughts, communications, languages, practices, beliefs, values, customs, courtesies, rituals, manners of interacting and roles, relationships and expected behaviors of a racial, ethnic, religious or social group; and the ability to transmit the above to succeeding generations. (p. 1)

To some extent, a person's cultural background defines his or her perceptions in the context of a larger group and influences how he or she behaves throughout a lifetime. Culture influences people's perceptions of their health; it also affects their health beliefs, attitudes, and actions such as diets and nutritional habits, self-care practices, communication, and health care–seeking behaviors (Nakamura, 1999; National Center for Cultural Competence, 2000). Thus, it is imperative that health educators recognize the importance of and apply the concept of culture in health education and prevention interventions.

In the past, health educators have relied on theories and models such as the health belief model, social cognitive theory, and the transtheoretical model, among others, to explain behavioral determinants of health. In addition, health educators have used planning models such as PRECEDE/PROCEED and MATCH to develop and implement health education and promotion programs. Although these commonly used theories and models emphasize logical and critical thinking in relation to health behaviors, they do not attend to the sociocultural determinants of health behaviors (Simon, 2006). Thus, the purpose of this chapter is to describe two theoretical models and two assessment frameworks that address the role of culture in the prevention of disease and promotion of health. The theoretical models, Purnell and Campinha-Bacote, specifically describe the role of culture and the concept of cultural competence among health care professionals. The assessment frameworks describe steps and concepts to use when developing health promotion and disease prevention programs.

Models for Assessing Cultural Competence

This section discusses two theoretical models: the Purnell model of cultural competence and the culturally competent model of care. Both models address and describe the role of culture and the concept of cultural competence among health care professionals.

Purnell Model for Cultural Competence

The *Purnell model* for cultural competence provides a comprehensive, systematic, and organized framework with specific questions and a format for learning and assessing the concepts and characteristics of culture (see figure 6.1) (Purnell, 2005, 2009; Purnell & Paulanka, 2003). With this model, health professionals across disciplines and settings can analyze the cultural data that will facilitate the development of culturally competent health promotion and illness and disease prevention programs.

Purnell model
A comprehensive, systematic, and organized framework with specific questions and a format for learning and assessing the concepts and characteristics of culture

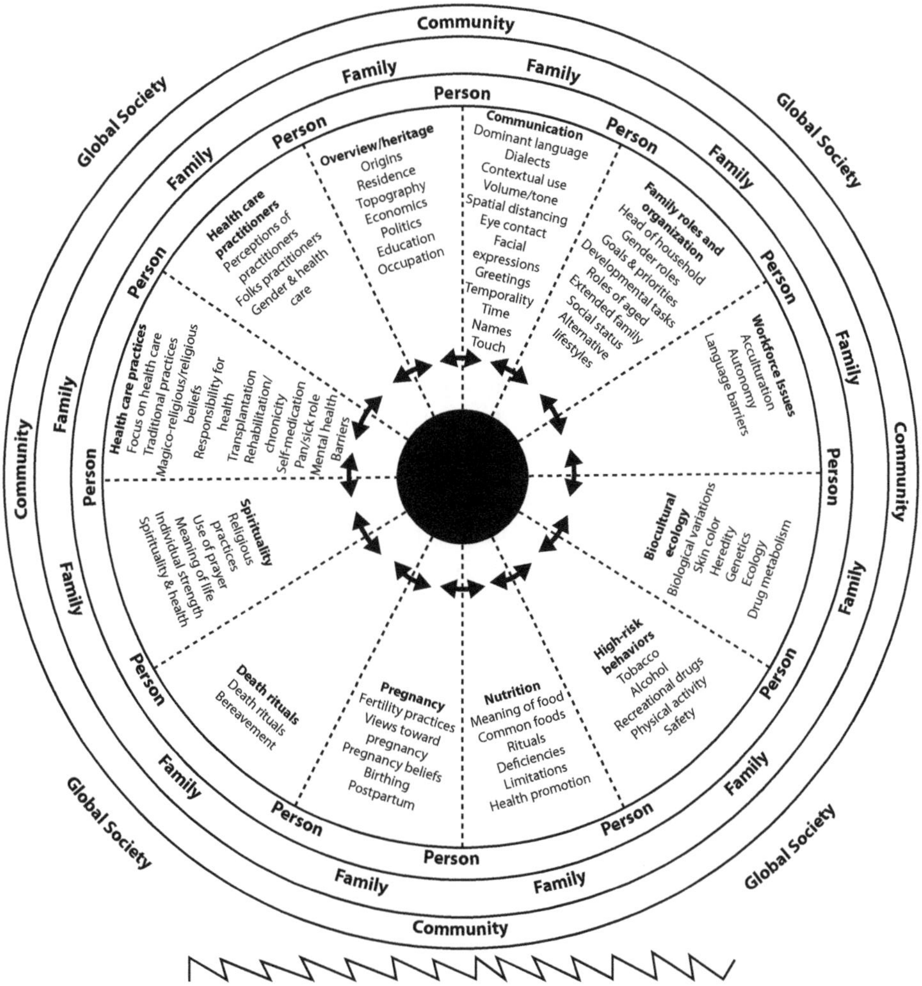

Unconsciously incompetent • Consciously incompetent • Consciously competent • Unconsciously competent

Primary characteristics of culture: age, generation, nationality, race, color, gender, religion

Secondary characteristics of culture: educational status, socioeconomical status, occupation, military status, political beliefs, urban versus rural residence, enclave identity, martial status, parental status, physical characterstics, sexual orientation, gender issues, and reason for migration (sojourner, immigrant, undocumented status)

Figure 6.1 Purnell Model for Cultural Competence

Source: Purnell (2005, p. 11). Reprinted with permission of the author.

Organization of the Model

The Purnell model is organized in a circle with four outlying rims representing the global society, the community, the family, and the person. The interior part of the circle is divided into twelve pie-shaped sections representing cultural domains and their concepts (Purnell, 2005, 2009; Purnell & Paulanka, 2003). It is important to understand that all these domains are interconnected (Purnell, 2009). In the center of the model is an empty circle representing unknown phenomena: the practices and characteristics of the individual or group of interest. This circle, which is difficult to measure, will expand or contract depending on the individual user's (in this case, the health educator's) understanding of and level of cultural competence with each ethnic and racial group. The model is based on several explicit assumptions and purposes. In addition, it displays a jagged line that illustrates the nonlinear process of acquiring cultural competence. Purnell (2005) explains that an individual progresses from unconscious incompetence (not being aware of lacking knowledge about other cultures), to conscious incompetence (being aware of lacking knowledge), to conscious competence (learning and providing culturally appropriate interventions), and finally to unconscious competence (automatically providing culturally competent services to everyone). Purnell warns that it is potentially dangerous to work from an unconscious competence level because it is difficult for any individual to address the needs of every racial and ethnic group when differences exist among individuals of each group. Thus, health educators must understand that cultural competence is a process and not an end point.

The outside rims, or macro aspect, of this model identify global society, community, family, and person. In thinking about the global society, users of this model consider world politics and communication, conflict and welfare, natural disaster and famine, and international exchanges, among other things, and also the expanding opportunity for people to travel around the world and interact with diverse societies. World events are broadly disseminated through television, radio, the Internet, social media, and newsprint and thus affect all societies. For example, diseases such as cholera and polio, which have been eradicated in the United States, continue to affect the lives of people in other parts of the world. As a result, people are forced to alter, consciously and unconsciously, their lifeways, worldviews, and acculturation patterns (Purnell, 2005; Purnell & Paulanka, 2003).

Community in this model is defined as a group of people having a common interest or identity and living in a specific vicinity. It also includes physical, social, and symbolic characteristics, such as mountains, economics, and history, that cause people to connect with one another. For example, people may define their community by their rural or urban environment, by social concepts such as politics and religion, or by symbolic characteristics such as art, music, and language.

Family refers to two or more people who are emotionally connected. It includes members of both the nuclear and extended family and close and distant blood and nonblood relatives and significant others. Family composition and roles change according to age, generation, marital status, relocation or immigration, and socioeconomic status, obligating each individual to rethink his or her beliefs and lifestyle.

Finally, a *person* is a human being who is constantly biologically, psychologically, sociologically, and culturally adapting to his or her community and environment. In general, in Western culture, an individual is thought of as a unique being and singular member of society, whereas in Asian culture, a person is identified first as a member of a family rather than a simple element of nature (Purnell, 2005; Purnell & Paulanka, 2003).

Model Domains

On the microlevel, the model displays a framework of twelve domains and sets of concepts common to all cultures. The domains are interconnected and have implications for organizing health promotion and disease prevention interventions in a manner that respects the differences among racial and ethnic groups. The twelve domains are (1) overview/heritage, (2) communication, (3) family roles and organization, (4) workforce issues, (5) biocultural ecology, (6) high-risk behaviors, (7) nutrition, (8) pregnancy and childbearing practices, (9) death rituals, (10) spirituality, (11) health care practices, and (12) health care practitioners (Purnell, 2005, 2009; Purnell & Paulanka, 2003).

Domain 1: Overview/Heritage The first domain involves concepts related to country of origin, current residence, the effect of the topographies of the country of origin and current residence, economics, politics, reasons for emigration, and educational status. These concepts are interconnected. For example, the social, political, and economic forces of the country of origin can often be the major reason for emigration. In addition, the value placed on education can influence the reason for emigrating among ethnic and racial groups (Purnell & Paulanka, 2003). For instance, second- and third-generation Mexican Americans have significant job skills and education; however, many current Mexican immigrants, especially from rural areas, have poor educational backgrounds and may not place a high value on education (Zoucha & Purnell, 2003). "Being familiar with the individual's personal educational values and learning modes allows health care providers, educators, and employees to adjust teaching strategies for clients, students, and employees" (Purnell & Paulanka, 2003, p. 13). Thus health educators need to consider and understand these concepts as part of any health needs assessment.

Domain 2: Communication The communication domain involves verbal and nonverbal interactions and considers the dominant language and use of language, dialects, paralanguage variations, eye contact, facial expression, and touch, among other variables likely to be distinctive in each cultural group. Health educators must be aware of these communication patterns because they can affect the educators' interactions with members of racial and ethnic groups. (See chapter 8 for further discussion of communication patterns.) For example, some groups may have limited English language ability; other groups may be willing to share personal thoughts and feelings only with family members and close friends and not with other people; and others may need to have their personal space respected (Purnell, 2009; Purnell & Paulanka, 2003). Public health educators also need to understand that communication issues are interrelated with issues in all the other domains.

Domain 3: Family Roles and Organization Issues in the family roles and organization domain affect issues in other domains and define what relationships will look like between insiders and outsiders. This domain addresses the views related to the head of the household and to gender roles; family roles including those for children, adolescents, and the elderly; and opinions about alternative lifestyles, such as single parenthood or same-sex sexual orientation (Purnell & Paulanka, 2003). For example, for many members of the Hispanic community, the family is the most important institution in life and in one's cultural and social existence, as it provides a strong feeling of loyalty, reciprocity, and solidarity among its members. Similarly, people with an Arab heritage have a strong patrilineal tradition and follow defined gender roles, which influence family structure and relationships among its members (Purnell, 2009).

Health educators targeting diverse racial and ethnic communities must understand the importance of traditional roles and expectations among members of these groups because they can affect group members' decisions about health care services and health-related behaviors.

Domain 4: Workforce Issues Workforce issues comprise language barriers, degree of assimilation and acculturation, and matters of autonomy. Moreover, concepts from the other domains, such as gender role, cultural communication, and health care practices, affect workforce issues in a multicultural work environment (Purnell & Paulanka, 2003). For example, Americans are expected to be punctual on the job and to use formal meetings and appointments in interacting with coworkers. For individuals from cultures where time is less important, such timeliness and punctuality are culturally based attitudes that can cause serious work problems. For example, a number of researchers have suggested that Hispanics can be considered present-oriented individuals; therefore, they do not demand punctuality and place more value on the quality of an interpersonal relationship than on the time during which this relationship takes place (Marin & Marin, 1991). Similarly, the poor English skills and workplace skills among first-generation Hmong immigrants can result in difficulties when performing their job (Purnell, 2009). Public health educators in administrative positions need to support cultural and diversity initiatives to diminish these possible problems.

Domain 5: Biocultural Ecology The domain of biocultural ecology is concerned with the physical, biological, and physiological variations among racial and ethnic groups. For instance, some racial and ethnic groups are more susceptible to and affected by certain illnesses and diseases than other groups. Moreover, health care professionals treating dark-skinned people for rashes, anemia, or jaundice need to employ assessments different from those they use with light-skinned people. In addition, differences among racial and ethnic groups in the way drugs are metabolized affect the prescription of medication for different groups (Purnell, 2009; Purnell & Paulanka, 2003). Health educators must be educated about these variations because they will affect the health care and health promotion interventions developed for specific groups.

Domain 6: High-Risk Health Behaviors Understandings of high-risk health behaviors such as tobacco, alcohol, and drug use; sexual practices; high-fat diets; and lack of physical activity differ among racial and ethnic groups (Purnell, 2009). For example, culture, rites, and customs may influence the use of alcoholic beverages among ethnic groups. For instance, the Roman Catholic Church uses wine during the celebration of Mass, and the French ingest larger amounts of alcohol than Americans do, a fact some have related to a lower mortality rate due to cardiovascular disease among the French (Purnell & Paulanka, 2003). When assessing alcohol use, health professionals must place this high-risk behavior within the context of the cultural group.

Domain 7: Nutrition The domain of nutrition looks at having adequate food, the meaning of food, common foods and rituals, food limitation and nutritional deficiencies, and the use of food for health promotion and disease prevention (Purnell & Paulanka, 2003). Cultural values and beliefs influence food choices, dietary behaviors, and the use of food for health promotion among racial and ethnic groups. For example, many racial and ethnic groups have theories that a balance of proper foods is needed for health maintenance and that selecting appropriate "hot" and "cold" foods can prevent and treat illnesses (Purnell & Paulanka, 2003; Spector, 2004). "Traditional Chinese Medicine divides medicines into four categories known as the four natures . . . hot, cold, warm and cool. The four natures . . . referred to as cold or hot relate to the effects on the body attributed to the food" (Liu et al., 2012, p. 64). In addition, dietary patterns and food selection are closely tied to health issues such as obesity, cardiovascular disease, and diabetes. Health educators need to understand the health behavioral patterns of different racial and ethnic groups to provide successful health promotion programs.

Domain 8: Pregnancy and Childbearing Practices Pregnancy and childbearing practices among multicultural groups are also determined by cultural influences. This domain considers culturally sanctioned and unsanctioned fertility practices; views about pregnancy; and prescriptive, restrictive, and taboo practices that are used during pregnancy, at birth, and after pregnancy (Purnell, 2009; Purnell & Paulanka, 2003).

Cultural beliefs and views regarding conception, pregnancy, and childbearing practices are passed down from generation to generation and are assimilated into each group's custom without being validated or completely understood. For example, Muslim and Orthodox Jewish groups expect limited involvement of the husband during the delivery of the baby and prescribe specific steps to protect the baby from evil spirits (Cassar, 2006). Other ethnic and racial groups follow traditional practices or avoid certain foods during pregnancy to prevent illness or harm to the baby (Purnell, 2009; Purnell & Paulanka, 2003). Health care providers must respect cultural beliefs surrounding conception, pregnancy, and childbearing when making decisions related to the health of pregnant women.

Domain 9: Death Rituals This and the next domain, spirituality, are interconnected with beliefs regarding life, religion, and death. Death rituals are the practices and views surrounding death and bereavement. These views are less likely than others to change over time within any cultural group and may cause concerns among health professionals (Purnell & Paulanka, 2003). For example, some racial and ethnic groups may not allow an autopsy or organ donation when asked to consider these possibilities.

For many racial and ethnic groups, rites surrounding death are connected to their beliefs about protecting the dead person and the family from evil spirits or ghosts and about preparing the dying person for his or her journey after death (Purnell, 2009). For example, many groups use candles in rituals surrounding death to illuminate the way for the spirit of the decease (Spector, 2004). Moreover, although the dominant American culture has a practice of burying the dead within few days, other cultural groups, such as the Mexicans, hold elaborate ceremonies in commemoration of the dead that may last for days. Among many groups, these rituals are influenced by religious beliefs and spirituality.

Domain 10: Spirituality The domain of spirituality is made up of religious practices, use of prayer, the meaning of life, and the relationship between spirituality and health care practices. For some people, religious beliefs, more than cultural beliefs, direct their other beliefs, values, and practices (Purnell, 2009; Purnell & Paulanka, 2003). Health educators must consider these religious and spiritual beliefs when developing health promotion programs. For example, the concept of spirituality has been used in health promotion to prevent early sexual behavior among African American adolescent girls (Doswell, Kopuyate, & Taylor, 2003) and has been associated with the development of resilience in African American children (Haight, 1998). (Given the importance of this domain among racial and ethnic groups, chapter 5 on spirituality and culture offers in-depth information in this topic.)

Domain 11: Health Care Practices This and the next cultural domain, health care practitioners, are also interconnected: they involve people's perceptions of health care practices and health care practitioners. This domain focuses on traditional, magicoreligious, and biomedical beliefs; individual responsibility for health; self-medicating; responses to pain; and views toward such medical issues as mental health and organ donation (Purnell, 2009).

For centuries, people have maintained their health by many different healing and medical practices. (Chapter 4 is dedicated to the cultural practice of complementary and alternative medicine and holistic health and the impact of this practice on the field of health education.) In addition it is important to recognize that cultural and religious beliefs influence views on organ donation and blood transfusion. Although some racial and ethnic groups favor organ donation, others (as well as some religious organizations) are against it because of fear of medical institutions or a belief that it will result in suffering in an afterlife (Purnell & Paulanka, 2003).

Health practitioners, including health educators, must explore health care practices and related beliefs among multicultural groups in order to provide culturally congruent health interventions.

Domain 12: Health Care Finally, culture also affects people's perceptions and use of traditional health care practitioners and folk healers, and it affects views on gender in relation to health care. Cassar (2006) has noted that Muslim and Orthodox Jewish women prefer a health care provider of the same sex during pregnancy and delivery. Some groups perceive older male physicians to be more knowledgeable and trustworthy than their younger counterparts, and others consider folk and magicoreligious healers to be superior to traditional physicians or nurses (Purnell & Paulanka, 2003). For example, members of the Hmong community obtain Western medical care, but they may also seek the use of traditional healers or shamans to address illness (Purnell, 2009). Public health educators and other health professionals need to understand these perceptions among multicultural groups, as they will influence people's use of traditional health prevention services.

A Culturally Competent Model of Care

Campinha-Bacote (1998, 1999, 2001, 2007) developed a conceptual model of cultural competence suggesting that cultural competence in delivering health care services is a process.[1] This process comprises five essential constructs: cultural awareness, cultural knowledge, cultural skills, cultural encounters, and cultural desire. Health educators can apply these constructs as they navigate through the process of cultural competence as the constructs presented are very applicable to their work.

Cultural Awareness

cultural awareness
The cognitive process through which health professionals become sensitive to the values, beliefs, and practices of different cultural groups

Cultural awareness is the cognitive process through which health professionals become sensitive to the values, beliefs, and practices of different cultural groups. This process involves an honest exploration of one's own cultural background and views, as well as a self-examination of one's own biases and prejudices toward other racial and ethnic groups. For example, some people may have some biases toward Mexican individuals due to their legal status, or against people from Haiti because of the color of their skin. Still, they may not realize these biases until they engage in a deep exploration of their feelings. This is only the first step on the journey toward cultural competence; health educators must go beyond awareness and develop other components of cultural competency (Campinha-Bacote, 1998, 2007, 2009).

cultural knowledge
An understanding of the biological and sociological factors that contribute to health disparities among racial and ethnic groups

Cultural Knowledge

As individuals move through the process of acquiring cultural competence, they must also go through a process of developing *cultural knowledge* in order to understand different racial and ethnic groups' worldviews. This cultural knowledge includes an understanding of the biological and sociological factors that contribute to health disparities among racial and ethnic groups.

The development of cultural awareness and knowledge is essential in the preparation of health educators and promoters (Luquis & Pérez, 2003), and resources for this awareness and knowledge are increasingly available. A growing literature exists on the cultural views of racial and ethnic groups, multicultural health, and diversity. Professional organizations have been formed to promote cultural competence (including the NCCC), and conferences are being held that offer opportunities to participate in workshops and presentations dealing with culture and health. In addition, a study of professional preparation programs in health education found that although most of these programs are not offering courses entirely devoted to cultural competency, they are adequately addressing content related to culture, race, ethnicity, and health in their existing courses (Luquis et al., 2006). Still, because cultures are constantly evolving, becoming completely familiar with all the cultural aspects of even one group is challenging at best; thus, health educators must also develop the cultural skills, encounters, and desire that allow them to obtain cultural knowledge directly from individuals.

Cultural Skills

The abilities to collect cultural relevant data regarding the individual or group presenting the health problem and to conduct culture-specific assessments are *cultural skills* (Campinha-Bacote, 2009). Health educators will benefit from developing these skills and applying them to develop, implement, and evaluate culturally appropriate interventions for people of diverse racial and ethnic groups (Luquis & Pérez, 2003). Developing such skills requires that health educators learn how to conduct a comprehensive cultural assessment to determine the explicit needs and appropriate intervention for the people being targeted (Campinha-Bacote, 1999, 2001, 2009). For example, Huff and Kline (1999, 2007) suggest that health educators collect cultural or ethnic group–specific demographic characteristics and cultural or ethnic group–specific epidemiological and environmental influences. Marin (1993) suggested that culturally appropriate health interventions reflect the cultural beliefs, values, cultural characteristics, and expected behaviors of members of the targeted racial or ethnic group. Thus, needs assessment conducted with a multicultural population must include a cultural assessment as well (Luquis & Pérez, 2003). Two such cultural assessments are discussed later in this chapter.

cultural skills
The abilities to collect culturally relevant data regarding the individual or group presenting the health problem and to conduct culture-specific assessments

Cultural Encounters

The term *cultural encounter* describes the process of engaging in multicultural interactions with people of a culturally diverse group (Campinha-Bacote, 1998, 2007, 2009). These interactions are opportunities for health

cultural encounter
The process of engaging in multicultural interactions with people of a culturally diverse group

educators to develop their understanding and beliefs regarding that particular racial or ethnic group. At times health educators may believe that because they have studied a specific racial or ethnic group and have interacted with three or four members of that group, they know everything they need to know about that group. However, three or four individuals probably do not fully represent the cultural beliefs and practices of the group. For instance, although Hispanics share many cultural values and beliefs, interaction with three or four members of the Hispanic population is not enough, because there are many Hispanic subgroups and they are culturally and socially diverse. Thus, culturally competent health educators must constantly make it a priority to have cultural encounters to prevent stereotyping and acquire the experiential knowledge needed to develop culturally relevant interventions.

Every day health educators have opportunities to interact with colleagues, clients, and other people with cultural backgrounds similar to and different from their own. These interactions will help them learn from each other as part of the process of achieving cultural competency, because learning from each other never ends. The more that health educators endeavor to seek out these encounters, the better equipped they will be to provide programs to racial and ethnic groups (Luquis & Pérez, 2003).

Cultural Desire

cultural desire
The genuine motivating force that makes one want to work with people from diverse cultural backgrounds and engage in the process of becoming culturally competent

Finally, *cultural desire* is the genuine motivating force that makes one want to work with people from diverse cultural backgrounds and engage in the process of becoming culturally competent (Campinha-Bacote, 1998, 2007, 2009). Health educators who have cultural awareness, knowledge, skill, and encounters must also develop a true motivation to work with people from different racial and ethnic backgrounds. Cultural desire is not something that can be taught in a classroom but something that health educators must have within themselves or develop during their journey toward becoming culturally competent. They must be inspired to work within a multicultural society. Health educators who "want to" (as Campinha-Bacote, 1999) says) and who have the desire to work with racial and ethnic populations are doing a good service not only to the community they serve but also to the profession.

Inventory for Assessing the Process of Cultural Competence among Health Care Professionals

In addition to this model of cultural competence, Campinha-Bacote (1998) developed the Inventory for Assessing the Process of Cultural Competence Among Healthcare Professionals (IAPCC) to measure the constructs presented in the model. In 2003, she revised this instrument (IAPCC-R) in order to add the construct of cultural desire. A sum of the scores of the five subscales shows whether a health professional is operating at a level of cultural proficiency (91 to 100), cultural competence (75 to 90), cultural awareness (51 to 74), or cultural incompetence (25 to 50). Higher scores represent a higher level of competence. Although the process of cultural competence model and the IAPCC-R were developed to be used with health care professionals, other health professionals can use them to understand the complexity of cultural competence and measure individuals' level of cultural competence. Luquis and Pérez (2005) used a modified version of the IAPCC-R to measure the level of cultural competence among professional health educators. For their study, they defined the levels of cultural competency used in the IAPCC-R as they apply to the field of health education:

> Culturally incompetent individuals can be described as those who lack an understanding of the difference among ethnic and cultural groups. They are at the lowest level of the cultural competence process. As they move through this process, the individual develops cultural awareness, or sensitivity to the values, beliefs and practices of different ethnic and cultural groups. Culturally competent individuals are not only culturally sensitive to the different groups, but are also able to respond appropriately to the needs of these groups. Finally, cultural proficiency can be described as the endpoint of cultural competence. An individual who is culturally competent has developed the ability to respond appropriately to groups of diverse ethnic and cultural backgrounds. (p. 159)

The results of this investigation showed that in general, health educators were operating at a level of cultural awareness. Moreover, 34 percent of the participants were operating at a level of cultural competency. Overall, the health educators in this study could be described as individuals who are sensitive to the values, beliefs, and practices of different ethnic and cultural groups and would be able to respond appropriately to the needs of these groups. Study results also showed that variables such as the race of the individual, encounters with diverse populations, and participation in a cultural diversity educational program influenced the level of cultural competency among health educators (Luquis & Pérez, 2005). Findings from this study demonstrate the role cultural competence education plays in developing culturally competent health educators, and they support the need for more research in this area for a better understanding of the complexity of cultural competency.

Models for Developing Health Education Programs

This section discusses two assessment frameworks, the cultural assessment framework and the PEN-3 model, which address the role of culture in the prevention of disease and promotion of health. These assessment frameworks describe steps and concepts to use when developing health promotion and disease prevention programs.

Cultural Assessment Framework

cultural assessment framework Five levels of assessment that should be included when planning health promotion programs for multicultural groups

The *cultural assessment framework*, developed by Huff and Kline (1999, 2007), contains five levels of assessment that should be included when planning health promotion programs for multicultural groups. The CAF categories and subcategories suggest areas of inquiry that are race, ethnicity, and culture specific. Huff and Kline also recommend employing these areas in assessment tools such as surveys, focus groups, and other formative evaluation processes. The five major categories of assessment are (1) cultural or ethnic group–specific demographic characteristics, (2) cultural or ethnic group–specific epidemiological and environmental influences, (3) general and specific cultural or ethnic group characteristics, (4) general and specific health care beliefs and practices, and (5) Western health care organization and service delivery variables.

Cultural or Ethnic Group–Specific Demographic Characteristics

The cultural or ethnic group–specific demographic characteristics include age, gender, social class and status, education and literacy, religion, language, occupation and income, residence and living conditions, and acculturation (Huff & Kline, 1999, 2007). The more that health educators and promoters know about these factors, the better they will be at targeting health education programs toward specific ethnic and racial groups and incorporating these characteristics into development, implementation, and evaluation processes. For example, when developing a program for a Hispanic population, it is important to note that although Hispanics as a group have some common demographic characteristics relating to such factors as socioeconomic status, educational level, and language, there are some differences among each subgroup. When the three main Hispanic subgroups in the United States are compared, for example, Mexicans are younger, have larger families, and have less income and educational attainment than Puerto Ricans and Central Americans (Ramirez & de la Cruz, 2002). Similarly, religion and religious practices are important components of many multicultural groups; thus, knowing how these affect their daily lives and behaviors will shape the development of a program (Huff & Kline, 2007). Such differences in demographic characteristics need to be taken into consideration when developing programs targeting specific multicultural groups and subgroups.

Epidemiological and Environmental Influences

Although most assessment models include epidemiological and environmental factors, Huff and Kline (1999, 2007) recommend that health education practitioners take a closer look at these factors. When epidemiological data are aggregated into larger categories of analysis, specific health issues in many racial and ethnic subgroups may be concealed. For example, a health educator who examines the aggregate data on the health status of Asians and Pacific Islanders might conclude that this group as a whole is healthy. However, a closer look at the same data by individual Asian and Pacific Islander subgroups would show that some of the subgroups have high incidences of breast, lung, and liver cancer and hepatitis B (Spector, 2004).

In addition it is important to assess environmental factors such as the presence of advertising, which might lead to the use of health-damaging products and stores that sell alcohol and fast food, as these might be associated with health disparities among racial and ethnic groups. LaVeist and Wallace (2000) found that liquor stores in the Baltimore area were more likely to be located in low-income African American communities than in other communities. The findings of this study, although not conclusive, suggest that the relative prevalence of liquor stores in low-income African American communities may be associated with the disproportionate share of alcohol-related problems experienced by residents of these communities.

While group-specific data gathering can be challenging and requires significant effort to obtain, these data provide rich and enlightening information about the group (Huff & Kline, 2007). To overcome this challenge, health educators must use primary data collection methods to gather epidemiological directly from the targeted group.

Cultural or Ethnic Group Characteristics

Throughout the health education literature, health educators (Huff & Kline 1999; Luquis et al., 2006; Luquis & Pérez, 2003; Stoy, 2000) have advocated that people in this profession need to become more culturally competent and sensitive to the racial and ethnic groups with which they work, and one level of the CAF is concerned with taking into consideration *specific cultural or ethnic characteristics*—cultural or ethnic identity, cosmology, time orientation, perceptions of self and community, social norms, values and customs, and communication patterns (Huff & Kline 1999, 2007).

Spector (2004) defines culture as the beliefs, practices, habits, norms, customs, and so on that individuals learn from their families. It is complex and dynamic, and although we can assume that for the most part, people's concept of their culture remains constant, cultural identity can change over time (Luquis & Pérez, 2003). As individuals from different racial and ethnic groups interact with members of other groups, new environments, and new situations, their cultural identity is reshaped (Bonder, Martin, & Miracle, 2001). Cultural identity influences the individual's behavior and health choices. Consequently, it is important for health educators to begin a cultural assessment by establishing how the targeted group identifies itself (Huff & Kline, 1999, 2007), as this identity will influence other cultural characteristics of the group.

Racial and Ethnic Health Care Beliefs and Practices

In conducting an assessment, health educators need to be aware of specific racial and ethnic health care beliefs and practices, which affect a group's interaction with the Western biomedical model and health promotion efforts (Huff & Kline, 1999, 2007). This level of the CAF includes assessment of a group's health and illness explanatory model, response to illness, perceptions and use of Western health care and health promotion services, and health behavior factors.

The Western biomedical model explains illness and disease in terms of pathological agents, whereas a racial or ethnic group might follow a diagnostic model that explains illness, disease, and course of treatment from a cultural point of view (Nakamura, 1999). For example, some racial and ethnic groups perceive and explain the cause of illness and disease in terms of "soul loss," "spirit possession," and "spells" (Spector, 2004). Similarly, some groups describe disease as the consequence of an individual's personal actions or interrelationship with family and community or as related to supernatural agents (Huff & Yasharpour, 2007); thus, members of these groups would be more likely to follow a nontraditional treatment modality to deal with the disease than they would be to visit a heath care provider. In addition, the perceptions an ethnic group has of the Western health care system will affect how they access health care and promotion services. "If target group members perceive the Western health care facility as a 'death house' where family or friends go in alive and come out dead, then they will be more likely to avoid contact with this type of facility except under the most dire situation" (Huff & Kline, 1999, p. 495). Health educators must be aware of racial and ethnic groups' understanding of health and illness, their health practices, and ways that group views can be incorporated into health promotion interventions.

Western Health Care Organization and Service Delivery System

Finally, this model proposes an assessment of the Western health care organization and the delivery system that provide services to multicultural groups. Although some may consider this area a separate assessment, Huff and Kline (1999, 2007) argue that the way the health care and promotion organization perceives and works with the target group plays a key role in the overall assessment process. This process must include assessment of the cultural competence and sensitivity of the agency and its staff, assessment of the extent to which organizational mission and policies enhance the process of cultural competence, and assessment of the evaluation processes in place to measure organizational efforts in this area. Although this process might be cumbersome, it is important for health promoters to understand the agency if they are to develop appropriate and effective health promotion programs.

The PEN-3 Model

The *PEN-3 model* was developed by Airhihenbuwa (1995) as a conceptual model for health promotion and disease prevention in African countries, specifically to guide a cultural approach to HIV/AIDS, and then it was adapted for use with African Americans. The model provides a functional method of addressing culture in the development, implementation, and evaluation of health education and promotion programs. Although it draws on theories and applications in cultural studies, it incorporates existing health education models, theories, and frameworks. Initially the model had three dimensions of health beliefs and behaviors: health education, educational diagnosis of health behavior, and cultural appropriateness of health behavior. The revised PEN-3 model, presented in figure 6.2, consists of three primary domains—relationships and expectations, cultural empowerment, and cultural identify—and three components (whose initial letters spell PEN) within each domain (Airhihenbuwa & DeWitt Webster, 2004). Once health educators and practitioners have identified a health issue, they can frame relevant sociocultural issues into the nine categories displayed in figure 6.2.

PEN-3 model
A conceptual model for health promotion and disease prevention in African countries, specifically to guide a cultural approach to HIV/AIDS, and adapted for use with African Americans

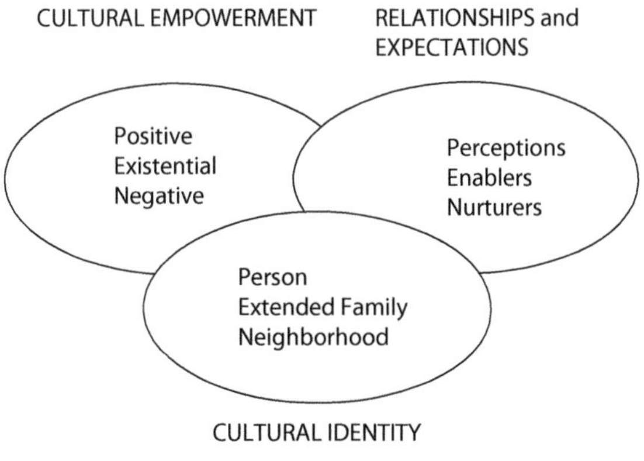

Figure 6.2 The PEN-3 Model

Source: *Airhihenbuwa (2007, p. 38). Reprinted with permission of author.*

According to Airhihenbuwa (2007, p. 37), "The PEN-3 model offers an opportunity to promote the notion of multiple truths by examining cultures and behaviors and by beginning with and identifying the positive—allowing us to examine and acknowledge the existential, which represents values that make a culture unique—before identifying the negative."

Relationships and Expectations Domain

The relationships and expectations domain assesses perceptions, enablers, and nurturers of behaviors from the cultural point of view. This dimension of the PEN-3 model has evolved from other theories and models, such as the health belief model (Rosenstock, 1974) and the PRECEDE-PROCEED framework (Green & Kreuter, 1999). However, this model places culture at the core of health promotion and disease prevention programs (Airhihenbuwa, 1995, 2007).

Among the three components of this domain, perceptions consist of the knowledge, attitudes, values, and beliefs that exist within a cultural context and that motivate or inhibit individual or group behavioral change. For example, knowledge and cultural beliefs about breast and cervical cancer can influence cancer screening and health and health care–seeking behaviors among Hispanic women (Allison, Duran, & Peña-Purcell, 2005; Garces, Scarinci, & Harrison, 2006; Luquis & Villanueva, 2006; Scarinci, Bandura, Hidalgo, & Cherrington, 2012). Enablers are resources, institutional support, and societal or structural factors that may enhance or hinder preventive health decision and actions. For instance, the role of government policy has been noted in the low incidence or even decline of new HIV cases in some African countries (Airhihenbuwa & DeWitt Webster, 2004). Similarly, trust in some community-based organizations, local churches, and community health advisors can serve as positive enabling factors in the prevention of cervical cancer among immigrant Latinas (Scarinci et al., 2012). However, distrust of research and medical care has had a negative influence on the recruitment of African American males for prostate cancer screening (Abernethy et al., 2005). Likewise, Garces et al. (2006) have suggested that lack of information, access to care, and medications prevents Latinas from seeking health care services. Nurturers are family, friends, and community members who have a positive or negative influence on health beliefs, attitudes, and actions. Abernethy and colleagues (2005) identify pastors, church leaders, and community leaders as individuals who can promote prostate cancer screening among African American males. Similarly, the cultural practice of caring for a sick relative at home has become an important aspect of HIV/AIDS care in Africa (Airhihenbuwa & DeWitt Webster, 2004).

Cultural Empowerment Domain

The cultural empowerment domain is an affirmation of the possibilities of cultural influences, which are positive, existential, and negative (Airhihenbuwa & DeWitt Webster, 2004). This dimension is crucial in the development of culturally appropriate health education and promotion interventions (Airhihenbuwa, 1995). As part of the development of such interventions, health educators must promote the good aspects and recognize the unique aspects of a culture and not merely focus on its negative aspects (Airhihenbuwa & DeWitt Webster, 2004).

Cultural empowerment is positive when it promotes the health behaviors of interest—for instance, the traditional healing modality for dealing with health problems such as sexually transmitted infections (Airhihenbuwa & DeWitt Webster, 2004). Similarly, eating a balanced diet, exercising, praying, and going to church are positive cultural aspects and behaviors that can be encouraged among Latinas (Garces et al., 2006). These behaviors will support other behaviors that help women to stay physically and spiritually healthy.

Existential aspects of a culture are the cultural beliefs, practices, and behaviors that are natural to a group and have no harmful effect on health. These should not be targeted for change and should not be blamed for the failure of a health education program. Garces et al. (2006) describe the use of alternative and complementary healing practices, such as home remedies, as an existential behavior among Latinas. The views of illness based on the principle of the balance between the yin and yang among members of the Chinese community illustrates another existential behavior (Yick & Oomen-Early, 2009). Health educators must be aware of and embrace these practices and beliefs because they can help to produce a holistic view that can inform the development of a health education program.

Finally, negative aspects are those based on values, beliefs, and relationships known to be harmful to health behaviors, for example, social actions that lay a foundation for inequality such as racism and differential housing and education (Airhihenbuwa & DeWitt Webster, 2004). Yick and Oomen-Early (2009) identified factors such as cultural attitudes about women, patriarchal authority, fear of shame and loss of face, and pressure to maintain harmony as negative behaviors affecting Chinese women. To be successful, health educators should develop programs that increase or support the naturally occurring positive behaviors while decreasing the negative behaviors and respecting the existential ones.

Cultural Identity

Finally, the cultural identity domain in the PEN-3 model seeks assessment of person, extended family, and neighborhood. It is important to understand that cultural identity, which represents an important intervention point of entry, is not defined by race and culture alone but refers to the multiple identities men and women experience in different cultures (Airhihenbuwa & DeWitt Webster, 2004). For example, "an African South African (such as Zulu) might out of necessity embrace the lived experiences of being Zulu (ethnicity), English (language), Afrikaans (oppressed experience) and poor person" (p. 8). Once the intervention point of entry, components of cultural identity, has been identified, the behavioral change can be addressed and promoted. It is also important to recognize that there could be multiple points of entry for addressing social context and behaviors (Airhihenbuwa & DeWitt Webster, 2004). In light of this fact, the individual can be provided with opportunities to acquire information and the skills needed to make good health decisions appropriate to his or her role in family and community (Airhihenbuwa, 1995). In addition, health education is concerned not only with the immediate nuclear family but also with the extended family. Family plays a key role in the lives of members of many racial and ethnic groups. For example, a husband's mother, given her influence on the expectations of the couple in such areas as sexual negotiation, might be the source of certain behaviors that need to be changed (Airhihenbuwa & DeWitt Webster, 2004). Finally, health education is committed to health promotion and disease prevention in neighborhoods and communities, as involvement of community members is critical in the provision of culturally appropriate interventions (Airhihenbuwa, 1995). For example, a community's ability to decide on billboard advertisement and communication about HIV/AIDS in its locality might be encouraged (Airhihenbuwa & DeWitt Webster, 2004). Health educators must develop interventions that target both the individual and the extended families and neighborhoods because of these interconnections.

Suggestions for Working with Diverse Groups

When working with diverse groups, health educators should consider the role of culture and cultural characteristics of the communities and individuals in order to be effective in addressing their needs. The following suggestions pertain to working with diverse groups:

- Health educators must examine their cultural awareness and knowledge in order to be responsive to the values, attitudes, and behaviors of diverse cultural groups. Both Purnell (2005) and Campinha-Bacote (1998) address cultural domains, concepts, and constructs that must be taken into consideration when creating awareness and knowledge of diverse groups. For example, Long (2011) used the Purnell model as a framework to provide examples on how to incorporate culture and spirituality in palliative and end-of-life care in a health care setting.

- By interacting (i.e., cultural encounters) with members of different ethnic or racial groups, health educators learn to understand and appreciate the diversity of values and belief systems that influence health and health-seeking behaviors among these groups. For example, as part of a multicultural health course, I used different activities to expose students to the practices, values, and beliefs among members from a racial and ethnic group different from their own. Students can choose to complete an interview with a member of a different ethnic or racial group or a health professional working with diverse populations, visit a traditional ethnic neighborhood or store, or attend a traditional racial or ethnic event. At the end of this activity, the student is able to learn and appreciate differences and commonalities between the specific racial or ethnic group and themselves.
- Both the CAF (Huff & Kline, 1999) and the PEN-3 (Airhihenbuwa, 1995) models describe frameworks that must be taken into account when assessing the needs of diverse groups as part of the development of health promotion and disease prevention programs. For example, Shoultz, Phillion, Noone, and Tanner (2002) used the CAF as a basis for a research study to develop reliable and valid (cultural-tailored) guidelines for the prevention of violence. Similarly, Scarinci et al. (2012) used the PEN-3 model to develop theoretical-based culturally relevant intervention for cervical cancer prevention among Latina immigrants.
- Health educators must use cultural assessment to gather data and information that would be beneficial in the development of cultural and linguistically appropriate health promotion programs. Yick and Oomen-Early (2009) applied the PEN-3 model to the topic of domestic violence within the Chinese American and immigrant community. By using this model, they provided suggestions for guiding domestic violence education and prevention among this community. Similarly, Huff and Kline (2007) provided suggestions on how to use the CAF when assessing cultural variables during program planning process.

Conclusion

Today's population growth and increasing population diversity validate health educators' efforts to incorporate cultural and linguistic competence into every aspect of planning, implementation, and evaluation of health education and promotion programs. In this process, it is essential to employ theoretical models that describe and explain culture and related concepts.

It is vital for health educators to apply these cultural constructs in every health education, promotion, and prevention intervention targeting diverse communities. In addition to considering the models and assessments discussed here that focus on the role of culture in the prevention of disease and promotion of health, health educators must also consider other theories discussed in this book when addressing the needs of the multicultural population in the United States.

Points to Remember

- Health educators need to consider the concept of culture and cultural factors during the development and implementation of culturally appropriate health education and promotion programs.
- The Purnell model for cultural competence provides a comprehensive, systematic, and organized framework with specific questions and a format for learning and assessing the concepts and characteristics of culture.
- Campinha-Bacote suggests that the process of cultural competence comprises five essential constructs: cultural awareness, cultural knowledge, cultural encounters, cultural skills, and cultural desire.
- The cultural assessment framework contains five levels of racial-, ethnic- and culture-specific assessments that should be conducted when planning health promotion programs for multicultural groups. These assessments can also be incorporated into such tools as surveys, focus groups, and other formative evaluation processes.
- The PEN-3 model provides a functional method of addressing culture in the development, implementation, and evaluation of health education and promotion programs. It also allows health educators to conduct culture-based research and develop effective interventions for combating illnesses in racial and ethnic groups.

Case Study

A group of health educators are in charge of developing community health education and promotion programs for the members of a diverse community. The population of this community is 45 percent white, 35 percent African American, 10 percent Hispanic, 5 percent Asian and Pacific Islander, and 5 percent members of other ethnic groups. Preliminary epidemiological data show differences in the incidence and prevalence of chronic illness among these groups. For example, the African American population has a significant higher mortality rate for heart disease, cancer, diabetes, and a higher rate of infant mortality.

1. What constructs could you use to assess the level of cultural competence among the team of health educators?
2. What steps would you follow to assess the health education needs of this community?
3. What cultural factors do you need to consider when developing a program?
4. What cultural factors will influence the risk behaviors among members of this community?
5. Which cultural theory or model would be more appropriate to use when assessing the needs of this community?

KEY TERMS

Cultural assessment framework
Cultural awareness
Cultural competence
Cultural desire
Cultural encounter
Cultural knowledge
Cultural skills
PEN-3 model
Purnell model

Note

1. For a graphical representation of this model, visit the Transcultural C.A.R.E. Associates website: http://www.transculturalcare.net.

References

Abernethy, A. D., Magat, M. M., Houston, T. A., Arnold Jr., H. L., Bjorck, J. P., & Gorsuch, R. L. (2005). Recruiting African American men for cancer screening studies: Applying a culturally based model. *Health Education and Behavior, 32*(4), 441–451.

Airhihenbuwa, C. O. (1995). *Health and culture: Beyond the Western paradigm.* Thousand Oaks, CA: Sage.

Airhihenbuwa, C. O. (2007). On being comfortable with being uncomfortable: Centering an Africanist vision in our gateway to global health. *Health Education and Behavior, 34*(1), 31–42.

Airhihenbuwa, C. O., & DeWitt Webster, J. (2004). Culture and African context of HIV/AIDS prevention, care, and support. *Journal of Social Aspects of HIV/AIDS Research Alliance, 1*(1), 4–13.

Allison, K. G., Duran, M., & Peña-Purcell, N. (2005). Cervical cancer screening practices among Hispanic women: Theories for culturally appropriate interventions. *Hispanic Health Care International, 3*(2), 61–67.

Bonder, B., Martin, L., & Miracle, A. (2001). Achieving cultural competence: The challenge for clients and healthcare workers in a multicultural society. *Generations, 25*(1), 35–42.

Campinha-Bacote, J. (1998). *The process of cultural competence in the delivery of healthcare services: A culturally competent model of care* (3rd ed.). Cincinnati, OH: Transcultural C.A.R.E. Associates.

Campinha-Bacote, J. (1999). A model and instrument for addressing cultural competence in health care. *Journal of Nursing Education, 38*(5), 203–207.

Campinha-Bacote, J. (2001). A model of practice to address cultural competence in rehabilitation nursing. *Rehabilitation Nursing, 26*(1), 8–12.

Campinha-Bacote, J. (2007). *The process of cultural competence in the delivery of healthcare services: A culturally competent model of care* (5th ed.). Retrieved from http://www.transculturalcare.net/Cultural_Competence_Modelhtm

Campinha-Bacote, J. (2009). A culturally competent model of care for African Americans. *Urologic Nursing, 29*(1), 49–54.

Cassar, L. (2006). Cultural expectations of Muslims and Orthodox Jews in regard to pregnancy and the postpartum period: A study in comparison and contrast. *International Journal of Childbearing Education, 21*(2), 27–30.

Doswell, W. M., Kopuyate, M., & Taylor, J. (2003). The role of spirituality in preventing early sexual behavior. *American Journal of Health Studies, 18*(4), 195–202.

Garces, I. C., Scarinci, I. C., & Harrison, L. (2006). An examination of sociocultural factors associated with health and health care seeking among Latina immigrants. *Journal of Immigrant Health, 8*, 277–385.

Green, L. W., & Kreuter, M. W. (1999). *Health promotion planning: An educational and environmental approach* (3rd ed.). Mountain View, CA: Mayfield.

Haight, W. L. (1998). Gathering the spirit at First Baptist Church: Spirituality as a protective factor in the lives of African American children. *Social Work, 43*(3), 213–221.

Huff, R. M., & Kline, M. V. (1999). The cultural assessment framework. In R. M. Huff & M. V. Kline (Eds.), *Promoting health in multicultural populations: A handbook for practitioners* (pp. 481–499). Thousand Oaks, CA: Sage.

Huff, R. M., & Kline, M. V. (2007). The cultural assessment framework. In R. M. Huff & M. V. Kline (Eds.). *Health promotion in multicultural populations: A handbook for practitioners and students* (2nd ed., pp. 125–145). Thousand Oaks, CA: Sage.

Huff, R. M., & Yasharpour, S. (2007). Cross-cultural concepts of health and disease. In R. M. Huff & M. V. Kline (Eds.), *Health promotion in multicultural populations: A handbook for practitioners and students* (2nd ed., pp. 23–39). Thousand Oaks, CA: Sage.

Joint Committee on Health Education and Promotion Terminology. (2012). Report of the 2011 Joint Committee on Health Education and Promotion Terminology. *American Journal of Health Education, 43*(2), 1–19.

LaVeist, T. A., & Wallace, J. M. (2000). Health risk and inequitable distribution of liquor stores in African American neighborhoods. *Social Sciences and Medicine, 51*(4), 613–617.

Liu, C., Sun, Y., Li, Y., Yang, W., Zhang, M., Xiong, C., & Yang, Y. (2012). The relationship between cold-hot nature and nutrient contents of foods. *Nutrition and Dietetics, 69*, 64–68.

Long, C. O. (2011). Cultural and spiritual considerations in palliative care. *Journal of Pediatric Hematology and Oncology, 33*(2), S96–101.

Luquis, R., & Pérez, M. A. (2003). Achieving cultural competence: The challenges for health educators. *American Journal of Health Education, 34*(3), 131–138.

Luquis, R., & Pérez, M. A. (2005). Health educators and cultural competence: Implications for the profession. *American Journal of Health Studies, 20*(3), 156–163.

Luquis, R., Pérez, M. A., & Young, K. (2006). Cultural competence development in health education professional preparation programs. *American Journal of Health Education, 37*(4), 233–241.

Luquis, R., & Villanueva, I. (2006). Knowledge, attitudes, and perceptions about breast cancer and breast cancer screening among Hispanic women residing in south central Pennsylvania. *Journal of Community Health, 31*(1), 25–42.

Marin, G. (1993). Defining culturally appropriate community interventions: Hispanics as a case study. *Journal of Community Psychology, 21*, 149–161.

Marin, G., & Marin, B. V. (1991). *Research with Hispanic populations*. Thousand Oaks, CA: Sage.

Nakamura, R. M. (1999). *Health in America: A multicultural perspective*. Boston: Allyn & Bacon.

National Center for Cultural Competence. (2000). *A planner's guide: Infusing principles, content and themes related to cultural and linguistic competence into meetings and conferences*. Retrieved from http://nccc.georgetown.edu/documents/ Planners_Guide.pdf

Purnell, L. D. (2005). The Purnell model for cultural competence. *Journal of Multicultural Nursing and Health, 11*(2), 7–15.

Purnell, L. D. (2009). *Guide to culturally competent health care*. (2nd ed.) Philadelphia, PA: F. A. Davis.

Purnell, L. D., & Paulanka, B. J. (2003). Transcultural diversity and health care. In L. D. Purnell & B. J. Paulanka (Eds.), *Transcultural health care: A culturally competent approach* (2nd ed., pp. 1–39). Philadelphia: F. A. Davis.

Ramirez, R., & de la Cruz, G. P. (2002). *The Hispanic population in the United States: March 2002* (Current Population Reports, P20–545). Washington, DC: US Census Bureau.

Rosenstock, I. M. (1974). Historical origins of the health belief model. *Health Education Monographs, 2*, 328–335.

Scarinci, I. C., Bandura, L., Hidalgo, B., & Cherrington, A. (2012). Development of a theory-based (PEN-3 and Health Belief Model), culturally relevant intervention on cervical cancer prevention among Latina immigrants using intervention mapping. *Health Promotion Practice, 13*(1), 29–40.

Shoultz, J., Phillion, N., Noone, J., Tanner, B. (2002). Listening to women: Culturally tailoring the violence prevention guidelines from the Put Prevention into Practice program. *Journal of the American Academy of Nurse Practitioners, 14*(7), 307–315.

Simon, C. E. (2006). Breast cancer screening: Cultural beliefs and diverse populations. *Health and Social Work, 31*(1), 36–43.

Spector, R. E. (2004). *Cultural diversity in health and illness* (6th ed.). Upper Saddle River, NJ: Pearson Prentice Hall.

Stoy, D. B. (2000). Developing intercultural competence: An action plan for health educators. *Journal of Health Education, 31*(1), 16–19.

US Census Bureau. (2008). *Projections of the population by sex, race, and Hispanic origin for the United States: 2010 to 2050.* Retrieved from http://www.census.gov/population/www/projections/summarytables.html

Yick, A. G., & Oomen-Early, J. (2009). Using the PEN-3 model to plan cultural competent domestic violence intervention and prevention service in Chinese American and immigrant communities. *Health Education, 109*(2), 125–139.

Zoucha, R., & Purnell, L. D. (2003). People of Mexican heritage. In L. D. Purnell & B. J. Paulanka (Eds.), *Transcultural health care: A culturally competent approach* (2nd ed., pp. 264–278). Philadelphia, PA: F. A. Davis.

CHAPTER 7

PLANNING, IMPLEMENTING, AND EVALUATING CULTURALLY APPROPRIATE PROGRAMS

Emogene Johnson Vaughn
Vickie D. Krenz

LEARNING OBJECTIVES

After completing this chapter, you will be able to

- Describe the relationship of the concepts of culture, health, and linguistics.
- Recognize the need for cultural and linguistic competence.
- Assess the essential use of needs assessments in culturally diverse groups.
- Examine cultural factors in the planning and implementation of culturally appropriate programs.
- Describe challenges and strategies used in the design of culturally appropriate evaluations.

This chapter explores the relationship between the concepts of culture and health to show the basis of one's understanding of the need for cultural and *linguistic competence*, the capacity of an organization and its personnel to communicate effectively and convey information in a manner that is easily understood by diverse audiences, including persons of limited English proficiency, those who have low literacy skills or are not literate, individuals with disabilities, and those who are deaf or hard of hearing. The concept of *cultural appropriateness* will be the focus of factors that are important to the effective planning, implementation, and evaluation of health education programs.

We examine the need for cultural and linguistic competence by addressing the attributes of health professionals who are expected, and often mandated, to apply professional and national standards such as culturally and linguistically appropriate services (CLAS) in the planning, implementation, and evaluation of programs appropriate for culturally diverse individuals and groups.

Concepts of Culture, Health, and Linguistics

Concepts of health, illness, and death are as phenomenal and multifaceted as the concepts of culture. The similarities among these concepts are that they are learned, acquired, and shared. The differences that exist among

linguistic competence
The capacity of an organization and its personnel to communicate effectively and convey information in a manner that is easily understood by diverse audiences, including persons of limited English proficiency, those who have low literacy skills or are not literate, individuals with disabilities, and those who are deaf or hard of hearing

cultural appropriateness
Denotes an approach that considers multiple cultural factors (e.g., beliefs, values, norms, language, experiences, gender, sexual orientation/gender identity, age, class, education) in the design and delivery of services, training, research, collaboration/partnerships, and community engagement

them are multitudinous and cultural. The essence of this diversity is realized when such differences find acceptance in our own concepts and, more important, when they are applied in the planning, implementation, and evaluation of culturally appropriate health programs. Edberg (2013) defines culture from such a multifaceted approach to include seven facets: classic, symbolic, ideologic, materialistic, linguistic, mental or cognitive, and cultural and biocultural. To highlight one of the facets, the mental or cognitive definition of culture, Edberg explains the concept of culture as something being primarily in the mind of people within a particular group—a kind of shared conceptual framework that organizes thought and behavior. It is from this facet that Edberg emphasizes "culture as not so much about what people do, but about what they think and how that determines what they do" (p. 11). In essence, "culture is man's way of finding acceptance and making sense of what he does" (p. 11).

Edberg's emphasis can be applied to the concepts of health and even illness and death as well. From a multicultural perspective, a variety of questions can be raised: Is health one's personal responsibility or illness one's own fault? Is health a divine reward, or is illness or death a due punishment? Is one's health, illness, or death due to sorcery or to be blamed on or caused by someone or something else? The responses to any one question are as diverse as the many health-related behaviors that result from one's cultural way of thinking and doing. For health professionals, the mental or cognitive perspective may require an assessment of the role that cultural-specific practices and beliefs, including race, ethnicity, socioeconomic status, age, gender identity, sexual orientation, education, and language, play in the concepts of health, illness, and death that culturally diverse individuals and groups hold.

Drawing again from one of Edberg's multifaceted perspectives, *linguistic culture* is defined as language that can make communication easier or difficult. It is interesting to observe persons from different geographies and faraway lands using similar expressions and phrases. Differences in cultures and language may exist, yet a conversation may be understood because the underlying message has a shared understanding. Expressions such as "a toast to your health" or "have a healthy day" or "the apple does not fall far from the tree" may have universal meanings. In contrast, cultural differences and languages may create confusions and misunderstandings. One's culture may dictate who speaks first or who extends a handshake. The cultural appropriateness of these behaviors may be interpreted as kind and friendly gestures or as rude and disrespectful actions. Cultural and language differences can help or hinder communication, compliance, and acceptance of information, products, or services. A useful suggestion is to improve one's cultural competence by learning about a community's history, resources, governance, and composition. Participating in community activities such as graduation ceremonies, community dinners, funerals of honored members, and special events such as neighborhood or block parties are recommended. A proactive strategy is to learn the language of the target audience or at least culturally appropriate phrases and expressions of the language. Such participation and interest build relationships and bonds of trusts that the health educator is accepted and welcomed in the community.

One of the tenets from the Office of Minority Health (OMH) strongly supports the importance and impact that communication and concepts of health and culture can have in the working relationships of health professionals and individuals and groups from diverse cultures. According to OMH (2013),

Culture and language may influence:

- health, healing, and wellness belief systems
- how illness, disease, and their causes are perceived by the patient/consumer
- the behaviors of patients/consumers who are seeking health care and their attitudes toward health care providers
- the delivery of services by the provider who looks at the world through his or her own limited set of values, which can comprise access for patients from other cultures (p. 3).

The impact of cultural beliefs serves as an example of the intersection between a cultural factor and health outcomes, for example, a simplistic view of an Asian cultural belief that the causes of diseases and illnesses come from an imbalance in hot and cold (yin/yang) or an Afro-Caribbean view that supernatural spirits when "vexed" can cause havoc in a person's mind and body. These beliefs are in direct contrast to the pathogenic theories of the biomedical system. How these contrasting beliefs are accommodated by both diverse individuals and groups and by health educators and health care providers highly influences decisions for program intervention strategies and their possible outcomes. The choice of program intervention may be with a healer using natural plants or herbs, or the choice may be toward the use of doctors using conventional medicines. Imagine the Asian or Afro-Caribbean aging patient engaging in the cultural practice of drinking an herbal tea along with the conventional practice of a daily low-dose aspirin to counteract his or her inflammatory condition such as arthritis or heart disease. Such an intervention becomes a culturally appropriate breakthrough in the integration of the acknowledgment and acceptance of cultural differences. The coexistence of the cultural diversity of the individual or group, along with the health educator or health care provider, is possible and feasible in that all sides acknowledge that all peoples have their own cultural knowledge and practices (Edberg, 2013). Furthermore, one's cultural knowledge and practices are neither right or wrong; they are just different.

The Need for Cultural and Linguistic Competency

Skills in cultural competency and linguistics are necessary for navigating health education programs that aim to address the goals of Healthy People 2020, which emanated from the 1985 Report of the Secretary's Task Force on Black and Minority Health (Department of Health and Human Services, 1985). Healthy People 2020 continues to promote the adoption of healthy behaviors for all Americans as a strategy to improve the quality of life, reduce health disparities, and extend life expectancy. However, the successes of this initiative continue to dim as health problems like obesity and lack of physical activity remain while the challenges continue to abound as measured by the initiative's long-standing goals. First, gaps in life expectancies and years of quality health still exist disproportionately and are threatened by ongoing observations that the life expectancy of young people today is projected to be shorter than that of their parents (Olshansky & Carnes, 2012). Second, access to and the availability of health care and services is still limited for minorities and made worse by inflationary health care costs and a lack of affordable health insurance even with the Affordable Care Act. And third, health disparities among cultural and ethnic groups remain a major concern.

Following the 1985 health report, Braithwaite and Taylor (1992) warned even then of too little focus being given to cultural competence as a strategy for effective health education or to close health gaps and disparities. Since 1999, with the launching of the Reach 2010 project (American Association for Health Education, 2004a) and initiatives from the Office of Minority Health (Johnston, Denboba, & Honberg, 1998), greater and growing interest has been directed toward culturally appropriate and community-driven strategies to address selected diseases and health problems that disproportionally affect specific racial and ethnic groups. To sum it up, the awareness and acceptance of the interrelatedness and connectedness of the concepts of health and culture as a strategy to improve quality of life for all peoples make clear the need for cultural and linguistic competence and should direct the planning, implementation, and evaluation of culturally appropriate health programs.

The future quality of health and wellness for all cultural groups depends not only on the quality of the health education for the diversity of the population, but also on the preparation of the new generation of health professionals for working with the diverse population. Professional organizations like the American Association for Health Education (AAHE) have responded to this challenge by publishing *Guidelines for Health Educators* (2004b) and a position statement on cultural competency (2006). Also, in a joint venture with the Health Resources and Services Administration, AAHE published a supplemental issue to its journal that highlighted cultural competence as a strategy for eliminating disparities for vulnerable populations (Schwartz, 2006). Whereas the composition of health professionals and health educators remains rather constant and homogeneous, the demographics of minority groups have diversified more rapidly. Consequently, the demand for health professionals to have diverse cultural and linguistic skills will become more challenging to meet.

In the interim, the emphasis still remains on program content with too little regard for culture-specific content, for the messenger, or how the message will be delivered. That is, the process for translating programs continues to be overlooked as a strategic action plan. Many community health promotion programs have failed due to lack of financial support, inability to reach target populations, especially those of high risk, and, of equal concern, an inability to design programs that are meaningful to the health beliefs, practices, and behaviors of the community to be served. The future realization of healthy lifestyles of specific target populations traditionally underserved, or yet to be served, and underrepresented may depend on the country's ability to effect changes in unhealthy lifestyles and in its efforts to prepare health professionals for working with racially and culturally diverse individuals and groups. When we ignore multicultural differences, a void exists in the health education process. Health gaps and disparities continue to widen because goals and behavioral outcomes may be set that are not shared by those of a different race or culture (Sue, 2001).

The goal of community engagement should be to build capacity and increase comfort levels when interacting with *diverse groups*. Within this goal, the aim is to provide multicultural training and experiences that challenge, stretch, and expand the health professional's world and local view in any health setting. Higher cultural competence is perceived when programs or services are culturally responsive, cultural differences are acknowledged and reframed, and images of color and racial blindness are projected (Atkinson, Thompson, & Grant, 1993).

diverse groups
A group of different or diverse people along the dimensions of gender, age, ethnicity, race, sexual orientation, socioeconomic status, physical abilities, political beliefs, religious beliefs, or other ideologies

Individually and collectively, addressing the cultural and linguistic competence of health professionals, particularly to include health educators, has gained some attention as another strategy to increase the adoption of healthy behaviors. Because health and social practices are usually manifestations of cultural beliefs and individual life experiences (Braithwaite & Taylor, 1992), understanding and developing cultural and linguistic competence should be of growing importance to health educators and other health professionals. Luquis and Pérez (2003) urge health educators to "assume their inherent responsibility" and to be proactive in forging a partnership and collaboration with federal agencies in establishing within the field of health education "discipline-specific" guidelines and interventions for cultural competence. In the academic areas of counseling, psychology, education, business, and advertising, the consensus is that through translators, culturally competent health professionals are likely to be the key to getting people to adopt healthy behaviors and creating supportive environmental conditions, thereby reducing the health gaps and disparities within the United States.

Program Planning Models and Cultural Diversity

The effectiveness of health education programs has focused on progress toward meeting the Healthy People 2020 outcomes. Program planning originated out of the Role Delineation Project of the 1970s. Over the subsequent decades, numerous planning models have emerged that address the health disparities of diverse populations. These models provide a systematic approach to identifying health issues and strategies and developing effective programs that lead to measurable health outcomes. Planning models provide structure, direction, and sequence to the planning process, thus allowing greater focus from the onset on program outcomes. The integration and linkage of concepts of cultural competence help to direct the focus of the planning model toward programs appropriate for the diverse population being served. Several planning models are commonly used in health education programming, and they are considered to have made the program planning process more effective in achieving desired program outcomes.

Planning models have been beneficial in providing structure and direction in the development of health programs. Models focus on the steps necessary for a comprehensive approach in addressing potential health issues within a particular community. However, a key element often missing from planning is the engagement of the targeted population as active participants in the process.

More recently, planning models have focused on the strengths of community-based partnerships to address health disparities at the local level. Community-based organizations can address the unique cultural factors that have an impact on the disparities of health outcomes. However, these organizations often lack the academic skills required to measure the outcomes of their interventions.

To address this issue, the *community-based participatory research* (CBPR) model was implemented to form partnerships among constituents that address program planning, implementation, and evaluation of outcomes. The CDC, OMH, National Institutes of Health, and state and nonprofit foundation funding sources initiated this approach to strengthen the collaborative research relationships between community-based organizations and academic institutions. As Minkler and Wallerstein (2003) noted, CBPR is a collaborative approach that recognizes the unique strengths that community-based and academic organizations bring to research endeavors. More specifically, "CBPR begins with a research topic of importance to the community with the aim of combining knowledge and action for social change to improve community health and eliminate disparities" (p. 4). Furthermore, Israel and colleagues (2003) point out that CBPR is presupposed by the genuine partnership of colearning between academic and community partnerships. As a result of this collaborative partnership, community members are trained and engaged in the research process, resulting in shared ownership of knowledge and findings. Most notable, CBPR is intended to build strong long-term commitments between community-based and academic partners in which the stakeholders equally and collaboratively address health disparities at the community level.

community-based participatory research
A partnership-based approach to research and evaluation

Sandoval and colleagues (2012) have pointed out that the CBPR approach has gained considerable attention and continues to be used to bring together community organizations and academic communities to address health disparities with culturally and linguistically appropriate programs that have measurable outcomes. Initiated by SOPHE, the Racial and Ethnic Approaches to Community Health program (REACH 2010) demonstrated the beneficial aspects of CBPR and identified forty funded community programs in collaborative partnerships to plan, implement, and evaluate strategies that addressed health disparities (Satcher, 2006). REACH 2010 demonstrated the symbiotic relationship that can result from collaborative partnerships between community and academic participatory research.

Collaborative partnerships have the potential to bring together the strengths of community-based leaders with the research strengths of academic professionals. This relationship has the potential to plan, implement, and evaluate culturally appropriate health promotion interventions that incorporate the strengths of all partners at all levels of the planning process.

Recognizing the roles and contributions that all partners bring to the planning process is important. Academic researchers bring the expertise of research methods and evaluation skills needed for evidence-based outcomes. These technical resources, which funders often require, provide credibility and accountability of program measures. However, academic partners often lack the cultural insights and nuances that community partners bring to the relationship. Thus, it is imperative that mutual respect for the contributions and expertise of all partners be established to ensure the successful development of culturally appropriate programs.

The culture of academic institutions can bias researchers' perceptions of culturally diverse populations. As Wallerstein and Duran (2006) noted, academic researchers are often driven by an institutional agenda that requires externally funded grants, a bias that can result in an overly zealous drive to pursue funding without inclusion of the targeted community. In addition, the potential exists that academic researchers will bring a paternalistic view that presupposes that they know what is best for the community. It is imperative that academic researchers closely evaluate their biases throughout the planning process to ensure that the targeted population is actively involved.

Planning, Implementation, and Evaluation of Culturally Appropriate Programs

In working with diverse community groups, health educators are charged with finding out more information about what is going on and why and how cultural issues may or may not influence a health problem or related risk behaviors. As information is gathered, a view of the community evolves that portrays what is and what is needed. This view becomes a picture of the community's strengths and resources and of its limitations, barriers, and areas of needed improvements. The tools of *needs assessments* help to paint this big picture (Hodges & Videto, 2005). The big picture is a social assessment, a term used to describe the quality of life and health status of a community group (Green & Kreuter, 1991). Painting the big picture guides the direction for targeting programs to specific populations. Succinctly stated, Hodges and Videto (2005) promote the use of needs assessments to assist health educators in investigating the web of factors that affect the health of the target population and the ability of health educators to have a positive influence on the cultural group through language and communication skills and through knowledge of health beliefs and practices.

needs assessments
Process by which the health educator identifies the health needs of the target population and decides whether these needs are being met

Edberg (2013) writes that gathering useful information that paints an accurate picture of community capacity and community needs starts with forming partnerships with key leaders and community organizations that can provide knowledge and expertise in collaborating on the conduct of a needs assessment. Edberg points out that partnering with the community draws on acceptance, participation, and involvement, which leads to a sense of connectedness and community ownership.

With this partnership, conducting a needs assessment acquires an added value in that "what is" and "what is needed" now become what "we" look like and what "we" need to do. This inward shift in attitudes eliminates the us/them evaluation and program attitude. Furthermore, it fosters the working relationship, team effectiveness, and team enthusiasm for each other's roles as equal program participants.

An underlying issue is the definition of *culture*, which is inherent at all levels of collaborative partnerships. As noted, culture reflects the organization of thought and behavior that has meaning and sense among a group of people (Edberg, 2013). The idea of culture is expansive and transcends a group's race/ethnicity. It is a complex and multifaceted set of experiences and personal histories that have meaning and sense to individuals. For example, there are shared language, symbols, behaviors, and experiences among young Americans that reflect a culture of youth. This group shares complex experiences in a technologically advanced world that cross racial/ethnic backgrounds. Their lives reflect the power of the Internet, social networking, smart and Android phones, high-definition television, and electronic learning systems. In comparison, their grandparents have journeyed through an existence of rotary land phones, party lines, tube televisions, transistor radios, and pencil and paper. Navas and colleagues (2005) propose that culture and the adaptation of social contexts involve a sociocultural reality, including religious, social, educational, political, labor, family relations, and ways of thinking (i.e., principles and values).

The academic community shares a pattern of thought and behavior that is reflected in the meaning and sense of research. The principles and values of the academic culture focus on sound research methodologies with statistical hypothesis testing to determine the effectiveness of programs for behavior change. The cultural thought values fidelity of programs with measures of reliability and validity. As Wallerstein and Duran (2006) pointed out, the culture of academic institutions focuses on being awarded external funding, along with concerns for tenure and promotion.

Conducting Culturally Appropriate Needs Assessments

Needs assessment tools and strategies provide primary, secondary, qualitative, and quantitative data helpful in painting the big picture. A general recommendation is that a combination of tools and strategies be used to ensure cultural appropriateness. The combination of approaches can provide a clearer picture than the initial view of the target population.

Primary information-gathering strategies have the advantage of providing a more accurate and specific baseline of information to describe uniquely what the community looks like. Qualitative means such as interviews of key leaders and community organizations, conducting forums and nominal and focus groups, and forming coalitions and advisory boards are helpful in discovering the community's own perception of the "way we look," of "having our needs met," and of the barriers to opportunities for "improving our community's quality of life." Shadowing "community-folk," an ethnographic, firsthand approach, and listening to the storytelling of key and lay members of the community can provide a rich and vast amount of information that often is overlooked or otherwise unavailable. Drawing qualitative data directly from the target community is strategic in that it provides specific information that gives insight into socioeconomic characteristics and cultural practices. Qualitative methods of information gathering are culturally appropriate for use with community groups where written language is a barrier and oral tradition is preferred. Key and lay members of a community may "talk your ears off" while they have a reluctance and a resistance to "filling out another written form." In situations where linguistics and education levels are not logistical issues, primary means to capture quantitative data have become more convenient, sometimes free or at low cost with the use of the Internet, to send out surveys, questionnaires, and checklists.

Secondary information-gathering strategies that help to paint the social assessment or big picture include information from and collected by external social, education, governmental, private, voluntary health, and humanitarian organizations. These external sources provide secondary information that represents studies of larger populations at national or state levels. Comprehensive health assessments and health status assessments can be obtained from a host of websites and other sources. Box 7.1 provides sources of information and websites for secondary data that can be used for needs assessments.

BOX 7.1 SOURCES OF INFORMATION AND WEBSITES

American Heart Association, www.americanheart.org/

Centers for Disease Control (CDC), www.cdc.gov/

Healthy People 2000/2010/2020 Report, www.healthypeople.gov/

Henry J. Kaiser Family Foundation, www.kff.org/

Morbidity and Mortality Weekly Report (MMWR), www.cdc.gov/mmwr

National Association of City and County Health Officers (NACCHO), sites available for each state

National Center for Health Statistics, www.cdc.gov/nchs

National Health Information Center, www/health.gov/nhic/

National Health Interview Survey (NHIS), www.cdc.gov/nchs/nhis.htm

National Institutes of Health (NIH), www.nih.gov/

Office of Minority Health, www.minorityhealth.hhs.gov/

Robert Wood Johnson Foundation, www.rwjf.org/

Rural Health Programs, www/ruralhealthweb.org/

Statistical Abstracts of the United States, www.census.gov/compendia/statab/

Youth Risk Behavior Surveillance System (YRBSS), www.cdc.gov/yrbs/

Population-based public health surveys have been widely used to provide prevalence and incidence data essential for needs assessments. Large-scale surveys typically reflect greater precision in sampling methodologies, representative sample sizes, and increased reliability and validity. However, problems arise with research methodologies that were developed with Anglo American populations and are applied to multiethnic survey samples. Pasick, Stewart, Bird, and D'Onofrio (2001) reported that the languages and cultures of multiethnic populations can affect survey results. They identified the following problems with multiethnic and multilingual survey data: questionnaire construct, diversity in cultural meanings, cultural appropriateness of survey items, nonequivalent connotations of translated items, and demographic characteristics of participants. Numerous other researchers (Burn, Sudman, & Wansink, 2004; Sudman, Bradburn, & Schwarz, 1996; Warnecke et al., 1997) have reported similar findings that the wording of multiethnic surveys can lead to misinterpretation by respondents.

Population-based public health surveys are often used to provide an understanding of racial/ethnic health outcomes. As a statistical construct, these surveys collapse broad ethnic groups into six categories: Caucasian (white), Hispanic/Latino (non-white and non-black), black or African American, Asian/Pacific Islander, Native American/Alaskan Native, and other. In this format, the categorical racial/ethnic groups are portrayed as homogeneous groups. In reality, there is tremendous diversity among the ethnic groups that are represented within these categories. For example, Hispanic/Latinos represent a wide range of ethnic backgrounds that have unique aspects of their culture, language, and experiences. And Asian/Pacific Islanders do not share a similar language, culture, or traditional experiences.

One the fastest-growing demographic groups in the United States is that of those who self-identify as two races. According to 2010 Census data, 2.9 percent of the population reported multiple races, with the most common reported multiple race combinations as white and black (1.8 million), white and some other race (1.7 million), white and Asian (1.6 million), and white and American Indian/Alaska Native (1.4 million) (Humes, Jones, & Ramirez, 2011). Furthermore, data from the American Community Survey revealed that 5.6 percent of children under 18 years are two or more races. California, Texas, New York, and Florida have the highest number of multiracial people (US Census Bureau, 2012).

Designing Culturally Appropriate Evaluations

Over the past several decades, greater attention has been given to the performance of public and nonprofit funded programs. Increasingly, the knowledge of what works and does not has led to program improvements, evidence-based policy decisions, and measurable health outcomes. Accountability of program funds has been a major factor for evaluation requirements in federally funded programs. Under the Government Performance and Results Act of 1993, federal agencies are required to establish annual quantitative performance targets with annual reporting (US Office of Management and Budget, 1993). Many state and nonprofit funders have followed this move to require evaluation of funded programs.

Considerable resources have been published in the field of *program evaluation*. Abundant volumes have been written on evaluation design methodologies and measurement issues. Attention has been focused on the level of evaluative precision, reliability, validity, and generalizability. However, the cost of an evaluation increases with the level of precision to measure program outcomes.

program evaluation
A process to determine if a program's goals and objectives have been achieved or to determine the effectiveness of a program

Evaluative research requires knowledge of research designs, including quantitative and qualitative methodologies, while keeping in mind that each program evaluation is unique and brings a set of challenges. The application of evaluation methodologies is as much art as it is science, so a cookie-cutter approach cannot be used to address all health programs. Evaluation methodologies require a balance of the program goals and objectives, the target population, and the resources available to implement the evaluation.

It is essential that evaluation planning begins at the inception of a potential program. Clear and measurable program goals and objectives are the basis for guiding the direction of a program. Evaluation begins at the start of the program with careful consideration as to the methodologies that will be used to measure whether the goals and objectives were met. This ensures that data can be collected at appropriate intervals, including preprogram assessments if they are required.

In addition, evaluation planning and evaluation do not occur in isolation but in a collaborative partnership with all program staff, including representatives of the target population. Successful collection of data relies on access to the targeted population throughout the funding period. Coordinated efforts between program and evaluation staff ensure this process is achieved.

There remains a dearth of published work on the evaluation of community-based public health programs. As interventions move from highly controlled settings to actual diverse settings, adherence to a new context can compromise the original program's fidelity. Achieving comparable control groups is often difficult in community-based setting. Furthermore, cultural adaptations may have an impact on the reliability and validity of evaluation instruments. These constraints have limited the publication of program results in the research literature.

Matching evaluation designs and assessments to diverse populations can be a challenging task. Diverse populations represent a constellation of considerations in determining how to design, adapt, or collect data. It is essential to consider a variety of factors that have a direct impact on the evaluation methods to be used. These factors include educational levels, verbal and written language constructs, cultural protocols, and acculturation.

Education

Education is an important consideration in program planning and implementation. As Ballantine and Spade (2008) and Durkheim (2008) noted, formal education has a socializing effect that imparts essential information about the values, skills, and information necessary to function within society. Students are prepared to engage in the social responsibilities of literate citizens in political and economic issues. Thus, formalized education is a mechanism by which individuals are taught how to function within the organization of society. The use of language and customs are integrated into how individuals are expected to participate in society (Bowles & Gintis, 2008; Sadovnik, 2008). As part of the educational process, students are familiarized with the structure of how information is organized and interpreted within our society. A literate citizen is expected to have the ability to communicate in verbal and written formats.

Western written format is generally organized in a linear and sequential manner. Print materials such as books and periodicals are read from the top (upper left) of the page and from left to right. The educational process instills in learners this organization to facilitate the efficiency of information in our society. This organization of information is evident in everyday experiences, from reading food labels to following a recipe.

In addition, the educational process provides opportunities for learners to be exposed to assessment constructs. Categorical constructions (gender, race/ethnicity, and so on) are "boxes" that students are taught the meaning of early in their educational training. As they progress, they are introduced to more advanced constructs that develop higher levels of cognitive skills. Thus, education provides opportunities to learn and practice assessment constructs that are commonly used in planning and measuring program outcomes.

Multicultural education research (Padilla, 2012) has demonstrated that the lack of formal Western education can compromise assessment constructs. Erroneous conclusions can result when the targeted population lacks the ability to understand written formats or the constructs used in program assessment and outcomes. Preliterate or low-literacy societies may have little or no experience with the abstract concepts of scaled intervals. Deyo (1984) found that errors can be introduced in conclusions when respondents are not able to perceive the meaning of intervals when asked, "On a scale of 1 to 5, with 1 being 'strongly disagree' and 5 being 'strongly agree,' how would you rate . . . ?" Singh-Manoux, Adler, and Marmot (2003) used a ten-rung ladder scale to depict perceptions of social status and health outcomes. Similarly, Chen, Gee, Spencer, Danziger, and Takeuchi (2009) assessed social standing among Asian immigrants in the United States using a ladder graphic representation:

> Think of this ladder as representing where people stand in the United States. At the top of the ladder are the people who are the best off—those who have the most money, the most education and the most respected jobs. At the bottom are the people who are the worst off—who have the least money, least education, and least respected jobs or no job. The higher up you are on the ladder, the closer you are to the people at the very top; the lower you are, the closer you are to the people at the bottom. What is the number to the right of the rung where you think you stand at this time in your life, relative to other people in the United States? (p. 862)

Language

Language is a reflection of the culture of a population and has specific meaning to that population. This brings a twofold challenge in designing culturally appropriate evaluations: words and concepts. Words can have totally different meanings between dialects of a same language. For example, the word *cake* is translated as *torta* in Peru, Colombia, and Venezuela, but a *torta* is a sandwich for people from Mexico. Similarly, geographic regions may have unique terms or phrases for the same action, object, or concept. For example, a cart used to transport groceries while shopping is called a "shopping cart" in California and a "buggy" in southern Louisiana.

The translation of words to other languages brings a greater challenge. As noted, language has specific meaning to a population. The meaning of a word in English may have no comparable translation in another language. For example, the mental health term *blue* could be interpreted as "sad" or "depressed" in English. However, the same term in German (*blau*) could be translated as "drunk" or "high." Nezami, Zamani, and DeFrank (2008) demonstrated that translation must accurately reflect a specific target population's language, standards, traditions, and culture.

Concepts are inherent in a cultural context and expressed in language. This poses a significant challenge in culturally appropriate evaluation designs. An anecdotal comment from a Hmong colleague reflected his experience in coming to the United States in the early 1980s as a refugee: "It was like getting on a plane in the 14th century and getting off in the 20th century." The concept of disease (cancer, mental illness, and so on) has shifted with acculturation to greater realization of a scientific basis (Fadiman, 1997). As Baker, Dang, Ly, and Diaz (2010) demonstrated, Hmong often blend traditional shamanism with Western medicine and may be distrustful of aspects of Western health care.

Precision of language has to be considered in culturally appropriate evaluations. Western languages are precise in terms of time sequencing. For example, the concept of last year or last month has precise time measurement. In comparison, the Hmong language does not have this level of precision. For example, elders often use such references to "rainy seasons" as a measure of time so that a child's age is measured in how many rainy seasons have passed since his or her birth.

Lack of written language or the inability to read is also a significant challenge in evaluation design. Preliterate ethnic groups may lack a written language and rely on spoken words and pictorial images to communicate. For example, the Hmong use hand-stitched storytelling tapestries to depict events or life. A Hmong tapestry, for example, depicts the invasion of the Hmong by communist soldiers in the Vietnam War and their journey to the Western world. The story portrayed has distinctive meaning and sequence with the older Hmong refugee culture. Oral administration of measurements such as face-to-face surveys has been used to accommodate these limitations with open-ended questions or the use of visual aids, or both (Jacobs, Karavolos, Rathouz, Ferris, and Powell, 2012). While face-to-face interview can result in high response rates, they typically are more costly to administer (Newcomer & Triplet, 2004).

Culturally appropriate surveys must take into consideration the wording and constructs of specific cultural groups. Pasick and colleagues (2001) investigated the effect of measurement in multiethnic surveys with Latina, African American, Chinese, and other races/ethnicities with cultural appropriateness and comparability of wording. Their findings reinforce the need for extensive qualitative and quantitative formative research, with attention to each culture to be studied. In addition, administration of multiethnic surveys must take into consideration literacy levels—both reading and writing skills. Researchers (Ashing-Giwa, Padilla, Tejero, & Kim, 2004; Berknaovic, 1980; Solomon, Card, & Malow, 2006) have highlighted the need to use qualitative data from key informant and focus group interviews to adapt instruments, back translation, and pilot test measures to be incorporated into a final instrument.

Cultural Protocols

Cultural protocols reflect the culturally sanctioned behaviors acceptable to a specific population. In many cultures, men carry dominant roles, and women refrain from expressing opinions in mixed company. Furthermore, sensitive topics such as sexual issues and male or female issues may be inappropriate to discuss with members of the opposite sex. Thus, evaluation measures (e.g., focus groups, interview surveys) that include both men and women together at one time may limit conclusions. Taylor and colleagues (2011) used gender-appropriate interviewers with Cambodian American men and women from the same household on hepatitis B knowledge and practices. However, differences between males (67 percent) and females (73 percent) were noted in the study response rates.

In many communities, cultural protocols may involve the manner in which community leadership is identified and engaged. Among American Indian communities, tribal leaders, councils, and other leaders are the culturally sanctioned facilitators of their communities. Researchers (Fisher & Ball, 2002; Unger, Soto, & Thomas, 2008; Wallerstein & Duran, 2006) have highlighted the importance of gaining approval by these official bodies prior to engaging in evaluation efforts and data collection. Furthermore, Letiecq and Bailey (2004) reported that face-to-face meetings are preferred in many American Indian communities rather than indirect forms for communication such as letters, telephone calls, and e-mails.

Cultural protocols are intrinsic in all communities. The patterns of behaviors pose considerable challenges in the planning, implementation, and evaluation of community-based programs. Engaging community partners as equal members of the research team contributes to understanding cultural norms, behavioral practices, and critical issues. Furthermore, community partners are essential for opening avenues for instrument adaptation, pilot testing, and participant recruitment.

Reflections on Cultural Appropriateness in Working with Diverse Individuals and Groups

Reflecting on Edberg's multifaceted perspectives of culture and specifically on his mental or cognitive definition that views culture as an outcome of what we think and how what we think influences what we do allows us to ponder the importance of trust and sensitivity in working with diverse individuals and groups. Trust and sensitivity are pillars in building positive working relationships and interactions between the health professional and cultural groups. As pillars, trust and sensitivity create and establish a connectedness that transcends the numerous factors (race, age, gender, economic difference, language) that are important to the effectiveness of health program interventions. Trust and sensitivity make engagement and empowerment realistic goals in making a difference in the quality of life of diverse individuals and groups.

Coupled with trust and sensitivity, cultural desire and cultural awareness are exemplified in the selection and design of health education program approaches and materials used to acknowledge and incorporate the existing knowledge, beliefs, and practices of diverse individuals and groups.

Fueled by cultural desire, strengthened by cultural awareness, and reinforced by cultural sensitivity, health professionals can develop the personal sensitivity, trust, and credibility that are pivotal for integrating cultural competence into the planning, implementation, and evaluation of health education programs.

Cultural appropriateness in working with diverse individuals and groups requires a collaborative partnership that recognizes and respects the skills of all parties. Community partners bring tremendous knowledge and experience within their cultural communities. They possess a practical intelligence that is not necessarily measured by academic degrees.

A strength of the CBPR model is capacity building in community partnerships. The collaborative relationship engages community partners in developing planning and evaluation skills that extend beyond the project. Culturally appropriate collaborative CBPR partnerships extend beyond one project. Relationships developed using this model can carry on to continued partnerships in other project areas and issues.

Conclusion

This chapter began by emphasizing the interrelatedness of culture, health, and linguistics. The interrelatedness was reflected as intersections that encompassed the complexity of these terms. This complexity was observed in the need for culturally and linguistically appropriate program planning, implementation, and evaluation.

The chapter closes with an equal emphasis on the interrelatedness of culture and evaluation. The common thread that intersects culture with evaluation is the concept of values. Culture shapes values, beliefs, and health practices. Evaluation attempts to measure the merit or impact of cultural values, beliefs, and health practices on the quality of life of diverse individuals and groups.

Several conclusions can be drawn from these discussions. First, in response to increasing demographic changes and persistent and emerging health problems in the nation's population, it is crucial that health education initiatives speak to the need for culturally and linguistically competent professionals and programs. Second, knowledge of the interrelatedness of culture, health, and linguistics and of the numerous factors that bear on this interrelatedness is essential to the health profession's ability to be effective in working with diverse individuals and groups. Third, to be skillful and effective in conducting needs assessments, using community participatory strategies, and designing health education programs, health professionals must have the desire, awareness, and sensitivity, along with ability, to build a sense of trust in the community being served. The attainment of our nation's health goals depends on culturally appropriate health education programs, health services, and health care.

Points to Remember

- The concepts of culture, health, and linguistics are interrelated, and the intersection of the three factors may serve as a bridge to providing culturally appropriate programs.
- Culturally competent health professionals are constantly examining their own culture-related views and always striving to improve the quality of health education programs for all people.
- Health education programs are more effective when they are designed and delivered with specific cultural factors in mind, using basic principles and practices appropriate for diverse individuals and groups.
- Collaborative partners between academic evaluation researchers, program staff, and community leaders (the CBPR model) can build on the strengths of all parties to address health disparities effectively.

- Needs assessments are the starting point for program planning, implementation, and evaluation of culturally appropriate programs.
- Program implementation and evaluation must take precautions to ensure cultural and linguistic appropriateness. Program evaluation occurs in a cultural context, and the process connects acceptable methodologies with the participants' customs and values.

Case Study

The rate of teen pregnancy is rising in a culturally diverse community in which an estimated 25 percent of the population are immigrants. In addition, the community is nearly 50 percent Latino and has a high number of at-risk youth. Its high school graduation rate is 73 percent, well below the state average of 82 percent. Statewide data estimate that 34 percent of the population 16 years and older in this community lack basic prose literacy skills.

1. Define the steps required to develop a needs assessment of the problem in this community, including primary and secondary data.
2. Who are the collaborative partners that need to be included in coalition to address the teen pregnancy problem?
3. What steps are needed to develop a program, implementation, and evaluation plan?
4. Describe the cultural considerations that must be addressed in the program plan, implementation, and evaluation design.

KEY TERMS

Community-based participatory research
Cultural appropriateness
Diverse groups
Linguistic competence
Needs assessment
Program evaluation

References

American Association for Health Education. (2004a). *Fact sheet: Eliminating racial and ethnic health disparities.* Retrieved from http://www.healtheducationadvocate.org/Summit2004/EliminHDREACH-2004_final.pdf

American Association for Health Education. (2004b). *Guidelines for Health Educators.* Reston, VA: Author.

American Association for Health Education. (2006). *A position statement of the American Association for Health Education: Cultural competency in health education.* Reston, VA: Author.

Ashing-Giwa, K. T., Padilla, G. V., Tejero, J. S., & Kim, J. (2004). Breast cancer survivorship in a multiethnic sample: Challenges in recruitment and measurement. *Cancer, 101,* 450–465.

Atkinson, D. R., Thompson, E. E., & Grant, S. K. (1993). Three-dimensional model for counseling racial/ethnic minorities. *Counseling Psychologist, 21*(2), 257–277.

Baker, D. L., Dang, M. T., Ly, M. Y., & Diaz, R. (2010). Perceptions of barriers to immunization among parents of Hmong origin in California. *American Journal of Public Health, 100,* 839–845.

Ballantine, J. H., & Spade, J. Z. (2008). Understanding education through sociological theory. In J. H. Ballantine & J. Z. Spade (Eds.), *Schools and society: A sociological approach to education* (3rd ed.). Thousand Oaks, CA: Sage.

Berkanovic, E. (1980). The effect of inadequate language translation on Hispanics' responses to health surveys. *American Journal of Public Health, 70,* 1273–1281.

Bowles, S., & Gintis, H. (2008). Schooling in capitalist societies. In J. H. Ballantine & J. Z. Spade (Eds.), *Schools and society: A sociological approach to education* (3rd ed.). Thousand Oaks, CA: Sage.

Braithwaite, R. L., & Taylor, S. E. (Eds.). (1992). *Health issues in the black community.* San Francisco: Jossey-Bass.

Burn, N. M., Sudman, S., & Wansink, B. (2004). *Asking questions: The definitive guide to questionnaire design—for market research, political polls, and social and health questionnaires.* San Francisco, CA: Jossey-Bass.

Chen, J., Gee, G. C., Spencer, M. S., Danziger, S. H., & Takeuchi, D. T. (2009). Perceived social standing among Asian immigrants in the US: Do reasons for immigration matter? *Social Science Research, 38,* 858–869.

Deyo, R. A. (1984). Pitfalls in measuring the health status of Mexican Americans: Comparative validity of the English and Spanish Sickness Impact Profile. *American Journal of Public Health, 74,* 569–573.

Durkheim, E. (2008). Moral education. In J. H. Ballantine & J. Z. Spade (Eds.), *Schools and society: A sociological approach to education* (3rd ed.). Thousand Oaks, CA: Sage.

Edberg, M. (2013). *Essentials of health culture and diversity: Understanding people, reducing disparities.* Burlington, MA: Jones and Bartlett.

Fadiman, A. (1997). *The spirit catches you and you fall down: A Hmong child, her American doctors, and the collision of two cultures.* New York, NY: Farrar, Straus, and Giroux.

Fisher, P. A., & Ball, T. J. (2002). The Indian Wellness Project: An application of the tribal participatory research model. *Prevention Science, 3,* 235–240.

Green, W., & Kreuter, M. W. (1991). *Health promotion planning: An educational and environmental approach.* Mountain View, CA: Mayfield.

Hodges, B. C., & Videto, D. M. (2005). *Assessment and planning in health programs.* Boston, MA: Jones and Bartlett.

Humes, K. R., Jones, N. A., & Ramirez, R. R. (2011). *Overview of race and Hispanic origin: 2010 (2010 Census Briefs).* Washington, DC: US Department of Commerce, Census Bureau.

Israel, B. A., Schulz, A. J., Y Parker, E. A., Becker, A. G., Allen, A. J., & Guzman, R. (2003). Critical issues in developing and following community based participatory research principles. In M. Minkler & N. Wallerstein (Eds.), *Community based participatory research for health* (pp. 53–76). San Francisco, CA: Jossey-Bass.

Jacobs, E. A., Karavolos, K., Rathouz, P. J., Ferris, T. G., & Powell, L. H. (2012). Limited English proficiency and breast and cervical cancer screening in a multiethnic population. *American Journal of Public Health, 95,* 1410–1416.

Johnston, L. L., Denboba, D. L., & Honberg, L. (1998). Reducing health disparities: Ideas for resource development and technical assistance. *American Journal of Health Education, 29*(5), S54-S58.

Letiecq, B. L., & Bailey, S. J. (2004). Evaluating from the outside: Conducting cross-cultural evaluation research on an American Indian reservation. *Evaluation Research, 28,* 342–357.

Luquis, R. R., & Pérez, M. A. (2003) Achieving cultural competence: The challenges for health educators. *American Journal of Health Education, 34*(3), 131–138.

Minkler, M., & Wallerstein, N. (Eds.). (2003). *Community based participatory research in health.* San Francisco, CA: Jossey-Bass.

Navas, M., Garcia, M. C., Sanchez, J., Rojas, A. J., Pumares, P., & Fernandez, J. S. (2005). Relative acculturation extended model (RAEM): New contributions with regard to the study of acculturation. *International Journal of Intercultural Relations, 29,* 21–37.

Newcomer, K. E., & Triplet, T. (2004). Using surveys. In J. S. Wholey, H. P. Hatry, & K. E. Newcomer (Eds.), *Handbook of practical program evaluation* (2nd ed.). San Francisco, CA: Jossey-Bass.

Nezami, E., Zamani, R., DeFrank, G. (2008). Linguistic translation of psychological assessment tools: A case study of the MMPI-2. *Evaluation and the Health Profession, 31,* 313–317.

Office of Minority Health (2013). *What is cultural competency?* Retrieved from http://www.minorityhealth.hhs.gov/templates/browse.aspx?lvl=2&lvlid=11

Olshansky, S., & Carnes, B. (2012). The paradox of immortality. *Gerontology, 59*(1), 85–92.

Padilla, A. M. (2012). Quantitative methods in multicultural education research. In J. A. Banks & C.A.M. Banks (Eds.), *Handbook of research on multicultural education* (2nd ed.). San Francisco, CA: Jossey-Bass.

Pasick, R. J., Stewart, S. L., Bird, J. A., D'Onofrio, C. N. (2001). Quality of data in multiethnic health surveys. *Public Health Reports, 116,* 223–243.

Sadovnik, A. R. (2008). Contemporary perspectives in the sociology of education. In J. H. Ballantine & J. Z. Spade (Eds.), *Schools and society: A sociological approach to education* (3rd ed.). Thousand Oaks, CA: Sage.

Sandoval, J. A., Lucero, J., Oetzel, J., Avila, M., Belone, L., Mau, J., . . . Wallerstein, N. (2012). Process and outcome constructs for evaluating community-based participatory research projects: A matrix of existing measures. *Health Education Research, 27,* 680–690.

Satcher, D. (2006). Working in and with communities to eliminate disparities in health. *Health Promotion Practice, 7,* 176S-178S.

Schwartz, R. H. (2006). Editor's notes. *Health Promotion Practice, 7,* 17S.

Singh-Manoux, A., Adler, N. E., & Marmot, M. G. (2003). Subjective social status: Its determinants and its association with measures of ill-health in the Whitehall II study. *Social Science and Medicine, 56,* 1321–1333.

Solomon, J., Card, J. J., & Malow, R. M. (2006). Adapting efficacious interventions: Advancing translational research in HIV prevention. *Evaluation and the Health Professions, 29,* 162–194.

Sudman, S., Bradburn, N. M., & Schwarz, N. (1996). *Thinking about answers: The application of cognitive processes in survey methodology.* San Francisco, CA: Jossey-Bass.

Sue, D. W. (2001). Multidimensional facets of cultural competence. *Counseling Psychologist, 29,* 790–821.

Taylor, V. M., Talbot, J., Do, H. H., Yasui, Y., Jackson, J. C., & Bastani, R. (2011). Hepatitis B knowledge and practices among Cambodian Americans. *Asian Pacific Journal of Cancer Prevention, 12,* 957–961.

Unger, J. B., Soto, C., & Thomas, N. (2008). Translation of health programs for American Indians in the United States. *Evaluation and the Health Professions, 31,* 124–144. doi:10.1177/0163278708315919.

US Census Bureau. (2012). *2010 Census shows multiple-race population grew faster than single-race population.* http://www.census.gov/newsroom/releases/archives/race/cb12–182.html

US Department of Health and Human Services. (1985). *Report of the Secretary's Task Force on Black and Minority Health.* Washington, DC: Author.

US Office of Management and Budget. (1993). *Budget baselines, historical data, and alternatives for the future.* Washington, DC: Executive Office of the President.

Wallerstein, N. B., & Duran, B. (2006). Using community-based participatory research to address health disparities. *Health Promotion Practice, 7,* 312–323.

Warnecke, R. B., Sudman, S., Johnson, T. P., O'Rouke, D., Davis, M., & Jobe, J. B. (1997). Cognitive aspects of recalling and reporting health-related events: Papanicolaou smears clinical breast examination, and mammograms. *American Journal of Epidemiology, 146,* 982–992.

CHAPTER 8

CULTURALLY APPROPRIATE COMMUNICATION

Raffy R. Luquis

This chapter discusses *communication models* and process; the communication patterns among racial, ethnic, and other groups; and the role of linguistic competence in delivering health education programs to these population groups. The discussion focuses on the health communication process and strategies, cultural and linguistic competence standards, historical perspectives on communication across cultures, communicating across cultures about health and disease, communication and persona and *community health*, communication and marketing techniques for various cultures, and communication patterns, barriers, and empowerment.

LEARNING OBJECTIVES

After completing this chapter, you will be able to

- Describe the components of the health communication model.
- Understand the importance of communicating across cultures about health and disease.
- Understand the effect of cultural communication on personal and community health.
- Explain the similarities and differences in communication and marketing techniques.
- Understand the language barriers minorities face in health education practice.
- Use the guidelines for effective communication and cultural competence in planning health education programs.

Communication Model

While there are numerous definitions of *health communication*, the 2011 Joint Committee on Health Education and Promotion Terminology (2012) defined it as "the art and science of using theory-based communication strategies and technologies to inform and influence individual and community decisions that advance health" (p. 12). Health communication involves more than just the production of messages and materials. For health communication to be successful, there must be an understanding of the intended audience's needs and perceptions. The National

I acknowledge the contribution of Matthew Adeyanu on this chapter in the first edition of this book and the contributions of Alba Lucia Diaz-Cuellar and Suzanne Evans, authors of chapter 2, to the section titled "The Importance of Verbal and Nonverbal Communication."

communication models
A graphical representation to help examine and understand the different parts of the communication process

community health
The health status of a defined group of people and the actions and conditions to promote, protect, and preserve their health

health communication
The art and science of using theory-based communication strategies and technologies to inform and influence individual and community decisions that advance health

Cancer Institute (NCI), which published "Making Health Communication Programs Work" (a document also known as the Pink Book), described the communication model in four distinctive phases: planning and strategy development; developing and pretesting concepts, messages, and materials; implementing the program; and assessing effectiveness and making refinements (NCI, 2008). These phases are arranged in a circular process that guides health educators through a continuous loop of planning, implementation, and improvement (see figure 8.1). (The description and explanation of each stage is beyond the scope of this chapter; thus, health educators are encouraged to review that document for more detailed information on how to use and implement this health communication process.)

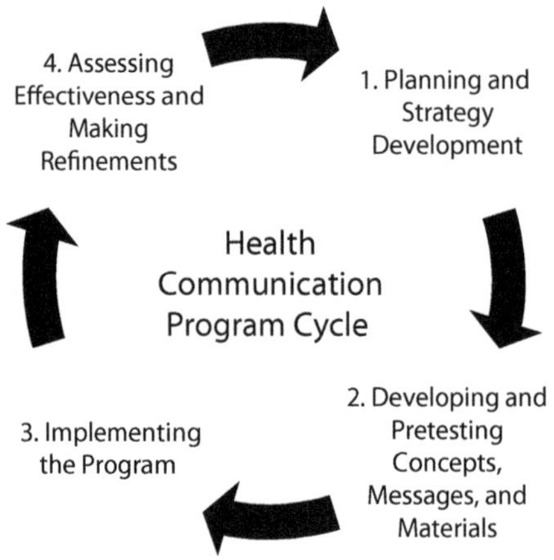

Figure 8.1 Stages of the Health Communication Process
Source: Modified from National Cancer Institute (2008).

It is imperative that when using this process, health educators take into account diversity and culture at each of these decision points when developing campaigns that target culturally diverse population subgroups. For example, during the planning and strategy development phase, health educators must identify the health problems and needs of the targeted group and determine if communication plays a role in addressing the problem. During the second phase, health educators must understand the ethnic/racial group cultural characteristics (language, acculturation, cultural values, and so on) and examine how these characteristics influence people's reaction to health messages (see more information in the "Strategies to Incorporate Cultural and Linguistic Competence in Health Education" section). As part of the implementation phase, health educators must put into action culturally relevant strategies designed to attract and keep the intended audience interest in the program, such as the use of language, dance, folklore, and music. Finally, when working with ethnic and racial subgroups, health educators must consider the use of mixed methods (i.e., qualitative versus quantitative) as part of the outcome evaluation to determine the effectiveness of the program (Young, 2011).

The Importance of Verbal and Nonverbal Communication

A way to explore cultural differences is to examine the concepts representative of all cultures, which include paralanguage, proxemics, and nonverbal behavior.

Paralanguage refers to language without the words, and it is more vast than the spoken word. It includes loudness, body language, looks, rate, inflections, the use of the active or passive voice, the frequency of the use of *I*, pauses, and silences. The analysis of paralanguage can reveal features of culture (Mehrabian, 1972, 1978). For example, some members of the European American culture feel uncomfortable with silence, while silence in other cultures, such as the Chinese and Japanese, is interpreted as a dignified expression, a desire to continue speaking after making a particular point, or a sign of respect to elders (Sue & Sue, 1990). In Latin American indigenous communities, silence is an expression of the beauty of being able to "have a dialogue with one's heart," to examine what is being said, and to reflect before responding. As health educators, it is important to understand that when individuals from other cultures are silent, it does not mean that they are not understanding what is being said; instead they are being respectful or thoughtful. Nonetheless, health educators must navigate a fine line between silence that implies respect and silence as lack of understanding.

Proxemics, which refers to the perception and use of personal and interpersonal space, is determined by cultural backgrounds (Sussman & Rosenfeld, 1982). Hall (1976) identified four interpersonal distance zone characteristics of US culture: intimate, personal, social, and public. In the United States, most people feel comfortable with a three-foot radius of public space, which is not the case in other cultures. Social space varies depending on the level of familiarity with the interaction group, personal space is the physical space around them, and intimate space is one that is shared with only close relatives, spouses, and children. When people from different cultures meet, the issue of proximity may lead to misunderstandings and confusion. For example, in mainstream America, an individual who enters another person's personal space without his or her permission may imply intimacy; in other cultures, individuals do not adhere to personal space and instead speak to each other in close proximity (Rose, 2011). Similarly, in some Hispanic subgroups, welcoming an acquaintance with a hug and kiss on the cheeks is acceptable, while in other cultures, this represents intimate behavior. Thus, understanding cultural parameters with regard to personal space will provide health educators with an insight into cultural norms and communication.

Although language, class, and cultural factors all interact to create problems in communication between health educators and ethnic and racial diverse communities, an often neglected area is nonverbal communication (Harrison, 1989). The power of nonverbal communication is that it tends to operate at an unconscious level of awareness but may be more trusted than words. It is therefore clear that the ways in which people communicate—the proximity, tone of voice, and directness—is related to a specific cultural and situational context.

Cultural knowledge comes through dialogue; it is intersubjective (Freire, 1987). One needs one's own cultural lenses to be able to have that dialogue. In this dialogue, the worlds of the interlocutors meet and partly overlap. This is the space where meaning is created and knowledge is generated (Ringe, 2008). To have a fruitful dialogue takes courage because it means making oneself vulnerable and putting one's own framework to question. The implications for health education practice are obvious. A culturally competent health educator is one who through a constantly inquisitive and self-critical mind is able to generate a wide repertoire of responses (verbal and nonverbal) consistent with the lifestyles and values of culturally different communities and can build bridges between cultures by going beyond the obvious, visible, and surface of his or her own worldview.

Standards for Cultural and Linguistic Competence in Health Education

In 2001, the Office of Minority Health (OMH) published the National Standards for Culturally and Linguistically Appropriate Services in Health Care (CLAS Standards), which provides the framework for all health care organizations to best serve the nation's increasingly diverse communities. In fall 2010, the OMH began an initiative to revise the CLAS to show the changes in the scope and advancements in this area. In April 2013, the OMH released the enhanced National CLAS Standards, which "are intended to advance health equity, improve quality, and help eliminate health care disparities by establishing a blueprint for individuals as well as health and health care organizations to implement culturally and linguistically appropriate services" (OMH, n.d.a, p. 1). These standards include a series of guiding principles to inform, direct, and make possible processes associated with culturally and linguistically appropriate health services (see box 8.1 and appendix). While the CLAS Standards are primarily directed to health care organizations, health educators can integrate and use the standards to make their health education and promotion programs more culturally and linguistically appropriate. Given this conceptual foundation, the enhanced standards are structured as follows: "Principal Standard (standard 1), Governance, Leadership, and Workforce (standards 2–4), Communication and Language Assistance (standards 5–8), and Engagement, Continuous Improvement, and Accountability (standards 9–15)" (OMH, n.d.a, p. 2). When working on health communication, health educators should place emphasis on the communication and language assistance standards, which are mandates for all recipients of federal funds (OMH, n.d.b). These standards specifically address the need to provide language assistance services, inform the individual of the availability of these services, ensure the competence of those who are providing language assistance, and provide health-related material in the group's preferred language.

BOX 8.1 NATIONAL STANDARDS ON CULTURALLY AND LINGUISTICALLY APPROPRIATE SERVICES

Principal Standard

1 Provide effective, equitable, understandable, and respectful quality care and services that are responsive to diverse cultural health beliefs and practices, preferred languages, health literacy, and other communication needs.

Governance, Leadership, and Workforce

2. Advance and sustain organizational governance and leadership that promotes CLAS and health equity through policy, practices, and allocated resources.
3. Recruit, promote, and support a culturally and linguistically diverse governance, leadership, and workforce that are responsive to the population in the service area.
4. Educate and train governance, leadership, and workforce in culturally and linguistically appropriate policies and practices on an ongoing basis.

Communication and Language Assistance

5. Offer language assistance to individuals who have limited English proficiency and/or other communication needs, at no cost to them, to facilitate timely access to all health care and services.

6. Inform all individuals of the availability of language assistance services clearly and in their preferred language, verbally and in writing.
7. Ensure the competence of individuals providing language assistance, recognizing that the use of untrained individuals and/or minors as interpreters should be avoided.
8. Provide easy-to-understand print and multimedia materials and signage in the languages commonly used by the populations in the service area.

Engagement, Continuous Improvement, and Accountability

9. Establish culturally and linguistically appropriate goals, policies, and management accountability, and infuse them throughout the organization's planning and operations.
10. Conduct ongoing assessments of the organization's CLAS-related activities and integrate CLAS-related measures into measurement and continuous quality improvement activities.
11. Collect and maintain accurate and reliable demographic data to monitor and evaluate the impact of CLAS on health equity and outcomes and to inform service delivery.
12. Conduct regular assessments of community health assets and needs and use the results to plan and implement services that respond to the cultural and linguistic diversity of populations in the service area.
13. Partner with the community to design, implement, and evaluate policies, practices, and services to ensure cultural and linguistic appropriateness.
14. Create conflict and grievance resolution processes that are culturally and linguistically appropriate to identify, prevent, and resolve conflicts or complaints.
15. Communicate the organization's progress in implementing and sustaining CLAS to all stakeholders, constituents, and the general public.

Source: Office of Minority Health: National CLAS Standards (n.d.a).

Moreover, health educators must become linguistically competent in order to address the needs of limited-English-proficient individuals. In doing so, they will be also fulfilling the requirements of Title VI of the Civil Rights Act of 1964, which requires all organizations that receive federal financial assistance, such as many health care organizations, to provide effective communication between the entity and the limited-English-proficient person (OMH, 2001). The National Center for Cultural Competence (NCCC) (2009) defined linguistic competence as

> the capacity of an organization and its personnel to communicate effectively, and convey information in a manner that is easily understood by diverse audiences including persons of limited English

proficiency, those who have low literacy skills or are not literate, and individuals with disabilities, and those who are deaf or hard of hearing. (para. 2)

Thus, health educators and health professionals must examine the capacity of their organizations to provide linguistic appropriate services included in the CLAS and NCCC documents. Box 8.2 provides a list of practices, procedures, and resources needed to support linguistic competence services and provide effective communication to diverse populations.

BOX 8.2 PRACTICES, PROCEDURES, AND RESOURCES THAT SUPPORT LINGUISTIC COMPETENCE SERVICES

- Bilingual/bicultural or multilingual/multicultural staff
- Cross-cultural communication approaches
- Cultural brokers
- Foreign language interpretation services, including distance technologies
- Sign language interpretation services
- Multilingual telecommunication systems
- Videoconferencing and telehealth technologies
- TTY and other assistive technology devices
- Computer-assisted real-time translation or viable real-time transcriptions
- Print materials in easy-to-read, low-literacy, picture and symbol formats
- Materials in alternative formats (e.g., audiotape, braille, enlarged print)
- Varied approaches to share information with individuals who experience cognitive disabilities
- Materials developed and tested for specific cultural, ethnic, and linguistic groups
- Translation services, including those of:
    - Legally binding documents (e.g., consent forms, confidentiality and patient rights statements, release of information, applications) and signage
    - Health education materials
    - Public awareness materials and campaigns
    - Ethnic media in languages other than English (e.g., television, radio, internet, newspapers, periodicals)

Strategies to Incorporate Cultural and Linguistic Competence in Health Education

communication strategy
Plans or methods for communicating information related to a specific issue, event, situation, or audience

Communication can be verbal (spoken) or nonverbal. Cultural differences in both of these areas can affect communication and self-understanding and serve as barriers to effective communication. For effective communication to take place, there must be a strong *communication strategy.* A communication strategy describes how a message will be framed and delivered to the target audience. It is based on a thorough understanding of the audience members and their knowledge, attitude, wants, beliefs, needs, values, traditions, and the like. The strategy describes the target audience, the action the audience members should take, the obstacles between the audience and the action to be taken, how audience members will benefit, and how to reach them with the message.

According to the NCI (2008), as part of the second phase of the communication model, when working with ethnic and racially diverse populations, health practitioners and educators must understand that culture influences how people view and react to health messages and materials. Thus, in order to develop a successful health communication strategy, health educators must understand how key aspects of culture influence the intended audience and build that understanding into communication strategy. NCI stated:

> Messages must take into account cultural norms in terms of what is asked (e.g., don't ask people to make a behavior change that would violate cultural norms), what benefit is promised in exchange (in some cultures, community is most important; in others, individual benefit is), and what image is portrayed. The symbols, metaphors, visuals (including clothing, jewelry, and hairstyles), types of actors, language, and music used in materials all convey culture. ("Developing Culturally Appropriate Communications," para. 2)

Although it is important to recognize culture within the intended group, developing distinctive messages and materials for each cultural group is not always necessary. Instead, health educators should carefully research the target audience to identify messages and images that will resonate across groups or situations in which different message messages or images work better.

Finally, the NCI (2008) shared information from the Center for Substance Abuse Prevention *Technical Assistance Bulletin* on considerations when developing culturally sensitive communication (see box 8.3).

BOX 8.3 DEVELOPING CULTURALLY SENSITIVE COMMUNICATION

- Acknowledge culture as a predominant force in shaping behaviors, values, and institutions.
- Understand and reflect the diversity within cultures. In designing messages that are culturally appropriate, the following dimensions are important:
  - Primary cultural factors linked to race, ethnicity, language, nationality, and religion
  - Secondary cultural factors linked to age, gender, sexual orientation, educational level, occupation, income level, and acculturation to the mainstream
- Reflect on and respect the attitudes and values of the intended audience—for example:
  - Whether the individual or the community is of primary importance
  - Accepted roles of men, women, and children
  - Preferred family structure (nuclear or extended)
  - Relative importance of folk wisdom, life experience, and value of common sense compared with formal education and advanced degrees
  - Ways that wealth is measured (material goods, personal relationships)
  - Relative value put on different age groups (youth versus elders)
  - Whether people are more comfortable with traditions or open to new ways
  - Favorite and forbidden foods
  - Manner of dress and adornment
  - Body language, particularly whether touching or proximity is permitted in specific situations
- Are based on concepts and materials developed for and with the involvement of the intended audience. Substituting culturally specific images, spokespeople, language, or other executional detail is not sufficient unless the messages have been tested and found to resonate with the intended audience. Formative research with audience members takes on added importance when planners and designers have cultural backgrounds different from those of the intended audience.
- Refer to cultural groups using terms that members of the group prefer. For example, many people resent the term *minority* or *nonwhite*. Preferred terms are often based on nationality, such as *Japanese* or *Lakota*.
- Use the language of the intended audience, carefully developed and tested with the involvement of the audience.

Source: National Cancer Institute (2008).

In addition, health educators should review information presented in the Gateway to Health Communication and Social Marketing Practices website (Centers for Disease Control and Prevention, 2011). This website gives health practitioners and educators access to resources to help build effective health communication campaigns and programs. This resource provides information on how to analyze an audience, how to choose the proper channels and tools, examples of health communication campaigns, and how to evaluate health communication messages and materials. The CDC provides examples of successful communication campaigns such as a multifaceted social marketing initiative ("Take Charge. Take the Test") designed to increase HIV testing among African American women, and a campaign to encourage black gay and bisexual men to get tested for HIV ("Testing Makes Us Stronger"). The website provides *Audience Insights*, in which the authors present information on different target audiences to use when developing effective communication messages. For example, the "Cultural Insights: Communicating with Hispanics/Latinos" describes information to help health professionals communicate more efficiently with this cultural group in order to change their behaviors. And "Audience Insight: Communicating to the Responsible Generation" addresses the characteristics and behaviors among those ages 64 to 84. Health educators should give special attention to the documents on the elderly and Hispanics, two of the fastest-growing populations in the United States (see chapter 1).

Communication and Culture

Culture is a complex concept that can be defined in many ways. As discussed in chapter 6, culture integrates "human behaviors that include thought, communications, languages, practices, beliefs, values, customs, courtesies, rituals, manners of interacting and roles. . .; and the ability to transmit the above to succeeding generations" (NCCC, 2000, p. 1). It is rooted in institutions such as families and schools and also in communication industries. In our daily lives, we are constantly making decisions about such matters as what foods to eat, what clothes to wear, how to greet others, what idiom of language to use when communicating with others, what behaviors to exhibit in a group, and how to perceive the world around us. Such decision-making processes are informed by our heritage and life experiences, and these lead us to develop our own cultural identity.

cultural identity
The identity of a group or culture or of an individual as far as one is influenced by one's belonging to a group or culture

Everyone comes from a culture, and individuals want to be associated with a culture. *Cultural identity* is made up of the specific and often unique ways that people think and act within the norms of their group. It encompasses a wide range of cultural influences on people's behaviors, beliefs, attitudes, and values. It is transmitted from generation to generation. Therefore, cultural identity is based primarily on a shared historical, linguistic, and psychological lineage. People with a common culture live in accord with a shared set of socially transmitted perceptions about the nature of the physical, social, and spiritual world, particularly as they relate to achieving life goals (Basch, 1990).

It is paramount that planners and evaluators of health education programs and services carefully examine the differences and the similarities in groups' cultural perceptions, so that they understand health beliefs, practices, knowledge, and attitudes more fully and hence address them appropriately within each group's particular context. Furthermore, they need to examine culture with a critical and open spirit. Culture is passed down from generation to generation. People have come before us, and people will come after us. Therefore, all individual moral and intellectual choices are superimposed on one's social and cultural environment and occur within a continuous, powerful, evolving belief system, faith, and set of values, customs, and traditions.

Cultural education with effective communication assists us in knowing the world better and the individual self better. Each individual person carries the cultural burden regardless of his or her personal background. Therefore, we have to come to an understanding of the cultural weight each of us carries and to empathize with the different loads borne by those of other cultures. This common knowledge and understanding will enrich us and free each of us from our culturally repressive ideas through *intercultural communication* (communication between or among people of different cultures).

intercultural communication
The process of communication between or among people of different cultures

Whether a health educator is serving a client at the microlevel (e.g., a family or small group unit) or working at a macrolevel (e.g., cooperating or collaborating with another service agency or health care facility), he or she is participating in intercultural communication. Whether the desired result is knowledge gain, behavioral change, attitude change, or skill acquisition, intercultural communication skills are needed. In fact, in health education practice, whether a client is seeking information for primary, secondary, or tertiary prevention, the ability to access information, persuade others, and participate in the selection of one's own health care protocols is essential. Intercultural communication proficiency empowers the individual or group in the decision-making processes of both personal (individual) and community (group) health.

Communication and Cultural Competence

Effective communication is the foundational building block for the health education profession. It cuts across all seven areas of responsibility for a health educator (National Commission for Health Education Credentialing,

2007), and it is the essential ingredient for conducting needs assessments and program planning, implementation, and evaluation. Effective communication is central to interacting with clients and community members and to serving as a resource person.

The communication model encompasses the message, the communication medium, the sender (teller or speaker) of the message, and the receiver (listener or audience) of the message. For effective communication to occur, the sender must send a concrete and clear message that the receiver understands with the same meaning intended by the sender (Rowe & Paterson, 2010). Barriers to effective communication can arise from the sender, the message, the channel of communication (medium), and the receiver of the message. Health educators need listening and speaking skills that will enable them to detect and remove these barriers. Roman, Maas, and Nisenholtz (2003) have addressed the issue of obstacles that stand between the audience (the receivers of the message) and the action taken (what the receivers should do) after receiving the message. When health educators know what real or perceived barriers stand in the way of clients' taking action, they have a tremendous opportunity to develop effective communication strategies. Understanding these barriers helps health educators select either implicit or explicit action messages to which audiences are most likely to be receptive. Rowe and Paterson (2010) recommend that health professionals can overcome *language barriers* by using very clear and simple English, relying on body language, repeating the information to reduce confusion, and reframing the question and providing the same information in different ways to ensure the receiver clearly understands.

language barriers
The difficulties that people who have no language in common face when trying to communicate with each other

Furthermore, many cultures have traditional ways of communicating among group members. Long ago, traditional news carriers were used to send messages from one place to another and announce special events in the community. In the Yoruba culture of southwestern Nigeria, the town crier is a good example of how messages are transmitted in the community. The oral tradition, that is, the spoken word, is one of the most common ways of transmitting information in many cultures. Symbols are also used as a medium of communication. Specific symbols mean different things. When a sender (a health educator) does not understand the culture of an audience and hence faces a communication barrier, serious communication breakdown can occur, which then affects the message. In many cultures, an oral tradition of storytelling plays an essential role in transmitting information to children and adults alike. However, exercising *cultural competence* also means that the health educator is aware of the ethical and cultural incongruence of assuming the role of the storyteller without proper training or education for that role and without a thorough

cultural competence
The capacity to work effectively across racial, ethnic, and linguistically diverse groups

understanding of the cultural implications of storytelling for learning in a specific cultural context.

When a health educator is adapting a communication to a specific community, it is imperative for the sender of the message to educate himself or herself in all aspects of the communication mechanisms (e.g., posters, flyers, pictorial symbols, storytelling) within the community's culture. The educator needs to be culturally competent in the community's cultural expressions before embarking on any health education and promotion intervention program planning, implementation, and evaluation. The health educator must be aware that even when the chosen methods and materials of communicating health are appropriate, questions about when and how they should be used may still need to be addressed. As Airhihenbuwa (1995) states, "Alternative methods of cross-cultural communication should be explored to ensure that the process does not dis-empower the target group" (p. 9).

A community is a group of individuals with a shared belief system, values, interests, or other attributes. Each cultural community has established particular codes, symbols, and strategies as methods of communication. These methods encapsulate the essence of meaning that such community groups bring to the development and acquisition of knowledge. Health educators and program planners should carefully examine these verbal and nonverbal communication methods as they relate to health behavior change processes and influence cultural values and beliefs. The power of the spoken word (oral tradition) is an ancient cornerstone of many cultures. Songs and dances too are found in the foundations of many cultures. Interpretations and decoding of the spoken word are embedded in storytelling, which may be expressed in songs and dances. Songs and dances are commonly used in different forms of rituals.

Historical Perspectives on Communication across Cultures

Communication across cultures has been a dominant and recurrent theme throughout human history. Misunderstanding and mistrust among communities due to lack of effective communication can result in internal or external conflicts. This can be seen in all the wars that have taken place throughout history to the present time. As Moroccan philosopher Mahdi Elmandjra (2003) said in discussing the prevention of such cultural conflicts or clashes of value systems that result in war, "We need people to communicate, to respect each other's systems and cultural diversity. The international community has no choice but to survive together" (p. 1). When a nation goes to war, the majority of its people label the people of the other nation with a single label. For example, prior to September 11,

2001, most American did not consider Arabs and Muslims to be terrorists; however, the "devastating terrorist attack of 9–11 caused a familiar and predictable response in the United States on two fronts: government policies specifically targeting Arabs and Muslims; and nationwide violence against Arabs and Muslims" (Akram, 2002, p. 79). It is a fact that the planners of the 9/11 catastrophe did inflict unprecedented damage to the people of United States; however, not everybody in the Arab or Muslim world is a terrorist or has plotted to attack America. Consequently, other people's cultures need to be viewed both as wholes and as made of their own diverse parts rather than stereotypically. Without this understanding, we will be enclosed by our own borders and become our own prisoners.

Communicating across Cultures about Health and Disease

Most cultures have culturally specific perceptions and conceptual explanations of health and disease. Hence, it is important to keep cultural competency in mind in discussions across cultures about health and disease. Examples of such conceptual explanations are the demonic (caused by a demon), celestial (caused by God or a higher being), phytogenic (caused by a plant), and miasmic (caused by an organism) theories of disease causation. When taboos and myths exist for certain populations, it is important for health educators to be familiar with them to effectively provide health education and promotion services to these clients. There are three factors to consider when communicating across cultures: the audience's degree of health literacy, the audience's level of knowledge about health and disease, and the audience's attitudes toward health, disease, and prevention.

Health Literacy

The degree of literacy, especially health literacy (the capacity to obtain, process, and understand basic health information), is important when communicating across cultures with brochures and other written educational materials because not everybody is at the same reading level. It does not make sense to use brochures written at the high school level when the majority of the population has not finished high school. Such materials create frustration and confusion. It is crucial to provide educational materials that are targeted toward the appropriate reading and comprehension level for each cultural group. In addition, it is necessary to consider using different communication strategies for different cultures. (Chapter 9 provides more information about health literacy.)

Level of Knowledge

The level of knowledge regarding health and disease is an important factor to consider when dealing with a diverse population. People from a small, rural community may be less educated than those who live in a large, urban area; therefore, health educators need to learn to communicate on the same level as the audience for ease of comprehension. This is imperative because in many instances, people with less knowledge are those who need health care and health education the most and may not be getting it due to their circumstances of health illiteracy.

Attitudes

Another consideration when communicating across cultures is cultural sensitivities or attitudes toward health. It is understandable that different cultures have different ways of explaining and interpreting health and disease concepts. Nonetheless, a majority of ethnic and racial diverse groups have little understanding of the medical concepts of disease process. Prevention is the key to living a healthy and quality life, and a lack of understanding of how to prevent illness can lead to devastating health effects. Taboos are especially important factors to consider when providing health care services to clients, both the well and the sick.

Communication and Personal Health

Health communication uses communication strategies to inform and influence individuals' and communities' health decisions. As such, it can raise individuals' awareness of health risks by informing them of potential hazards they may face. One of the seven areas of responsibility for health educators is to serve as a resource person (National Commission for Health Education Credentialing, 2007). Communicating how to avoid health risks is therefore an essential role for health educators.

Health risk communication is a two-way process: delivering a message to an interested party about the nature, significance, and management of the risk and the receipt of such a message for the ultimate use of the information provided (message) for decision making (by the intended audience) in disease prevention, health protection, health promotion, and health maintenance. Therefore, both health educators and their intended audience have responsibilities and high stakes in the avoidance of health risks. Health educators provide the health information, and the clients need to comprehend that information to make informed decisions about their health. The communication must be a two-way process for any meaningful, positive health outcome to occur. It is the duty of health educators to pass along health risk communication as new data and research arise. Health educators may discuss risks individually with a client or may provide information through the mass media and thereby communicate with a community (Nicholson, 1999). For example, from time to time, there are commercials telling people of warnings about and recalls of pharmaceutical products due to the availability of new research and data on the adverse health effects of these products. A health educator aware of such recall or warning information might discuss with a client the risks in the use of such a product. The ultimate decision is for the client to make. The role of the health educator is to assist in providing available science-laden information. In addition, the health educator can direct the client in enriching her health by promoting a better quality of life for her and preventing disease occurrence.

personal health
An individual's health status

In communicating *personal health* (health of the individual) information, the health educator must be mindful of the influence of cultural factors on the client's knowledge base, attitude, and behavior. Communicating personal health information must result in changes in the individual's belief system. Knowledge and attitude changes alone will not lead directly to a behavioral change. In order to change a personal health behavior, a person must have motivation to change (Glanz, Rimer, & Lewis, 2002). This has been demonstrated through the stages of a health behavior change model known as the transtheoretical model, which is fully discussed in other health education textbooks (Prochaska & DiClemente, 1983; Prochaska, DiClemente, & Norcross, 1992). Health educators are better able to motivate an individual and reduce a risk when they are able to determine in which stage the person is. For example, a person in the precontemplation stage does not intend to change within the next six months. If this is the case, having a health educator discuss with him the potential risks of not changing his behavior may move him along to the contemplation stage. Sometimes people need just a little push to get started. The health educator can apply communication strategies to that little push to start this person on the path to behavioral change.

Health communication can help individuals find other people who are in situations similar to theirs by encouraging them to attend group therapy or other meetings. Group therapy, such as that offered through Alcoholics Anonymous, can help some individuals overcome obstacles by providing support. However, people from certain cultural groups (e.g., indigenous people from Oaxaca in Mexico) prefer not to discuss personal issues in public settings; thus, health educators must be aware of this preference in order to provide them with the proper counseling therapy. Having support for a person in a difficult situation can enable that person to change his or her behavior and be less likely to slip back to the old behavior. Ultimately it will reinforce a new attitude toward changing a behavior to a healthier lifestyle. Group therapy is a positive aspect of health communication.

Public health is constantly changing, which means that the needs of individuals are changing also. One community may need a specific service, whereas another community may not. Communicating with individuals in a community can help health specialists decide which services are needed and which are not. A poor and underserved community may need assistance such as the WIC program in providing young children in the area with nutritional food, whereas a privileged community may not need such assistance. It is the responsibility of the health educator to serve as the resource person in assisting individuals and groups to find the needed resources for health promotion, health protection, and disease prevention.

Communication and Community Health

Community health refers to the "health status of a defined group of people and the actions and conditions to promote, protect, and preserve their health" (Joint Committee on Terminology, 2012). Community health communication can be powerful when it is approached correctly. It has the ability to influence the public agenda, advocate for policies and programs, promote positive changes in the community, improve health care delivery services, and create supportive partnerships within the community.

As a community becomes more informed through health education, its members begin to recognize the health-related problems occurring in the community. When the goal is to bring change to policies and programs, a community is much more powerful than individuals are alone. A community has the ability to make its public and commercial buildings smoke free, for instance. However, it must get a majority of the community to agree with a smoking ban in order to implement that change. The only way to change the minds of the people on such a subject is to influence them through health communication. A strong community is built by strong individuals; therefore, it is important to get through to the individuals by using diffusion of innovation and mass communication theories. Among the different ways to get a message across to a large population are news releases, radio and TV commercials, newspapers, magazines, and advertisements.

Community health communication can also promote other positive changes in the community, such as changes in the physical environment. Communicating to a population about the benefits of exercise and well-being may make people realize that their environment does not provide easy access to exercise. Some communities do not facilitate nonvehicular transportation. Successful community health education in this area could promote a change of scenery (Pérez, Weiller, Morrow, Martin,

Caldwell, & Jackson, 1999). One contemporary example of such change is building a bike path or sidewalks so that people can transport themselves in more vigorous ways. One of the ways health communication can translate into advocacy is through social organization and action. *Social action* is the empowerment or mobilization of community members to take matters into their own hands, in this case for the improvement of their mutual health and the protection of their environment. The health educator is the change agent for such a mobilization, using effective communication strategies to begin and support the process.

Communication and Marketing Techniques

When dealing with various cultures, it is of primary importance for health educators to identify their target audience before proceeding to communicate and market products or ideas to them. Doing this first will save the health educator precious time and money. It will also enable the health educator to be more effective in communicating and marketing (responsiveness to the needs, demands, and wants of target audience) because he or she will understand the culture of the people he or she is working with.

Many different techniques are used in marketing public health to promote social change (Siegel & Lotenberg, 2007). Some of the common methods are brochures, mailings, advertisements (in magazines, newspapers, billboards, and so on), commercials, websites, and social media. Although these are all effective techniques, it is necessary to determine the target audience prior to selecting a method. Marketing professionals who were trying to market a health product to a poor, rural village in a developing country using a website or e-mail would not be effective because the villagers most likely do not have access to computers.

Health education professionals should realize that there are differences in the ways people learn and think. Even in the developed world, not everybody thinks the same way. Cultures are unique, and in order for health educators to be effective in communicating with the public, they need to identify the differences in learning and thinking patterns among the various cultures. Making false assumptions about a culture and *stereotyping* are common and can have negative effects when they are used in marketing a new product to the target population. It is important to consider not only a country's dominant culture but also its subgroup cultures. Knowledge and understanding of such subcultures can make health educators more accepted by the public when planning programs for them.

stereotyping
Oversimplified standardized image of a person or group

A given message will not be equally effective in all cultures. In order to understand why this is so, health educators need to be aware of the different communication strategies and their uses. Communication strategies are tied to effective program planning and marketing techniques. Understanding a community's culture is one way to establish good marketing techniques for that community. This cultural understanding makes it easier to transmit information to the community. For example, Japanese audiences prefer indirect verbal communication and symbolism as the source of information; the Yoruba people of southwestern Nigeria prefer spoken words embedded in language codes, symbols, images, songs, and metaphors; and American advertising primarily relies on the spoken and written word as the source of information. Marketing techniques have strategic elements that are often described as the four Ps: product, price, place, and promotion. In order to address cultural differences it is necessary to adjust at least one of the four Ps. The most commonly changed P is promotion, which is basically the language of the advertisement.

Marketing techniques and strategies must frequently be revised when marketing to multiple cultures (Siegel & Lotenberg, 2007). Translating a message should be entrusted only to a professional translator or advertiser. Also, as suggested earlier, symbols and icons may not have meanings in one culture but may have very strong meanings in another. When marketing to various cultures, keep in mind that each culture holds different values, and some strategies will not be as effective as others.

Communication Patterns and Language Barriers

According to the US Census (2011), 60 million people ages 5 and older (21 percent of the population) in the United States speak a language other than English at home, and 25 million have limited English proficiency. This typically makes it difficult for these individuals to access health care, and health educators face major problems when planning, implementing, and evaluating health education services or programs for these individuals. Because of these problems, these individuals' quality of care can deteriorate. The language barrier makes it difficult for the patients and health care providers to communicate effectively. It is the responsibility of health educators in the health care setting to ensure that translators are sought for such patients in order to provide them with optimal health care.

Some studies (Flores, 2006; Luquis & Pérez, 2005; Murty, 1998; Peinkofer, 1994; Ponterotto, 1995; Velde, Wittman, & Bamberg, 2003; Wang, 2005) on the issues of communication patterns, cultural competence, and the language barriers minorities face in the delivery of health care in general and health education services in particular were reviewed for this chapter. These reviews make it clear that language issues play a major role in the quality of all health care delivery services, including health education services. Effective communication is a cornerstone of the delivery of health care services. The importance of developing listening and speaking skills cannot be overemphasized for all those involved in health care delivery services. Health care providers (including health educators) must demonstrate skill in listening, speaking, empathizing, probing, advocating, confronting, conveying immediacy, caring, and showing concern while responding to the health care needs of their clients and clients' families. They must understand the literacy levels of their clients and promote cross-cultural understanding. They should be prepared to recognize and meet the physical, social, emotional, mental, and spiritual needs of their clients.

Client confidentiality (as set out in the Health Insurance Portability and Accountability Act), informed consent, and client rights are extremely important in the delivery of care. The more that effective communication occurs between the provider and the client, the better the care is that is provided and the healing process. To stimulate health care discussions between provider and client, a brief introduction of the provider with reference to his or her qualifications, care philosophy, cultural background, interests, and relevant health topics to the client's well-being will be in order. Communication barriers impede the delivery of care and the healing process.

In conclusion, the language barrier among ethnically and racially diverse groups needs to be addressed. The issue is getting more attention, but it appears that rural and underserved areas and special populations in particular need help urgently. Although this is a relatively small population, these people are the ones who need health care the most. A greater percentage of ethnically and racially diverse groups live in metropolitan areas, but they are mainly being targeted by existing interventions. It may seem impossible, but this issue must be addressed everywhere in the world, in large cities like New York and in small towns in rural America, Southeast Asia, Africa, and elsewhere. In addition, efforts should be directed toward helping all diverse groups—whatever their difference, disability, or ethnic or racial identity—overcome their language barriers.

Conclusion

The chapter highlights health educator guidelines for effective health communication as part of the planning, implementation, and evaluation of health education and intervention programs. Health educators working with clients whose health knowledge, beliefs, practices, and attitudes differ significantly from those of the health educator should be aware that such cultural factors influence clients' responses to health education and health communication and that these clients require culturally and linguistically appropriate health education programs to influence their knowledge, attitudes, and behaviors. It is imperative that health educators demonstrate through their communication skills that they respect and value cultural diversity and encourage others to do so as well, while also unobtrusively observing clients' verbal and nonverbal behaviors and cues. Such behaviors and cues may be obstacles to effective communication.

Furthermore, it is crucial for health educators to exemplify how health practitioners in general are supposed to communicate with different clients, demonstrating how to interact with racially and ethnically diverse populations in order to provide them with adequate health information to encourage clients to make decisions concerning their health and health care.

Culture-specific and sensitivity training will assist health educators in becoming more flexible in inferring motives or attributing meanings to another's behavior, thereby increasing their communication effectiveness and cultural competency. They must continually advocate for effective cross-cultural communication and remember to focus on the important elements of communication, cultural sensitivity, marketing techniques, and language barriers as they carry out their roles and functions in their various practice environments.

Points to Remember

- The communication model described four phases that can guide health educators to work through a continuous loop of planning, implementation, and improvement of health communication.
- It is imperative that health educators take into account the diversity and culture of the population when developing health communication campaigns that target culturally diverse populations.
- Health educators should acknowledge the group culture and diversity within the culture, including language, images, values, and attitudes, when developing culturally appropriate health communication strategies.
- Health educators should always be willing to analyze and select effective communication channels that are likely to reach and influence the program participants that are sensitive to those participants' cultural underpinnings and use multicultural message strategies appropriate and relevant to the cultural environment.
- Health educators must possess active listening and speaking skills so that effective communication ensues.

Case Study

As a health educator, you have been invited to participate in a project on breast cancer prevention among immigrant women. Data from national studies show that while breast cancer screening has increased among white women, barriers for screening remain among women from Asian, Arab, and Latin countries. Latina, Asian, and Arab immigrant women are less likely to participate in clinical breast examination and mammography than white women. In addition to socioeconomic factors, cultural and religious beliefs may be barriers to breast cancer screening among these women. You are in charge of developing a health communication campaign to increase breast cancer screening among these groups.

1. What cultural and religious factors must you take into consideration when developing this campaign?
2. What other factors must you consider when developing an effective health communication message for these groups?
3. What communication strategies would you consider using as part of this campaign?
4. What are the implications of this case study for health education practice?

KEY TERMS

Communication model
Communication strategy
Community health
Cultural competence
Cultural identity
Health communication
Intercultural communication
Language barrier
Personal health
Stereotyping

References

Airhihenbuwa, C. O. (1995). *Health and culture: Beyond the Western paradigm.* Thousand Oaks, CA: Sage.

Akram, S. M. (2002). The aftermath of September 11, 2001: The targeting of Arabs and Muslims in America. *Arab Studies Quarterly, 24*(2/3), 61–118.

Basch, P. F. (1990). *International health.* New York, NY: Oxford University Press.

Centers for Disease Control and Prevention. (2011). *Gateway to health communication and social marketing practice.* Retrieved from http://www.cdc.gov/healthcommunication/

Elmandjra, M. (2003, October 20). Moroccan philosopher says cultural communication prevents war. *Asian Political News*. Retrieved from http://www.findarticles.com/p/articles/mi_m0WDQ/is_2003_Oct_20/ai_109021640

Flores, G. (2006). Language barriers to health care in the United States. *New England Journal of Medicine, 355*(3), 229–231.

Freire, P. (1987). *Pedagogy of the oppressed*. New York, NY: Continuum Press.

Glanz, K., Rimer, B. K., & Lewis, F. M. (Eds.). (2002). *Health behavior and health education: Theory, research, and practice* (3rd ed.). San Francisco, CA: Jossey-Bass.

Hall, E. (1976 *) Beyond culture*. Garden City, NY: Anchor Press.

Harrison, R. P. (1989). Non-verbal communication. In S. Sanderson King (Ed.), *Human communication as a field of study: Selected contemporary views* (pp. 113–126). Albany, NY: SUNY Press. Joint Committee on Health Education and Promotion Terminology. (2012). Report of the 2011 Joint Committee on Health Education and Promotion Terminology. *American Journal of Health Education, 43*(2), 1–19.

Joint Committee on Health Education and Promotion Terminology. (2012). Report of the 2011 Joint Committee on Health Education and Promotion Terminology. *American Journal of Health Education, 43(2), 1*–19.

Luquis, R., & Perez, M. A. (2005). Health educators and cultural competence: Implications for the profession. *American Journal of Health Studies, 20*(3), 156–163.

Mehrabian, A. (1972). *Nonverbal communication*. Chicago, IL: Aldine-Atherton.

Mehrabian, A. (1978). How we communicate feelings nonverbally. *Psychology Today*. Recording No. 20170. New York, NY: Ziff Davis.

Murty, M. (1998). Healthy living for immigrant women: A health education community outreach program. *Canadian Medical Association Journal, 159*(4), 385–387.

National Cancer Institute. (2008). *Making health communication programs work*. Retrieved from http://www.cancer.gov/cancertopics/cancerlibrary/pinkbook

National Center for Cultural Competence. (2000). *A planner's guide: Infusing principles, content and themes related to cultural and linguistic competence into meetings and conferences*. Retrieved from http://nccc.georgetown.edu/documents/Planners_Guide.pdf

National Center for Cultural Competence. (2009). *Definition of linguistic competence*. Retrieved from http://nccc.georgetown.edu/documents/Definition of Linguistic Competence.pdf

National Commission for Health Education Credentialing. (2007). *Responsibilities and competencies*. Retrieved from http://www.nchec.org/aboutnchec/rc.htm

Nicholson, P. J. (1999). Communicating health risks. *Occupational Medicine, 49*(4), 253–258. Retrieved from http://occmed.oxfordjournals.org/cgi/reprint/49/4/253.pdf

Office of Minority Health. (2001). *Standards for cultural and linguistic competence in health education*. Retrieved from http://minorityhealth.hhs.gov/templates/browse.aspx?lvl=2&lvlID=15

Office of Minority Health (n.d.a). *National CLAS Standards: Fact sheet*. Retrieved from https://www.thinkculturalhealth.hhs.gov/pdfs/NationalCLASStandardsFactSheet.pdf

Office of Minority Health (n.d.b). *What are the National CLAS Standards?* Retrieved from https://www.thinkculturalhealth.hhs.gov/Content/clas.asp

Peinkofer, J. R. (1994). HIV education for the deaf, a vulnerable minority. *Public Health Reports, 109*(3), 390–396.

Pérez, M. A., Weiller, K., Morrow, J. R., Martin, S., Caldwell, P., & Jackson, A. (1999). Project PEAK: Physical education and activity for kids. *Strategies, 13*(1), 13–16.

Ponterotto, J. G. (1995). A multicultural competency checklist for counseling training programs. *Journal of Multicultural Counseling and Development, 23*(1), 11–20.

Prochaska, J. O., & DiClemente, C. C. (1983). Stages and processes of self-change in smoking: Toward an integrative model of change. *Journal of Consulting and Clinical Psychology, 5*, 390–395.

Prochaska, J. O., DiClemente, C. C., & Norcross, J. C. (1992). In search of how people change. *American Psychologist, 47*, 1102–1114.

Ringe, H. A. (2008). *Participatory action research: Cultural perspectives.* Master's thesis, Free University, Amsterdam, Holland.

Roman, K., Maas, J., & Nisenholtz, M. (2003). *How to advertise* (3rd ed.). New York, NY: St. Martin's Press.

Rose, P. R. (2011). *Cultural competency for health administration and public health.* Sudbury, MA: Jones and Bartlett.

Rowe, J., & Paterson, J. (2010). Culturally competent communication with refugees. *Home Health Care Management and Practice, 22*(5), 334–338.

Siegel, M., & Lotenberg, L. (2007). *Marketing public health: Strategies to promote social change.* Sudbury, MA: Jones & Bartlett.

Sue, D. W., & Sue, D. (1990). *Counseling the culturally different. Theory and practice.* (2nd ed.). New York, NY: Wiley.

Sussman, N. M., & Rosenfeld, H. M. (1982). Influence of culture, language, and sex on conversational distance. *Journal of Personality and Social Psychology, 42*(1), 66–74.

US Census. (2011). *Selected social characteristics in the United States: 2011 American Community Survey 1-year estimates.* Retrieved from http://factfinder2.census.gov/faces/tableservices/jsf/pages/productview.xhtml?pid=ACS_11_1YR_DP02&prodType=table

Velde, B., Wittman, P., & Bamberg, R. (2003). Cultural competence of faculty and students in a school of allied health. *Journal of Allied Health, 32*(3), 189–195.

Wang, S. (2005). Developing an innovative cross-cultural strategy to promote HIV/AIDS prevention in different ethnic cultural groups of China. *AIDS Care, 17*(7), 874–891.

Young, K. (2011, March). *Health disparities, the role of cultural competencies and community based participatory research in health education research.* Paper presented at the American Alliance for Health, Physical Education, Recreation, and Dance National Convention. San Diego, CA.

CHAPTER 9

FOUNDATIONS FOR HEALTH LITERACY AND CULTURALLY APPROPRIATE HEALTH EDUCATION PROGRAMS

Miguel A. Pérez

LEARNING OBJECTIVES

After completing this chapter, you will be able to

- Define literacy.
- Define and discuss health literacy.
- Explain the impact of health literacy in the health status of individuals.
- Discuss health literacy in relationship to the Healthy People 2020 goals.
- Discuss the importance of health literacy to health educators.
- Discuss the relationship between health literacy and cultural competence.

Literacy has been defined as the ability to comprehend written and oral messages and includes the ability to apply received information to mundane activities such as reading maps, understanding warranty information, and balancing a checkbook (Irving, 1991). It is presumed that literacy represents a fundamental skill necessary to fully enjoy life and function in today's information society (United Nations Educational Scientific and Cultural Organization, 2003, 2005).

The National Adult Literacy Survey of 1993 (NALS) is a seminal national initiative designed to measure Americans' literacy at three distinct levels: prose literacy, document literacy, and quantitative literacy. Each of these domains is designed to ascertain an individual's ability to decode written and oral messages. Data from the NALS indicate that approximately 21 percent of Americans had a relatively low literacy level (level 1 on a scale from 1 to 5) and an additional 27 percent had a level 2 literacy level. "While there are no exact grade equivalents, Level 1 literacy is generally defined as less than fifth-grade reading and comprehension skills, and Level 2 is generally defined as fifth through seventh grades reading and comprehension skills" (Federal Highway Administration, 2012, para. 3). It

---

I express my appreciation to Sinsakchon "Tony" Aunprom-me and Carmen Chapman for their review, comments, and editing on earlier drafts of this chapter.

literacy
The ability to comprehend written and oral messages and to apply received information to mundane activities such as reading maps, understanding warranty information, and balancing a checkbook

should be noted that in the NALS sample, all adults with a level 1 literacy level experienced some dysfunction in their ability to read, write, and perform everyday functions such as completing an employment application, reading a food label, or reading a story to a child. "While most of these adults are not considered 'illiterate,' they do not have the full range of economic, social, and personal options that are open to Americans with higher levels of literacy skills" (Federal Highway Administration, 2012, para. 3).

A follow-up study, the 2003 National Assessment of Adult Literacy (NAAL), found that 14 percent of American adults were below basic levels in the prose domain (National Assessment of Adult Literacy, 2009). The study also found that 66 percent of adults age 60 and over have either inadequate or marginal literacy skills, a finding similar to what was noted in the 1993 NALS, which impairs their ability to fully function in the information age (Kutner, Greenberg, Jin, Paulsen, & White, 2006). Table 9.1 presents demographic characteristics of the NAAL sample, as well as the percentages scoring below the basic prose level.

Table 9.1 NAAL Sample Demographics

Characteristic	Percent in Below Basic Prose Population	Percent in Total NAAL Population
Did not graduate from high school	55	15
No English spoken before starting school	44	13
Hispanic adults	39	12
Black adults	20	12
Age sixty-five and over	26	15
Multiple disabilities	21	9

Source: National Assessment of Adult Literacy (2009).

Health Literacy

health literacy
The degree to which individuals have the capacity to obtain, process, and understand basic health information and services needed to make appropriate health decisions

Health literacy is the result of a symbiotic relationship of the health care system, educational systems, and social and cultural factors that take place at home, at work, and in the community. It allows individuals to read, understand, and apply information designed to improve their quality of life, including the weighing of risks and benefits associated with personal behaviors.

The definition of health literacy continues to evolve (Nutbeam, 2008). It can be defined as "the degree to which individuals have the capacity to obtain, process, and understand basic health information needed to make appropriate health decisions" (National Network of Libraries of Medicine, n.d., para. 2). This is the definition used in Healthy People 2020. Similarly, in 2012, the Joint Committee on Health Education and Promotion Terminology (2012, p. 13) defined *health literacy* as "the degree to which individuals have the capacity to obtain, process, and understand basic health information and services needed to make appropriate health decisions."

The 2003 NAAL (2009) identified four levels of health literacy: below basic, basic, intermediate, and proficient. Box 9.1 provides a definition for each of these levels as well as an example of the limitations that may be experienced by a person in each of them.

BOX 9.1 HEALTH LITERACY LEVELS

Below Basic Level

Adults at the below basic level have the most elementary literacy skills. These skills range from being nonliterate in English to being able to locate easily identifiable information in short, commonplace prose text. An adult at this level might be able to locate and circle the date of a medical appointment on a hospital appointment slip.

Basic

Adults at the basic level have the skills necessary to perform simple, everyday activities such as reading and understanding information in short, commonplace texts. An adult at this level might be able to state two reasons a person with no symptoms of a disease should be tested for the disease, based on information in a clearly written pamphlet.

Intermediate Level

Adults at the intermediate level have the literacy skills necessary to perform moderately challenging activities, such as summarizing written text, determining cause and effect, and making simple inferences. An adult with this level of skill might be able to determine a healthy weight range for a person of a specified height on the basis of a graph that relates height and weight to body mass.

Proficient Level

Adults at the proficient literacy level have the skills to perform complex activities, such as integrating, synthesizing, and analyzing multiple pieces of information. An adult might find the information required to define a medical term by searching through a document.

Source: Kutner et al. (2007).

Health Literacy Impact

The 2003 NAAL found that 90 percent of Americans lack the health literacy levels necessary to understand primary prevention strategies and may also lack the ability to follow medical directives designed to improve their health status. Individuals with low health literacy levels are unable to understand information necessary for properly using safety equipment, reading food labels, or making informed decisions when it comes to vote on a proposal for a local smoking ban. In addition, low health literacy levels also prevent individuals from becoming engaged in advocacy efforts designed to improve their health status. This alarming fact led former US Surgeon General Richard Carmona to conclude, "We must close the gap between what health professionals know and what the rest of America understands" (Carmona, n.d., para. 6).

In its 2004 report, *Health Literacy: A Prescription to End Confusion*, the Institute of Medicine (IOM) identified self-management/health literacy as a national priority. The IOM concluded that unless changes were implemented at all levels, efforts to transform the health care system and manage increasing health care costs would fail. Despite the relevance of health literacy to the nation's health care system, questions have been raised about efforts to improve it (Parker & Kindig, 2006).

The 2003 NAAL identified specific characteristics of adults who possessed below basic health literacy levels. Its data suggest that men have lower health literacy than women, Hispanics have the lowest health literacy of all ethnic groups in the United States, adults living below the poverty level had lower health literacy levels, and adults age 65 and older had the lowest health literacy levels. It also found differences in health literacy levels by ethnic group. Whites tend to have higher levels of health literacy than nonwhites in the United States (National Center for Education Statistics, 2009). The study also found that health literacy declined dramatically with age, even after researchers made adjustments for years of school completed and cognitive impairment (Paasche-Orlow, Parker, Gazmararian, Nielsen-Bohlman, & Rudd, 2005). As Carmona had suggested, below basic health literacy levels contribute to health disparities, lack of access to preventive services, and poor health outcomes due to lack of compliance with health care directives.

Health Literacy and Healthy People 2020

The mounting evidence establishing the integral relationship between high health literacy levels and good health status provides the foundation for the incorporation of health communication and health information technology as one of the goals of Healthy People 2020 (box 9.2).

BOX 9.2 HEALTHY PEOPLE 2020 HEALTH LITERACY GOALS

HC/HIT-1 (Developmental) Improve the health literacy of the population

HC/HIT-1.1 Increase the proportion of persons who report their health care provider always gave them easy-to-understand instructions about what to do to take care of their illness or health condition

HC/HIT-1.2 Increase the proportion of persons who report their health care provider always asked them to describe how they will follow the instructions

HC/HIT-1.3 Increase the proportion of persons who report their health care providers' office always offered help in filling out a form

Source: National Institutes of Health (2012).

While Healthy People 2020 focuses its attention on increasing the proportion of persons who report their health care provider always gave them easy-to-understand instructions about what to do to take care of their illness or health condition (e.g., HC/HIT-1.1), these goals have an impact on health literacy and present an opportunity for health educators to assist Americans to improve their health status.

Health educators' attention is specifically called to goal HC/HIT-1, which calls for the improvement of health literacy levels among the general population. This challenge, coupled with the areas II and VII of the Responsibilities and Competencies for Health Education Specialists (National Commission for Health Education Credentialing, 2008), provides a clear mandate for health educators to take specific steps.

Similarly, HC/HIT-13 calls for increasing social marketing in health promotion and disease prevention programs. The ease of diffusion of social messages underscores the need for the development of clear, up-to-date, and easily understood messages that provide accurate information and do not perpetuate misunderstanding that can be too easily distributed to mass audiences. (Chapter 8 contains a more detailed discussion on communication.)

Health Literacy and Health Status

In the United States, five chronic diseases—heart disease, cancer, stroke, chronic obstructive pulmonary disease (e.g., asthma, bronchitis, emphysema), and diabetes—cause more than two-thirds of all deaths each year, making primary prevention a key domain for health educators, who often work with individuals to prevent the onset of disease and infirmity. Given the leading morbidity and mortality indicators in the United States, it should be surprising that prevention programs are designed to strengthen protective factors and reverse or reduce risk factors.

Acknowledging the symbiotic relationship of prevention and health literacy, the National Prevention, Health Promotion, and Public Health Council developed the National Prevention Strategy in 2011. This initiative focuses on increasing life expectancy and quality of life and emphasizes four areas:

- Building healthy and safe environments
- Expanding quality preventive services
- Empowering people to make choices
- Eliminating health disparities, using prevention strategies and health education strategies that use appropriate health literacy levels

One tenet of the National Prevention Strategy is that prevention is not an added component to wellness but rather a foundation that should be woven into every aspect of daily life. Efforts are currently under way to ensure that the plan's seven priority areas are implemented in a way that addresses low health literacy levels. According to the plan,

> Information needs to be available to people in ways that make it easy for them to make informed decisions about their health. Providing people with accurate information that is culturally and linguistically appropriate and matches their health literacy skills helps them search for and use health information and adopt healthy behaviors. For example, providing people with information about the risks and benefits of preventive health services can motivate them to seek preventive care. Providing people with information (e.g., nutrition information on menus and food product labels) can help increase demand for healthy options and may influence supply, because companies are more likely to provide healthy options when they perceive consumer demand for such products. (National Prevention Council, 2011, p. 22)

Primary prevention efforts are predicated on the public's ability to receive, process, and apply interventions designed to prevent the onset of medical conditions. Adequate levels of health literacy assist individuals in understanding directions, adhering to medication schedules, and, most important, engaging in health-protective behaviors. Individuals with low health literacy may not be able to engage in self-assessment activities (e.g., glucometer, peak flow meter, blood pressure monitoring), engage in self-treatment (e.g., insulin, steroids, diuretics), or engage in correct health care utilization (e.g., insurance coverage, knowing when to seek a specialist).

The research literature shows that individuals with low health literacy levels not only experience preventable medical problems, but may also contribute to the congestion of emergency rooms and unwillingly contribute to increasing health care costs (Baker, 2006; Berkman, Pignone, DeWalt, & Sheridan, 2004; Weiss & Palmer, 2004). The estimated additional health care expenditures due to low health literacy skills were over $70 billion in 1998 dollars.

Studies have found that people at the lower end of the health literacy spectrum experience a large number of health conditions, many of them preventable (Berkman, Pignone, DeWalt, & Sheridan, 2004; Gazmararian, Williams, Peel, & Baker, 2003; Weiss, Hart, McGee, & D'Estelle, 1992) (see box 9.3). Additional issues that can be affected by limited health literacy include misunderstanding and misapplication of health warnings regarding food safety, missed opportunities to avail oneself of preventive screenings including vaccinations, misapplied information about emergency preparedness, and misunderstanding important information such as the quality of water in a given community. The National Prevention Strategy clearly calls for health educators to not only be knowledgeable about health literacy but to apply skills ensuring that their clients obtain accurate, up-to-date, and easy-to-understand information.

BOX 9.3 SELECTED HEALTH ISSUES THAT INDIVIDUALS WITH LOW LITERACY LEVELS ENCOUNTER

- Difficulty taking medications appropriately and interpreting labels and health messages
- Higher rates of hospitalization, emergency care visits, and lower rates of flu immunizations
- Less health knowledge and comprehension of health information
- More likely to report their health as poor
- For seniors, worse health status and quality of life and early mortality

Source: Berkman et al. (2004).

Health Literacy and Cultural Competence

Health literacy must be understood and addressed in the context of race, culture, and language. Cultural background encompasses communication patterns, behavior, language preference, customs and beliefs, and self-care. Culture is a multilayered and dynamic process that includes body language, religious affiliation, approach to problem solving, decision-making processes, and the balance between individual rights and the collective good. It is influenced by a person's education and, in the case of immigrants, affected by their acculturation levels.

cultural competence
A developmental process defined as a set of values, principles, behaviors, attitudes, and policies that enable health professionals to work effectively across racial, ethnic, and linguistically diverse groups

Cultural competence is a concept designed to facilitate communication between health care providers, including health educators, and the populations they serve. It requires that individuals and organizations have a clearly defined, congruent set of values and principles, and demonstrate behaviors, attitudes, policies, structures, and practices that enable them to work effectively cross-culturally. It has been suggested that cultural competence requires three components: the head, hands, and the heart: the head to understand that people think, believe, behave, perceive, and understand; hands to implement the skills and knowledge to work effectively with those who are different; and a heart to comprehend (not necessarily accept) the differences and similarities between and among people (National Resource Center for Family Centered Practice, 2009).

In some instances, culture may be perceived as an adverse partner in health education efforts. Cultural practices such as the use of alternative medicine, different time orientation, and a family rather than individual orientation present challenges that many health educators are ill prepared to address. However, culture cannot be discounted, no matter how assimilated a target group may be. In fact, it could be argued that until the health educator identifies the cultural factors that shape an individual's health status, his or her health education efforts will have limited impact.

Public health professionals in general and health educators in particular have their own culture—one that is defined by their educational level, commitment to help others, and educational level. An honest assessment of the health educator's own cultural values will enable him or her to deliver health education and primary prevention programs more effectively.

Improving Health Literacy

Data from the 2003 NAAL suggest that individuals with limited health literacy experience a number of preventable health issues and may experience adverse effects in chronic conditions (Bryan, 2008; Clement, Ibrahim, Crichton, Wolf, & Rowlands, 2009; Eichler, Weiser, & Brügger, 2009). It is therefore easy to conclude that by improving health literacy levels, improving communities' access to health information, and enabling individuals to use it correctly, we empower disenfranchised populations (Howard, Sentell, & Gazmararian, 2006; Nutbeam, 2000; Nutbeam & Kickbusch, 2000; Office of the Education Council, 2010).

Health educators have a responsibility not only to assess needs, assets, and capacity for health education programs but also to implement those programs among high-risk populations (National Commission for Health Education Credentialing, 2008). Health literacy, however, is often not considered part of health educators' responsibilities, which leads to the erroneous assumption that clients fully understand delivered messages.

The medical profession has taken specific steps to address health literacy among patients. The Newest Vital Sign, the Rapid Estimate of Adult Literacy in Medicine, and the Test of Functional Health Literacy in Adults are some of the tools at the disposal of health care professionals (Baker, Williams, Parker, Gazmararian, & Nurss, 1999; Cotugna, Vickery & Carpenter-Haefele, 2005; Ryan et al., 2008; Shea et al., 2004). More recently, physicians have been encouraged to use the Ask Me 3 approach when dealing with their patients (National Patient Safety Foundation, 2007). It is time for health educators to adopt specific strategies designed to improve health literacy.

The North Carolina Program on Health Literacy (2011) has identified a number of health literacy assessment instruments designed to ascertain patient health literacy levels. Box 9.4 lists and briefly describes these instruments. Health educators are encouraged to become familiar with these tools and employ them in their daily activities.

BOX 9.4 SELECTED HEALTH LITERACY TOOLS

Adult Basic Learning Examination (ABLE)

The ABLE is designed to measure the functional abilities in adults, specifically those whose education does not exceed the eighth-grade level. No time limits have been set for this test, which is divided into levels based on the years of formal education the patient has completed.

Literacy Assessment for Diabetes (LAD)

This diabetes-specific literacy assessment is a word recognition test that has three graded word lists ordered by difficulty for the patient. It measures the patient's ability to pronounce terms related to health care. The terms are on a fourth-grade level or on a sixth- to sixteenth-grade reading level. It can be administered in three minutes or less.

Newest Vital Sign (NVS)

The NVS consists of a nutrition label with six questions to assess literacy. It takes approximately three minutes to administer and is meant to help health care providers make a quick assessment of a patient's literacy, which can help them adapt their communication to the client to achieve better outcomes. It assesses literacy and numeracy and is available in English and Spanish versions.

Nutritional Literacy Scale (NLS)

The NLS, which consists of twenty-four questions, is designed to evaluate patients' understanding of current nutrition labels. The test uses actual nutritional labels that the patients refer to. The first twelve questions are open-ended in nature, and the last twelve require the patient to decide between two response options. The test can be administered without a time limit.

Rapid Assessment of Adult Literacy in Medicine (REALM)

The REALM is a screening tool designed to measure adults' ability to read common medical words or lay terms that correspond to anatomy or illnesses. It is a word recognition test and so does not assess comprehension. However, it is highly correlated with other tests of comprehension. It takes approximately three minutes to administer and score.

Rapid Assessment of Adult Literacy in Medicine–Revised (REALM-R)

This shortened version of the REALM is used to help identify adult patients' literacy levels. It consists of eight items and is used to measure how well individuals can read words they will encounter in a medical setting.

Short Assessment of Health Literacy for Spanish-speaking Adults (SAHLSA)

This is both a word recognition and a comprehension test that employs multiple-choice questions. It was designed to assess the health literacy for adults who speak Spanish.

Single Item Literacy Screener (SILS)

This single-item instrument is designed to identify patients who need help reading health-related information. The question is: "How often do you need to have someone help you when you read instructions, pamphlets, or other written material from your doctor or pharmacy?" Responses range from 1 (never) to 5 (always). The authors identified the cut-off point of 2 to capture all patients potentially in need of assistance.

Slosson Oral Reading Test

The Slosson, which consists of tests from preschool to adult levels, is meant to be a quick estimate to target word recognition levels for children and adults. It takes three to five minutes to complete and assesses the level of oral word recognition, or reading level. It is meant only to measure certain aspects of literacy.

Test of Adult Basic Education (TABE)

This exam, which is divided into three sections (English language, math, and reading), determines the skill of a test taker in each one of the three areas. The results can help in placing test takers into adult education programs. It measures academic skill up to the twelfth grade.

Test of Functional Health Literacy in Adults (TOFHLA)

The full test consists of a reading comprehension section and a numeracy section. The former is composed of fifty questions, the latter of seventeen items. The entire test usually takes up to twenty-two minutes to administer. The reading passages and numeracy question are from common medical scenarios. The s-TOFHLA is a truncated version that uses questions only from the reading comprehension subsection of the full test. There are thirty-six items that are administered in seven minutes. The scoring categorizes respondents into inadequate, marginal, or adequate levels of health literacy.

Wide Range Achievement Test (WRAT)

The WRAT measures literacy in reading recognition, spelling, and arithmetic computation. It takes twenty to thirty minutes to complete. There is a level for children ages 5 to 11 and another level for ages 12 to 64. In health-related research, most investigators have used only the reading recognition subtest, which takes about five minutes to administer.

Source: Cecil G. Sheps Center for Health Services Research (2011).

Written Communication

An important step in improving health literacy is found in Public Law 111–274, the Plain Writing Act of 2010, which requires all levels of the federal government to develop written materials in easy-to-understand language. (Examples of federal efforts to implement this law may be found at http://www.plainlanguage.gov/examples/before_after/index.cfm.)

The NIH's Office of Communication and Public Liaison is taking the lead in this "clear communication" initiative to "cultivate a growing health literacy movement by increasing information sharing of NIH educational products, research, lessons learned, and research in the area of health literacy" (National Institutes of Health, 2012, para. 4).

One of the most frequently employed educational tools that health educators used is written material. Unfortunately, often those materials are developed without much thought about the health literacy of the target populations (Friedman & Hoffman-Goetz, 2006; Hoffmann & McKenna, 2006). Box 9.5 provides a summary of the NIH's tips for using plain language in health education messages.

The literature has identified incorrect readability levels in the development of both written and oral prevention messages as contributors to low health literacy (Kirkpatrick & Mohler, 1999; Ratzan, 2001; Taylor, Skelton, & Czajkowski, 1982). Aguilera, Perez, and Alonso Palacio (2010) found that the majority of education materials for clients with diabetes reviewed as

BOX 9.5 RECOMMENDATIONS FOR PLAIN LANGUAGE MESSAGES

Engage the Reader

- Consider who the audience is (e.g., by gender, educational level). Often there is more than one reader.
- Consider what the reader needs to know. Organize content to meet these needs.
- Write for the appropriate reading level.
- Use common, everyday words whenever possible.

WORD CHOICES

- Use common, everyday words
- Use other personal pronouns such as *you*.
- Use *must* instead of *shall*.
- Avoid using undefined technical terms.
- Use positive rather than negative words.
- Avoid using gender-specific terminology.
- Avoid long strings of nouns.

VERB FORMS

- Use the active voice.
- Use action verbs.
- Use the present tense.

STRUCTURE

- Use parallel construction.
- Be direct.

Display Material Correctly

Appearance is an important aspect of clear communication. A document that is pleasing to the eye will be more likely to attract readers' attention. Appearance can also be an aid to readers by improving their comprehension and retention. Appearance has several aspects:

- *Organization*. Strong, logical organization includes an introduction followed by short sentences and paragraphs. Organize messages to respond to reader interests and concerns.

- *Introduction*. In lengthier documents, use an introduction and a table of contents to show the reader how the document is organized.
- *Short sentences and paragraphs*. Sentence length should average fifteen to twenty words. Sentences that are simple, active, affirmative, and declarative hold the reader's interest. Generally each paragraph should contain only one topic. A series of paragraphs may be used to express complex or highly technical information. The more that writing deviates from a clear and to-the-point structure, the harder it will be for readers to understand.
- *Layout*. Layout refers to how material appears on a page; it encompasses, for example, margins, headings, and white space. Provide white space between sections to break up the text and make it easier for readers to understand. Use headings to guide readers; the question-and-answer format is especially helpful. Try to anticipate readers' questions and pose them as your readers might. Use adequate margins.
- *Tables*. Tables make complex information readily understandable and can help readers see relationships more easily. They may require fewer words than straight text.
- *Typography:* Typography relates to the fonts chosen and typographical elements used for emphasis, such as bullets or italics.

Evaluate Your Document

To ensure that you are communicating clearly, evaluate the document or have another person read it and offer suggestions for clarification. They should look over the document for:

- Correct spelling, grammar, and punctuation
- Inclusion of appropriate devices, such as dating, page numbering, and consistency
- Visual appeal
- Consistency and effectiveness of layout and typographical devices (avoid overuse)
- Line breaks that inadvertently separate part of a name or date in a way that reduces clarity.

Source: NIH (2012).

part of their study did not reach their intended audience because of the high readability levels of those materials.

Many times the oversight in ascertaining readability levels is unintentional; in fact, most health education programs lack a health communication course in their undergraduate or graduate curriculum. Nevertheless, health educators are encouraged to ascertain the readability levels for all education materials they develop and use in their education (Adkins, Elkins, & Singh, 2001; Schillinger et al., 2002; Sondra, 2006). Box 9.6 provides an overview of some commonly used assessment tools.

BOX 9.6 COMMON TOOLS FOR ASSESSING READABILITY LEVELS

Simplified Measure of Gobbledygook (SMOG) Readability Formula

To use the SMOG formula, researchers do not have to evaluate the entire written document; a sample of thirty sentences is sufficient. The sample consists of ten sentences from the beginning of the material, ten from the middle, and another ten from the end. In this sample, any word with more than three syllables is circled. The circled words are tallied, and the nearest number that equals a perfect square root of this figure is found. Finally, the square root is added to a constant that is equal to 3. The number that is the sum is the grade level required to understand the reading material (McLaughlin, 1969).

Readability Assessment Instrument (RAIN)

This instrument measures the readability of health-related materials comprehensively; it looks at components of text unity, graphic placement, font color and size, coherence, vocabulary, cultural appropriateness, and so on. To start the evaluation process, investigators must list all the components to be evaluated. Studies found this method effective and easy to administer (Adkins et al., 2001; Kirkpatrick & Mohler, 1999).

Fry Readability Method

In this method, researchers obtain three samples of one hundred words from a document, omitting headings, and determines the number of syllables in the sample. The average numbers of syllables and sentences are calculated from the three samples and the results used to plot a point on the Fry graph. The *x*-axis represents the number of syllables in the sample average, and the *y*-axis represents the number of sentences in the sample average. The graph has a curve with markers that represent grade levels, permitting researchers to identify the grade level of the plotted point that represents the sample (Taylor et al., 1982).

Flesch-Kincaid Readability Formula (FK)

The FK readability formula (Flesch, 1945) measures vocabulary difficulty. The literature shows that this formula has been used to test the readability of health information materials, although it was not designed to evaluate health materials only. The result of the application of the formula is identification of the grade-school level at which a person can read and understand the text (Cotugna et al., 2005).

Flesch Reading Ease Score (FRE)

The FRE measures the average number of syllables per word and the average number of words per sentence. The score ranges from 0 to 100. It is widely available through a built-in Microsoft Word adequate readability tool. This feature is not turned on by default; therefore, the user must be sure to check the "show readability statistics" function (Friedman & Hoffman-Goetz, 2006).

Gunning Fog Index

This index measures the average number of words per sentence and percentage of words with more than two syllables. It requires less time to administer than the FRE and FK Readability formula. However, it cannot measure the reading difficulty of text in tables (Friedman & Hoffman-Goetz, 2006).

The New Dale-Chall Readability Formula

This formula measures the number of syllables per sentence and the percentage of difficult words. It is developed primarily for health education materials with the highest validity when tested for reader comprehension. It is not available in word processing software (Wang, Capo, & Orillaza, 2009).

Suitability Assessment of Materials

This tool measures the suitability of print, media, and audiovisual tools. It appears to be the only tool that can assess the influence of illustrations on comprehension. Completing the assessment process can exceed thirty minutes (Hoffmann & McKenna, 2006; Wallace, Turner, Ballard, Keenum, & Weiss, 2005).

Sources: Aguilera (2006); Aunprom-me and Aunprom-me (2009).

In addition to using the tools described in box 9.6, health educators are encouraged to use a variety of other simple yet effective tools to improve the readability levels of their educational materials:

- *Large font.* Assists individuals with visual impairments to read. It is much easier to read a 14 point font than it is to read a 10 point font.
- *Use clear headings.* Short subheads in bold break up the text and have a greater visual appeal than a sea of paragraphs without any breaks.
- *Simple words.* It is worth repeating that easy-to-understand terminology (e.g., *cancer* rather than *carcinoma*) improves the understanding of written material.
- *White space with pictures.* The use of culturally appropriate graphics encourages readers to stay with the materials. Be sure to obtain copyright permission before including graphics in your materials; availability on the Web does not mean it is free.
- *Bright contrasting colors.* The use of color increases the visual appeal of written materials, although it also increases reproduction costs.

- *Short sentences.* While professors and bosses may be impressed with complex and long sentences, the literature suggests that short sentences are better for health education messages.
- *How to.* Don't forget to include a how-to section to enable the reader to practice the skills that have been introduced.

Presentations

Group presentations are an easy way to reach large audiences, though poor planning, implementation, and delivery can limit their impact. The following suggestions are designed to improve delivery:

- *Be comfortable.* Good public speaking skills are the result of much practice and do much to allay anxiety. Be sure to practice your presentation several times—in front of a friend or other trusted individual, for example.
- *Face people at all times.* It is too easy to turn your back to the audience when using visual cues such as a slide presentation. If necessary, keep a small stack of cards with salient notes, but never read the slides to the audience.
- *Speak slowly, clearly, and loudly.* A group presentation is not an opportunity to develop your rapid speaking skills. The speaker needs to be aware of the audience's engagement and response to the tempo and loudness of the presentation and adjust them accordingly. A good rule of thumb to use is to think you are speaking to the last person in the farthest part of the room.
- *Reduce background noise.* The audience should be able to focus on the speaker and not be distracted by ambient or extraneous noise whenever possible.

Many health educators employ slide presentations to assist in the delivery of their messages. The following recommendations can improve these presentations:

- *Decide on the goal of the presentation.* Are you trying to inform or influence the audience?
- *Use large fonts.* Using sizes lower than 24 points is rarely advised.
- *Select colors with high contrast.* Noncontrasting colors or pictures may make it difficult to read the materials, especially for those sitting in the back.
- *Use bullet points* as opposed to complete sentences.

- *Present one bullet point at a time.* This can be accomplished by using the simple animation effect.
- *Avoid excessive animations* during the presentation, which tends to be confusing to the audience.

Bridging Health Literacy and Culture

Low health literacy affects all segments of society, and language limitations compound problems associated with it. The following recommendations are designed to ameliorate the impact of culture and language on health literacy levels:

- *Differentiate among culture, race, and ethnicity.* As we have seen throughout this book, the terms *culture, race,* and *ethnicity* are not synonyms. This erroneous classification may lead to erroneous assumptions about people; for instance, we might think a person to be of a given race given his or her skin color, but that person's cultural identity or ethnicity may not correspond to that color. Health education interventions that have no relevance to the target community will not succeed. Along with information gathered from Western-style medicine, we need to include information that is relevant to the community. Whenever possible, provide a contrast between the Western and non-Western approach to health and illness, beliefs, and practices. Be careful not to show reverence for one and disdain for the other.

- *Avoid stereotypes.* Low health literacy affects individuals regardless of their race, culture, or ethnicity. It also affects individuals regardless of their educational level and even their ability to read and write. Health educators will do well to ascertain individuals' literacy levels at the beginning of all their interventions.

- *Be cognizant of language preference.* Generally first-generation immigrants require translation of materials and spoken words into their native language; less obvious is the need to provide materials in different languages to those who are second and subsequent generations in the United States. Language preference, however, is a key factor in delivering culturally appropriate health education programs since it allows people to communicate their needs and wants in an appropriate format. Language preference also refers to selecting and using the terminology employed by the target population rather than the technical language we are used to. Finally, language preference refers to having qualified personnel, regardless of cultural or ethnic background, proficient in the language. Do not assume that all Nisei speak Japanese.

- *Understand what translation and interpretation are.* Simple translation of materials from one language to another without interpretation may result in inadequate educational tools. Cultural interpreters are necessary in the development of written and visual materials to ensure they are relevant to the diverse populations that health educators reach. Using plain language, eliciting cultural beliefs and attitudes, and using the teach-back method are all effective tools to reaching diverse populations. Use a medically trained interpreter or translator as needed.

- *Incorporate CLAS standards.* The standards were re-released in 2013. A list is provided in the appendix .

- *Avoid jargon.* The excessive use of technical terminology has been found to be detrimental to implementing effective health education programs. Using simple language (e.g., *painkiller* rather than *analgesic*) and defining technical terms, using the active voice, breaking down complex information into understandable chunks, and organizing information so the most important points come first are useful tools in working with diverse populations.

- *Ascertain acculturation levels.* Acculturation has been defined as the degree to which an immigrant adopts the culture and behaviors of the host country. Income, education, and language preference are all proxies for acculturation but do not represent the complete picture. A highly educated English-proficient first-generation immigrant may still practice alternative medicine while proficiently navigating the US health care system.

- *Incorporate diversity in teaching methods.* Inadequate incorporation of multiple learning modalities produces less-than-desirable outcomes. Health educators need to incorporate a variety of teaching methods (e.g., lecture, role play, case studies) into their interventions (Clement et al., 2009).

- *Use narratives.* The use of anecdotes relevant to the audience enables the assimilation and practice of the materials being discussed.

Health Literacy and the Electronic Frontier

The number of people turning to electronic resources for health-related information has increased exponentially in the past two decades. There is, however, a significant digital divide between the haves and have-nots, which affects the ability to access reliable and current health information. Health educators intending to use the Web or social media to educate their target populations should consider how well their clients can use these materials, and indeed whether they have access to a computer.

The Research-Based Web Design and Usability Guidelines developed by the US government (available at http://www.usability.gov) provide a road map for health educators who want to use electronic media as an educational tool. The guidelines, which health educators would do well to become familiar with, include information on design process and evaluation, the optimization of the materials for users, accessibility, page layout and navigation, usability testing, and text appearance among others.

While many health educators may take for granted the use of technology in their day-to-day activities, not everyone in the audience will have the same level of competency in using the technology the health educator employs. The two recommendations that follow are provided to improve health literacy through the use of technology:

- Supplying the hardware and software is insufficient. While one of the goals of Healthy People 2020 is to increase the number of people who use technology, including the Web, to obtain health-related information and to communicate with their health care providers, health educators using technology as part of their arsenal need to provide training and technical assistance on computer and Internet use.
- Support staff must be provided for computer maintenance and troubleshooting. Certainly technology opens a world of possibilities, but it can and will break from time to time. Health educators need to provide gatekeepers to use technology with their clients.

Conclusion

In today's information society, a healthy person is also a health-literate person. Health educators have a responsibility to convey easy-to-understand messages that may be acted on, are easily understood, and are easily applied. Ascertaining a person's health literacy level may be difficult because it is not directly related to a person's educational level, race, or language preference. The literature indicates, however, that improving health literacy levels will in fact result in more effective primary prevention messages.

Points to Remember

- The ability to understand and apply health-related information, including verbal, written, and electronic messages, is key to living a healthy life.
- Health educators have a responsibility to understand the health literacy levels of the populations they work with and tailor their interventions to meet those needs.
- A number of tools are designed to improve the health literacy levels of materials that health educators develop.

Case Study

A health educator is assigned to work in a nonprofit agency serving farmworkers. Ms. Rodriguez, a native-born English speaker with a fourth-grade education, expresses her frustration with her fourth pregnancy after indicating she has unsuccessfully tried several birth control methods. She says she has spoken to both doctors and nurses who have "lectured" her about the efficacy of the methods she employs but have never truly answered her questions. The last time she saw a health care provider, she was given a series of pamphlets on birth control to read. She tries to avoid coming to the clinic where her doctor is located because she has trouble navigating the large medical complex. Since she cannot get straight answers from her medical providers, she usually turns to friends for questions related to contraceptives.

1. What cultural elements are present in this situation, and how might they affect health literacy?
2. What are the health issues that must be considered as priorities in this case?
3. What steps can you as a health educator take to assist Ms. Rodriguez?
4. How can you improve Ms. Rodriguez's health literacy levels?

KEY TERMS

Cultural competence

Health literacy

Literacy

References

Adkins, A. D., Elkins, E. N., & Singh, N. N. (2001). Readability of NIMH easy-to-read patient education materials. *Journal of Child and Family Studies, 10*(3), 279–285.

Aguilera, C. (2006). *Readability assessment of written diabetes education materials.* Master's thesis, California State University, Fresno.

Aguilera, C., Perez, M. A., & Alonso Palacio, L. M. (2010). Readability of diabetes education materials: Implications for reaching patients with reading materials. *SaludUninorte, 26*(1), 12–26.

Aunprom-me, S., & Aunprom-me, M. (2009). *Knowledge and experiences in health literacy among fourth year nursing students enrolled in the Bachelor of*

Nursing Science Program in nursing colleges under the direction of Phraboromarajchanok Institute, Ministry of Public Health, Thailand.

Baker, D. W. (2006). The meaning and the measure of health literacy. *Journal of General Internal Medicine, 21,* 878–883.

Baker, D. W., Williams, M. V., Parker, R. M., Gazmararian, J. A., & Nurss, J. R. (1999). Development of a brief test to measure functional health literacy. *Patient Education and Counseling, 38,* 33–42.

Berkman, N., Pignone, M. P., DeWalt, D., & Sheridan, S. (2004). *Health literacy: Impact on health outcomes.* Rockville, MD: Agency for Healthcare Research and Quality.

Bryan, C. (2008). Provider and policy response to reverse the consequences of low health literacy. *Journal of Healthcare Management, 53*(4), 230–241.

Carmona, R. (n.d.) *Health literacy: Key to improving Americans' health.* Retrieved from http://www.medicinemagazine.us/medicine/articles/march2004/health_literacy.asp

Cecil G. Sheps Center for Health Services Research. (2011). *Literacy assessment instruments.* Retrieved from http://nchealthliteracy.org/instruments.html

Clement, S., Ibrahim, S., Crichton, N., Wolf, M., & Rowlands, G. (2009). Complex interventions to improve the health of people with limited literacy: A systematic review. *Patient Education and Counseling, 75,* 340–351.

Cotugna, N., Vickery, C. E., & Carpenter-Haefele, K. (2005). Evaluation of literacy level of patient education pages in health-related journals. *Journal of Community Health, 30*(3), 213–219.

Eichler, K., Wieser, S., & Brügger, U. (2009). The costs of limited health literacy: A systematic review. *International Journal of Public Health, 54,* 313–324.

Federal Highway Administration. (2012). *How to engage low-literacy and limited-English-proficiency populations in transportation decisionmaking.* Retrieved from http://www.fhwa.dot.gov/planning/publications/low_limited/lowlim04.cfm

Flesch, R. F. (1945). A new readability yardstick. *Journal of Applied Psychology, 32* (3), 221–231.

Friedman, D. B., & Hoffman-Goetz, L. (2006). A systematic review of readability and comprehension instruments used for print and web-based cancer information. *Health Education and Behavior, 33,* 352–373.

Gazmararian, J. A., Williams, M., Peel, J., & Baker, D. (2003). Health literacy and knowledge of chronic disease. *Patient Education and Counseling, 51,* 267–275.

Hoffmann, T., & McKenna, K. (2006). Analysis of stroke patients' and carers' reading ability and the content and design of written materials: Recommendations for improving written stroke information. *Patient Education and Counseling, 60,* 286–293.

Howard, D. H., Sentell, T., & Gazmararian, J. A. (2006). Impact of health literacy on socioeconomic and racial differences in health in an elderly population. *Journal of General Internal Medicine, 21,* 857–861.

Institute of Medicine. (2004). *Health literacy: A prescription to end confusion.* Washington, DC: National Academy of Sciences.

Irving, P. M. (1991). *National Literacy Act of 1991: Major Provisions of P.L. 102–73.* Washington, DC: Congressional Research Service. Library of Congress.

Joint Committee on Health Education and Promotion Terminology. (2012). *Report of the 2011 Joint Committee on Health Education and Promotion Terminology. American Journal of Health Education, 43*(2), 1–19.

Kirkpatrick, M. A., & Mohler, C. P. (1999). Using the readability assessment instrument to evaluate patient medication leaflets. *Drug Information Journal, 33,* 557–563.

Kutner, M., Greenberg, E., Jin, Y., Boyle, B., Hsu, Y.-C., & Dunleavy, E. (2007). *Literacy in everyday life: Results from the 2003 National Assessment of Adult Literacy.* Retrieved from http://nces.ed.gov/pubs2007/2007480.pdf

Kutner, M., Greenberg, E., Jin, Y., Paulsen, C., & White, S. (2006). *The health literacy of America's adults: Results from the 2003 national assessment of adult literacy.* Washington, DC: National Center for Health Statistics.

McLaughlin, G. H. (1969). SMOG grading: A new readability formula. *Journal of Reading, 12,* 639–646.

National Assessment of Adult Literacy. (2009). *Demographics: Overall.* Retrieved from http://nces.ed.gov/naal/kf_demographics.asp

National Center for Education Statistics. (2009). *Basic reading skills and the literacy of America's least literate adults: Results from the 2003 National Assessment of Adult Literacy*(NAAL). Retrieved from http://nces.ed.gov/pubs2009/2009481.pdf

National Center for Education Statistics. (n.d.). *National Assessment of Adult Literacy.* Retrieved from http://nces.ed.gov/naal

National Commission for Health Education Credentialing. (2008). *Responsibilities and competencies for health education specialists.* Retrieved from http://www.nchec.org/credentialing/responsibilities/

National Institutes of Health. (2012). *Plain language.* http://www.nih.gov/clearcommunication/plainlanguage.htm

National Network of Libraries of Medicine. (n.d.). *Health literacy.* Retrieved from http://nnlm.gov/outreach/consumer/hlthlit.html

National Patient Safety Foundation. (2011). *Ask Me 3.* Retrieved from http://www.npsf.org/for-healthcare-professionals/programs/ask-me-3/

National Prevention Council. (2011). *National Prevention Strategy: America's plan for better health and wellness.* Retrieved from http://www.healthcare.gov/prevention/nphpphc/strategy/report.pdf

National Resource Center for Family Centered Practice. (2009). *Supervising cultural competence family support practice.* Retrieved from http://www.uiowa.edu/~nrcfcp/training/documents/PPTSupervisingCulturallyCompetentPractice.pdf

North Carolina Program on Health Literacy. (2011). North Carolina Program on Health Literacy. Retrieved from http://www.nchealthliteracy.org/

Nutbeam, D. (2000). Health literacy as a public health goal: A challenge for contemporary health education and communication strategies into the 21st century. *Health Promotion International, 15*(3), 259–267.

Nutbeam, D. (2008). The evolving concept of health literacy. *Social Science and Medicine, 67,* 2072–2078.

Nutbeam, D., & Kickbusch, I. (2000). Advancing health literacy: A global challenge for the 21st century. *Health Promotion International, 15*(3), 183–184.

Office of the Education Council. (2010). *Guidelines of the Health Literacy Development for Children, Youths, and Families Using the Empowered Education Networks.*

Paasche-Orlow, M. K., Parker, R. M., Gazmararian, J. A. Nielsen-Bohlman, L. T., & Rudd, R. (2005). The prevalence of limited health literacy. *Journal of General Internal Medicine, 20,* 175–184.

Parker, R., & Kindig D. (2006). Beyond the Institute of Medicine Health Literacy Report: Are the recommendations being taken seriously? *Journal of General Internal Medicine, 21*(8), 891–92.

Plain Language.gov. (n.d.). *Before-and-after comparisons.* Retrieved from http://www.plainlanguage.gov/examples/before_after/index.cfm

Ratzan, S. C. (2001). Health literacy: Communication for the public good. *Health Promotion International, 16*(2), 207–214.

Ryan, J. G., Leguen, F., Weiss, B. D., Albury, S., Jennings, T., Velez, F., & Salibi. N. (2008). Will patients agree to have their literacy skills assessed in clinical practice? *Health Education and Research, 23,* 603–611.

Schillinger, D., Grumbach, K., Piette, J., Wang, F., Osmond, D., Daher, C., . . . Bindman, A. B. (2002). Association of health literacy with diabetes outcomes. *Journal of the American Medical Association, 288,* 475–482.

Shea, J. A., Beers, B. B., McDonald, V. J., Quistber, A., Ravenell, K. L., & Asch, D. A. (2004). Assessing health literacy in African American and Caucasian adults: Disparities in rapid estimate of adult literacy in Medicine (REALM) scores. *Family Medicine, 36,* 575–581.

Sondra, C. (2006). Following the physician's recommendations faithfully and accurately: Functional health literacy, compliance, and the knowledge based economy. *Journal for Critical Education Policy Studies.* Retrieved from http://www.jceps.com/PDFs/04-2-10.pdf

Taylor, A. G., Skelton, J. A., & Czajkowski, R. W. (1982). Do patients understand patient education brochures? *Nursing and Health Care, 3,* 305–310.

United Nations Educational Scientific and Cultural Organization (2003). *Literacy as freedom: A UNESCO roundtable* [Electronic version]. Paris: Literacy and Non-Formal Education Section, Division of Basic Education, UNESCO. Retrieved from http://unesdoc.unesco.org/images/0013/001318/131823e.pdf

United Nations Educational Scientific and Cultural Organization. (2005, June). *Aspects of literacy assessment: Topics and issues from the UNESCO Expert Meeting*, Paris.

Wallace, L. S., Turner, L. W., Ballard, J. E., Keenum, A. J., & Weiss B. D. (2005). Evaluation of web-based osteoporosis educational materials. *Journal of Women's Health, 14*, 936–945.

Wang, S., Capo, J. T., & Orillaza, N. (2009). Readability and comprehensibility of patient education material in hand-related Web sites. *Journal of Hand Surgery, 34*(7), 1308–1315.

Weiss, B. D., Hart, G., McGee, D. L., & D'Estelle, S. (1992). Health status of illiterate adults: Relation between literacy and health status among persons with low literacy skills. *Journal of the American Board of Family Practice, 5*, 257–264.

Weiss, B. D., & Palmer, R. (2004). Relationship between health care costs and very low health literacy skills in a medically needy and indigent Medicaid population. *Journal of the American Board of Family Medicine, 17*, 44–47.

CHAPTER 10

THE AGING US POPULATION

An Increasing Diverse Population

William H. Dailey Jr.
Bertha Felix-Mata

Despite increasing research on the graying of America, most people continue to view aging as a mysterious and fearsome process, surrounded in myths and stereotypes extending from health to economics; there is an almost universal fear of getting old. Regardless of how we define aging or when we believe it starts, there is one truth: we cannot escape the aging process. If we live long enough, we are all bound to experience what Walt Whitman poetically romanticized as one of the four seasons in our lives.

We tend to measure age along a chronological continuum, viewing individuals as aging in distinct cohorts that share similar birth years; go through infancy, childhood, adolescence, adulthood, and midlife; and then reach their retirement years, signifying old age. For example, the baby boomers' age cohort was born between 1946 and 1964 (Alwin, McCammon, & Hofer, 2006).

This chapter addresses the older adult population as members of a generation who share a unique culture and life experiences that shape their individual identities as older adults. It also addresses the building of an *interprofessional collaboration,* among practitioners in health education, health care roles, and gerontologist. In addition, Kemp states that the foundation for public health is rooted in the pioneer work of C.E.A. Winslow (1920), who stated that public health

LEARNING OBJECTIVES

After completing this chapter, you will be able to

- Describe the characteristics of the aging population.
- Understand why health promotion efforts and priorities for aging populations should be developed through interactive interprofessional collaboration among health education practitioners, gerontologists, and health care professionals.
- Understand the importance of culturally competent programs for aging minority older adults.
- Understand the importance of providing primary prevention programs for older adult populations.
- Identify the scope of health promotion practices affecting older adults who wish to maintain their individual quality of life.

interprofessional collaboration An innovative strategy where two or more professionals learn about, from, and with each other to enable effective collaboration and improve health outcomes, as well as better response to the health needs of those they service as practitioners

> is the science and art of preventing disease, prolonging life, and promoting physical health and efficiency through organized community efforts for the sanitation of the environment, the control of community infections, the education of individuals in principles of personal hygiene, the organization of medical and nursing for the early diagnosis and preventive treatment of disease, and the development of the social machinery which will ensure to every individual in the community a standard of living adequate for the maintenance of health.

Professionals in the areas of health and aging provide a wide range of programs, services, and support systems for assisting older adults. The overall aging process can create significant challenges and opportunities for gerontologists, health educators, and public health practitioners (Atchley & Barusch, 2004; Hillier & Barrow, 2010). Health educators play an important role in the lives of the older individuals they come in contact with (Keller & Fleury, 2000).

According to Kemp (2012), "Public health has been the driving force in the United States in creating an infrastructure and programs for protecting the population's well-being" (p. 3). Kemp notes as well that the discipline of public health and health care roles differs among health care practices, programs, services, and resources for the general population. Often practitioners represent their distinct field of practice. For example, public health educators may focus on the environment, community health, or health care administration, whereas gerontologists may focus on chronic disease, health prevention options, long-term care necessity, and end-of-life aspects of aging. Thus, building an interprofessional collaboration effort among health educators in partnerships with practitioners in the field of aging to address the challenges of living longer, being healthier, and remaining independent is imperative. Practitioners have many opportunities to incorporate new ideas, programs, and services from older adults' life experiences, perceptions, and overall ideals about aging overall to promote the concepts of managing health and safety, promoting improved health, preventing the consequences and suffering associated with chronic disease as we age, and developing coping strategies toward successful aging.

Many older adults face major losses: loss of independence, economic status, social position, and loss of one's spouse, family, and friends. Other challenges include health difficulties, limited transportation, affordable housing options, affordable health care resources, and personal care resources to allow older adults to age in place (Albert & Freedman, 2012; Hillier & Barrow, 2010).

This chapter presents an overview of the older adult population demographics, a brief summary of the health status of its members, and a focus on older adults' interactions with health educators, gerontologists, and the health care professions in general serving older adults.

Demographic Characteristics of Older Americans

According to the Profile of Older Americans (Administration for Community Living, 2012), some 41.4 million Americans, or approximately 18 percent of the population, are over the age of 65. Adults age 65 and over are expected to reach 74.4 million by 2040 and 92 million by 2060. Currently the older adult population represents one in eight Americans, that is, 13.3 percent of the population; in 2030, older adults will represent one in five adults over the age of 65, representing 20 percent of the total population.

In 2012, approximately 21 percent of older adults represented racial and ethnic minority populations, totaling 8.5 million, and are projected to reach 20.2 million in 2030, representing 28 percent of older adults. A significant demographic projection shows a tenfold increase among those 65 years of age and older since the 1900s Older adults represented 3.1 million compared to the projections for 2060 representing 92 million older adults.

The population pyramids in figure 10.1 provides health educators, gerontologists, health care professionals, and community stakeholders a picture of an increasing older adult population from 2010 to projections for 2030 and 2050.

Future population pyramids will include centenarians, who represents a new age cohort of older adults experiencing increased life expectancy. According to Hillier and Barrow (2010), the population pyramids show that "the proportional changes in the 85+ group as well as all age groups age 65+ represent dramatic growth in numbers and population" (p. 18).

In 2010 there were 49,121 centenarians age 100 to 104, 3,893 age 105 to 109, and 330 age 110 and over living in the United States (US Census Bureau, 2010). In fact, it has been suggested that the impact of the baby boomer generation will be equal to that of immigration during the first part of the twentieth century. The majority of health educators seem ill equipped for dealing with these demographic changes affecting the US population (Albert & Freedman, 2012; Wallace, 2005).

Current and future demographic changes among the population of older adults require an examination of the racial and ethnic composition of that population group. In 2000, a majority of the individuals aged 65 years and over (84 percent) were non-Hispanic whites. As we view the fastest-growing segment of older adults reaching 85 and older, we see that race and

Population Pyramid for 2000

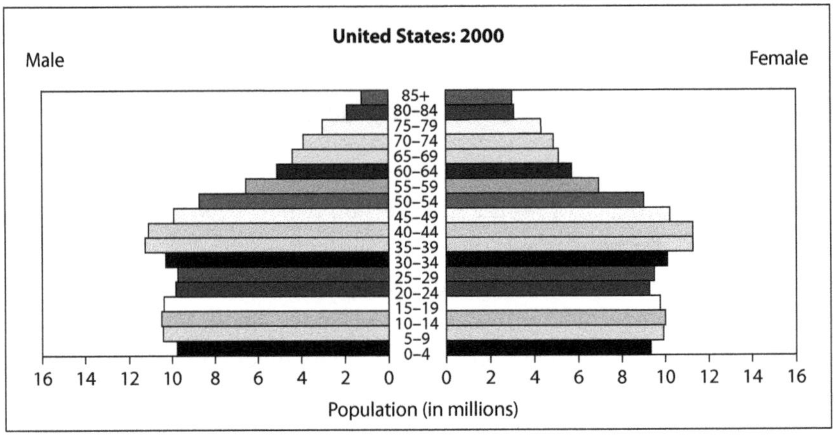

Projected Population Pyramid for 2025

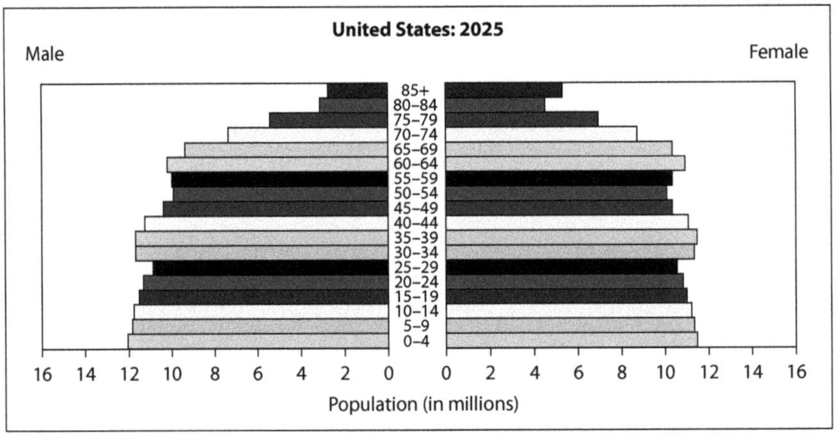

Projected Population Pyramid for 2050

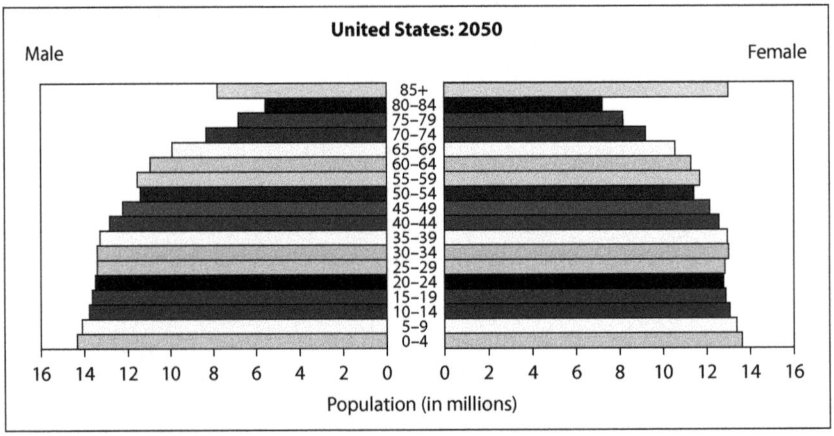

Figure 10.1 Gender and Age of the US Population, 2010 and Projected for 2030 and 2050

Source: U. S. Census Bureau International Database.

ethnic diversity add challenges for meeting the needs facing older adults. Table 10.1 shows significant increases among race and ethnic minorities' reaching this aging milestone in their lives as older adults.

Table 10.1 Projected Distribution of the Population Aged 85 and Older, by Race and Hispanic Origin, 2010, 2030, and 2050 (in thousands)

	2010	2030	2050
85 years and over	5,751 (100.0)	8,745 (100.0)	19,041 (100.0)
White alone	5,189 (90.2)	7,542 (86.2)	15,491 (81.4)
Black alone	397 (6.9)	701 (8.0)	1,982 (10.4)
American Indian and Alaska Native alone	20 (0.4)	62 (0.7)	180 (0.9)
Asian alone	113 (2.0)	356 (4.1)	1,145 (6.0)
Native Hawaiian and Other Pacific Islander alone	3 (0.1)	11 (0.1)	35 (0.2)
Two or more races	29 (0.5)	74 (0.8)	208 (1.1)

Source: U.S. Census Bureau, 2008.

Note: Parenthetical entries are percentages. Data are middle-series projections of the population. All data refer to the resident US population. Hispanics may be of any race.

As might be expected, the older adult population is not evenly distributed over the fifty states. In 2011, eleven states reported comparatively high proportions of older adults in their populations: California, Florida, New York, Texas, Pennsylvania, Ohio, Illinois, Michigan, North Carolina, New Jersey, and Georgia (Administration on Aging, 2012, p. 6).

One of the reasons for the large number of individuals in the age 65 and older category is the increase in life expectancy for US residents. For instance, individuals born in 2000 can expect to live an average of twenty-nine years longer than someone born in 1900. Better access to health care, advances in medical science, and less dangerous occupations account for the increases in life expectancy. One thing that has not changed much since the turn of the century, however, is the difference by gender. In general, women tend to live longer than men (51 years on average in 1900 and 85 years in 2011 for females and 48 years in 1900 and 82 years in 2011 for males).

Minority ethnic groups constitute the fastest-growing segment within the US aging population. Yet health and health care disparities continue to disproportionately affect these minority communities across the US health care system. Older adults who are members of ethnic minority groups face higher morbidity and mortality rates for such diseases as diabetes, cancer, and heart ailments. The impact of race and ethnic minorities among older adults is projected to increase significantly during the next four decades. For example, in 2010, non-Hispanic whites accounted for 80 percent of the

US elderly population, while 9 percent were African Americans, 3 percent Asians, and 7 percent Hispanic (any race). By 2050, the proportion of non-Hispanic whites will decrease to 58 percent, while other ethnic groups will continue to increase; projections are that the relative percentages then will be 20 percent Hispanic, 12 percent African Americans, and 9 percent Asians. In addition, the number of the oldest old will increase significantly among all racial groups. Vincent and Velkoff (2010) concluded, "Although each race and ethnic group is projected to increase in the proportion age 65 and over between 2010 and 2050, the percent 65 and over varies by race and Hispanic origin. Some groups will see increases of nearly 13 percentage points, while others will see increases less of than 3 percentage points" (p. 6).

Figure 10.2 shows the percentage distribution of adults age 65 and up by race and Hispanic origin in 2010 and projected for 2050.

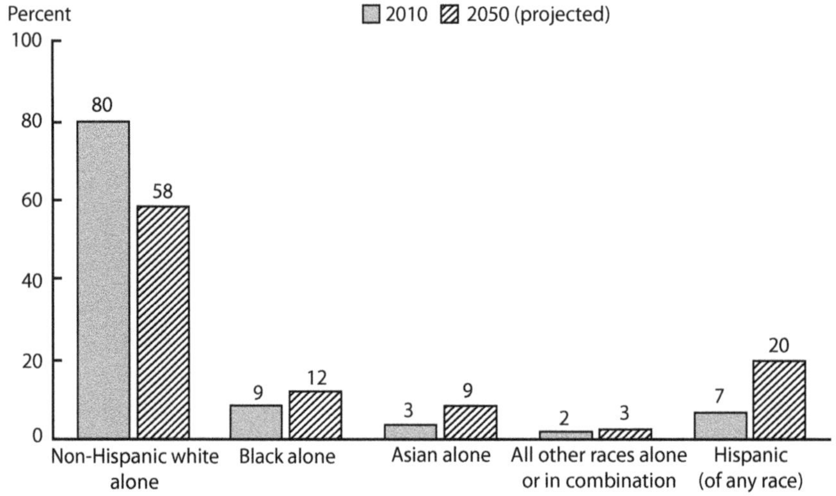

Figure 10.2 Population Age 65 and Over, by Race and Hispanic Origin, 2010 and 2050 (Projected)

Source: U.S. Census Bureau, 2011. 2010 Census Summary File 1; U.S. Census Bureau, Table 4: Projections of the population by sex, race, and Hispanic origin for the United States: 2010–2050. Interagency Forum on Age-Related Statistics (2012).

Note: These projections are based on Census 2000 and are not consistent with the 2010 Census results. Projections based on the 2010 Census will be released in late 2012. The term "non-Hispanic White alone" is used to refer to people who reported being white and no other race and who are not Hispanic. The term "Black alone" is used to refer to people who reported being black or African American and no other race, and the term "Asian alone" is used to refer to people who reported only Asian as their race. The use of single-race populations in this figure does not imply that this is the preferred method of presenting or analyzing data. The U.S. Census Bureau uses a variety of approaches. The race group "All other races alone or in combination" includes American Indian and Alaska Native alone; Native Hawaiian and Other Pacific Islander alone; and all people who reported two or more races. Reference population: These data refer to the resident population.

Issues Facing Older Adults

The academic literature and research on aging that focuses on challenges, barriers, and overall health status suggest that the major issues facing older people in the United States today are loss of independence, loss of economic or social position, changes in marital status including loss of spouse, and changes involving loss of family members and friends (Albert & Freedman, 2012; Hillier & Barrow, 2012; Novak, 2012). Additional challenges to *healthy aging* are a higher likelihood of developing chronic diseases and the limited availability of affordable transportation resources, housing options, health care options, and personal care to help people remain independent (Bernstein et al., 2003; Hogson & Chi, 2001).

healthy aging
The development and maintenance of optimal physical, mental, and social well-being and overall functional health among older adults

One group within the older adult population that requires specific discussion is the baby boomer generation, which markedly affects the proportions of the elderly and the "oldest old" in the total population (Eggebeen & Sturgeon, 2006). It is projected that one in five people will be 65 years old or older by 2030 (Federal Interagency Forum on Aging-Related Statistics, 2012). Clearly health educators must become more educated in strategies designed to reach the older population.

Ageism refers to negative stereotypes and discrimination based on age (Bahr, 1994; Moody, 2006; Stallard, Decker, & Sellers, 2002). When directed toward older adults, it tends to be based on negative assumptions about the expected biological slowdowns that occur naturally with advancing age. Ageism tends to be experienced mostly by aging populations but is also exhibited toward teenagers (Hagestad & Uhlenberg, 2006). The term *ageism* when attributed to the elderly accentuates negative stereotypes, placing this population as out of touch, unable to learn, and unwilling to adapt to an ever-changing world. These stereotypes, added to the health needs of diverse seniors, call on medical care providers to take an interprofessional collaborative management approach.

ageism
Discrimination against those who are in the later period of adulthood. For example, media articles, cartoons, and greeting cards illustrate some aspects of ageism focusing on negative aspects of the aging process

Findings from the National Health Interview Survey (NHIS) show that a majority of Americans aged 65 and over report having good to excellent health (Albert & Freedman, 2012; Schiller & Bernadal, 2004). This trend is supported by older individuals' increasing years of active life, increasing participation in prevention activities, and fewer complications from previously fatal health conditions (Bernstein et al., 2003; Centers for Disease Control and Prevention, 2004).

As they develop new public health strategies and community models for the older adult population seeking a healthy lifestyle as they age in place, health education and gerontological practitioners will need to address issues of health literacy, cultural competencies, disease prevention, and *health promotion.* Any planned combination of educational, political, environmental, regulatory, or organizational mechanisms that support the actions and conditions of living conducive to the health of individuals, groups, and communities, resources targeting needs, expectations, as well as positive health outcomes to maintain older adults' overall quality of life and their personal well-being.

health promotion
Any planned combination of educational, political, environmental, regulatory, or organizational mechanisms that support the actions and conditions of living conducive to the health of individuals, groups, and communities

Building Culturally Appropriate Health Promotion Programs

For some time, health care professionals have focused on three distinct health care models (Novak, 2012), each with specific approaches for caring for individuals:

- *The medical model* views health care as sickness. It requires a diagnosis, a treatment plan, and rehabilitation to meet the needs of patients seeking medical treatment.
- *The social model* defines health care more broadly and refers to it as more than the absence of disease. It focuses more on an individual's abilities to function with the support of family and community in the social world where they are most comfortable.
- *The health promotion model* focuses on disease prevention and delaying disability.

A continuum level of care is vital as we explore the incorporation aspects of each of these models.

In the health care professions, as well as in academia, the foundations of health care training, education, and health care outcomes have been rooted in the medical model. In recent years, health care professionals, gerontologists, and health care professions have started to recognize a need for interprofessional collaboration to incorporate improved outcomes through working together. The World Health Organization in 2010 noted that "interprofessional collaboration in education and practice is an innovative strategy that will play an important role towards the integration of the overall health care work force" (p. 8).

A study conducted by Bainbridge, Nasmith, Orchard, and Wood (2010) found that interprofessional collaboration in health care education revolves around six domains that contribute to interprofessional patient-related care and interprofessional communication among health care professionals:

1. Role clarification
2. Patient/client/family community context
3. Team functioning
4. Collaborative leadership
5. Interprofessional communication
6. Dealing with interprofessional conflicts

These six domains establish the foundation for interprofessional collaboration in health care work focusing on patient safety, health, shortages in human resources, and effective and efficient care. A focus on healthy aging strategies to improve quality of care as well as keeping one's independence is vital for *successful aging.*

successful aging
A superior quality of life; in other words, older adults should be able to engage completely in their lives by maintaining their physical strength, cognitive functions, and positive relationships throughout their life

In the field of public health, aging and social work have focused on similar health-related topics and research and addressed the overall challenges, issues, and resources of the increasing numbers of older adults. The American Public Health Association's Task Force on Aging (TFA) established guidelines and objectives to guide its work. Among its recommendations, it noted that efforts to connect community and public health agencies working on aging issues should consider population diversity that includes ethnic identification, socioeconomic status, and age groups 75 years of age and older. The TFA's report, "Scope of Public Health and Aging" (2004), identified eight key focus points:

1. An emphasis on healthy aging, health promotion, disease prevention, and injury risk reduction initiatives at the individual, community, state, and national levels
2. Partnerships among public health departments, area agencies on aging, state units on aging, and disease-specific voluntary organizations in carrying out health promotions
3. An awareness of the critical role played by family, neighbors, and friends and informal caregivers in dealing with chronic disease management and access to community resources
4. Health care workforce and research
5. Health regulations, consumer protections, and access to services
6. Population-based interventions
7. Community orientation
8. Health and disease orientation

Also, in 2003, the Centers for Disease Control (CDC), in partnership with the Administration on Aging (AOA) and the US Department of Health and Human Services (DHHS), launched a collaborative research project, The Aging States Project: Promoting Opportunities for Collaboration between the Public Health and Aging Services Network. This project gathered significant data and resulted in a wide range of recommendations for building interprofessional collaboration to meet the needs of an increasing older adult population. This research study also described older adult attitudes and beliefs regarding wellness, self-care, and participation in health promotion activities. And it identified these key factors for developing collaboration efforts among health educators and health care practitioners (Vincent & Velkoff, 2003):

1. Promote improved collaboration between state health departments and state units on aging
2. Support health promotion/disease prevention for older adults
3. Promote needed training and technical assistance
4. Promote collaboration and communication among agencies

There are challenges for partnerships in learning and collaborative efforts to develop effective programs. They include cultural limitations (e.g., lack of available language interpreters), low levels of health literacy, not enough printed media resources, socioeconomic restraints (e.g., low-income resources, lack of transportation, poverty), health care access, and transportation barriers. The perceptions of elders of participation in and acceptance of community endeavors involves other considerations too: their willingness to accept community support, financial constraints, and lack of previous knowledge about community resources available to them. Wallace (2005) has identified three components important for public health educators to focus on in their efforts: "an emphasis on health rather than disease, a proactive rather than a reactive approach, and the focus on the population rather than the individual" (p. 5).

In establishing new guidelines for health promotion and disease prevention through the Healthy People 2020 Initiative, the US Department of Health and Human Services (2000) identified a major goal for older adults as to "improve the health, function, and quality of life for older adults" (p. 1). In its overview of older adults, the initiative states that "60 percent of older adults, age 65 and over, will have at least one chronic condition by 2030" (p. 2). Older adults have a higher risk for developing chronic diseases and disabilities that include diabetes mellitus, arthritis, congestive heart failure, and dementia.

A key health indicator among older adults is their quality of life, which is affected by increased hospitalizations, nursing home admissions, and loss of their ability to live independently. The objectives of Healthy People 2020 for adults age 65 and older address a number of important factors for this age group: overall quality of life, understanding the health of older adults, the impact of social environments, and quality of health care community-based resources and social services care management. It identified emerging issues as well: coordinated care options, self-care management, and quality measures and training opportunities for health care workers.

Smith (2003) has stated that "we'd likely either group public health with the medical profession or define it as the local health department. Public health (care) professionals work on ways to prevent health problems that affect large segments of the population" (p. 9). Furthermore, wrote Smith, public health professionals are associated with ten essential public health services that include the interprofessional roles of public health professionals, medical personnel, and gerontologists as they share responsibilities for dealing with preventive health problems that affect the larger population. Finally, Smith also stated the benefits in public health partnering with health care education:

- Teaching students about health and how it affects society and history
- Strengthening the connection between students and their school or community
- Encouraging an interdisciplinary integrated approach to health
- Exposing students to careers in public health

Finally, Albert and Freedman (2012) have shown that the focus of the overall goals of public health and aging are to "create circumstances under which a population is likely to achieve health through health promotion and disease prevention" (p. 34). The roles of public health and aging overlap on social and clinical aspects of health, the human aging process, social needs, and maintaining health.

Health Literacy among Older Adults

Health literacy may be defined as "a multidimensional issue encompassing the ability to read, understand, and use health information to make appropriate healthcare decisions and follow instructions for treatment that allow patients to manage their health and improve the quality of their lives" (Brown et al., 2004, p. 150). It is a key issue to consider when dealing with older populations because it influences patient-provider interactions, including compliance with treatment (Greene, Hibbard, & Tusler, 2005; National Institute on Aging, 2006; Osborne, 2005).

Results from the 2003 National Assessment of Adult Literacy (NAAL) show that 29 percent of the adult population 65 years old and older had a health literacy proficiency of 30 percent and were at the basic level, 38 percent were at the intermediate level, and only 3 percent of the participants were at the proficient health literacy level (Kutner, Greenberg, Jin, & Paulsen, 2006; National Institute on Aging, 2006). According to these findings, adults age 65 and older have the lowest health literacy level when compared to the other age groups (Kutner et al., 2006; National Institute on Aging, 2006).

Lee, Gazmararian, and Arozullah (2006) conducted a study "examining health literacy, social support, and their relations to health status and health care use among older adults" (p. 324). They noted that older adult populations with low health literacy tend to be comparatively isolated from the society in which they live; therefore, they obtain less social support, and their health tends to diminish as a consequence. Similarly, findings from the NAAL indicate that adults categorized as being in the below basic range of health literacy have difficulties reading documents, filling out medical forms, and navigating the health care system (Osborne, 2005; Powell, Hill, & Clancy, 2007).

Osborne (2005) discusses the importance of considering a person's background before starting to convey information. For example, health educators should be aware of clients' personal health, such as the presence of chronic illnesses, complications, and medications, because this knowledge will be important to implementing health promotion programs. Health educators can meet the needs of older adults by determining the health literacy of the target population and then employing good communication skills and well-written instructions that are at the appropriate level for this population.

Osborne (2005) also suggests that information presented to older adults should be limited to a few important points, adjusted according to the audience's attention span, and repeated to ensure understanding. Nakasato and Carnes (2006) suggest that health promotion programs targeting older adults address three key needs of these individuals: maintaining a low risk of experiencing disease and disease-related disabilities, maintaining a mentally and physically active lifestyle, and maintaining their engagement in life. The following strategies can be applied in these health promotion programs:

- *Create a shame-free atmosphere where older adults can comfortably acknowledge when they do or do not understand the materials being presented to them.* Group participants can be encouraged to draw from their vast experiences and share their lifelong learning about health. Health educators can work to update the information clients have when it does not conform to established scientific standards.
- *Create an environment conducive to learning and good communication,* with large visual aids, well-lit rooms, and quiet spaces to talk. Culturally apt and age-appropriate graphics that are easy to read and follow can facilitate the learning process. Health educators working with older adult populations need to be mindful of their voice projection to ensure they can be heard without shouting or sounding condescending.

- *Make spoken information concrete and concise.* Voice projection is important in delivering information to and discussing issues with older adult populations. Health educators should also seek to decrease their use of jargon and technical language that their target audience may not understand. Examples should be placed within a context that is familiar to the target population.
- *Engage in short trips "down memory lane."* Older adults enjoy recalling facts they have learned, the experiences they have had, and the people with whom they shared these experiences.
- *Incorporate social activities into health education and promotion programs.* Active learning must be encouraged and promoted throughout health promotion programs.
- *Using a geragogy model of teaching when teaching older adults.* Build on adult learning theory and teaching patients interventions designed to accommodate physical, sensory, and cognitive deficits.

Cultural Competence with Older Adults

Betancourt, Green, Carrillo, and Ananeh-Firempong (2003) find that health care can be considered culturally competent when it is based on an understanding of the ways in which patients' society and culture influence their health behaviors and health beliefs. Hillier and Barrow (2010) noted that *culture competence* refers to "the ability to honor and respect styles, attitudes, behaviors, and beliefs of individual families, and staff who receive and provide services among older adults" (p. 6).

Health education practitioners can build cultural competence with aging populations by using the core curriculum in ethnogeriatrics, examining the aging, health, and ethnicity of an elderly individual with respect to his or her culture, beliefs, and practices that influence choices and behavior when it comes to health care services. The Stanford Ethnogeriatrics teaching curriculum model was developed in 1999 and 2000 by the Stanford Geriatric Education Center (SGEC). The center collaborative noted that there are flaws and limitations in the US Census data that affect our ability to learn about cultural and demographic groups (Yeo, 2000).

The SGEC is a widely recognized leader in the field of ethnogeriatrics—that is, health care for elders from diverse populations. Since its inception in 1987, the center has provided extensive training in medicine, nursing, social work, psychology, occupational therapy, pastoral counseling, and related fields. It has established a set of ethnogeriatric competencies for training health providers:

1. Assess and describe their own cultural and spiritual/religious values and discuss the effect of those values on their health care beliefs and behavior.

2. Identify and understand the heterogeneity within categories and groups of elders and their families.
3. Assess their clients' position on the continuum of acculturation in relation to their preferences, perceptions, and definitions and their explanatory models of physical and mental health and illness, their health literacy, and their health behaviors.
4. Demonstrate interviewing skills that promote culturally appropriate decision making and mutual respect between health care providers and ethnic clients and their families in patient-centered care throughout their lives, including end-of-life care.
5. Communicate effectively, and elicit information from elders of any ethnic background and their families, particularly those who speak little or no English, with appropriate use of interpreter services and information technology.
6. Communicate with ethnic elders and their families using oral and written strategies that are mindful of health literacy levels and abilities.
7. Explain the importance of cultural and historical experiences (e.g., historical trauma from racism and discrimination).
8. Describe their effect on older clients' help-seeking behaviors and their access to and use of health care services, including emergency preparedness.
9. Identify the resources for older individuals, their families, and their communities for promoting and maintaining elders' physical, mental, and spiritual health, and support those resources in a respectful way.
10. Advocate for policies and practices that facilitate cultural humility and ethnically sensitive and proficient health care within patient-centered medical homes, institutions, organizations, and professions.
11. Maintain up-to-date knowledge of health disparities in geriatric care and the effect of ethnicity and culture on the physical and mental health care of older adults.

Yehieli, Grey, and Werff (2004) cited three critical questions to ask in their report to establish a comprehensive knowledge base for health professionals working with diverse aging groups:

1. What are the cultural backgrounds of some of the most significant minority and newcomer elder populations in the United States?
2. How do the cultural, religious, and socioeconomic backgrounds of these minority seniors affect their perspectives on health and the health care system? How do these seniors from different cultures define health?

3. What should health care providers know about these minorities and newcomers that will help them provide the best possible care to those who are aging?

Demographic data and ethnic and cultural perspectives affect the educational community programs developed to meet the needs of our growing population of older adults. Acknowledging ethnogerontological educational resources may provide the context for better collaborative efforts among aging populations and health education practitioners and thus better learning outcomes

A study in rural Florida found that even physicians showed ageist perceptions, especially toward people 85 years of age and older and those living in nursing homes (Gunderson, Tomkowiak, Menachemi, & Brooks, 2005). Health promotion programs need to reduce this type of discrimination, which can be achieved by creating culturally competent programs with linguistically appropriate educational materials.

Figure 10.3 depicts the context of ethnogeriatrics for working with older adult populations. It emphasizes the interrelations of aging, ethnicity, and health, transculture health in all human cultures—"a transcultural ideal of freedom embracing all the peoples of the world" in collaboration with the field of geriatrics and ethno gerontology.

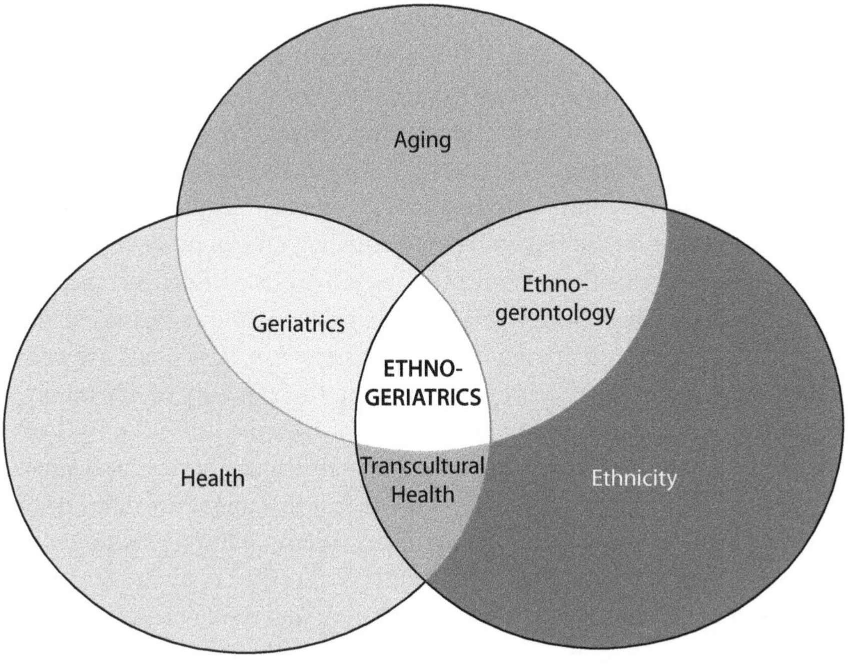

Figure 10.3 The Context of Ethnogeriatrics

Source: Stanford Geriatric Education Center (2012).

Healthy Aging and Health Education

The expected economic impact on the nation's health care system resulting from population increases among individuals aged 65 and over demands that additional prevention services be developed and implemented for that population group (Wallace, 2005). According to the Federal Interagency Forum on Age-Related Statistics (2012), the projected increase in the size of the population 65 and older will translate into even higher levels of health care service demands and expenditures for this population group. The average health care expenditures for older non-Hispanic blacks, for example, were $19,839 compared to a health care cost for older Hispanics of $15,362 in 2008. Overall health care cost varies among older adults experiencing no chronic disease compared to older adults with five or more multiple medical issues costing on average $24,658. Elders living in long-term care facilities cost $61,318 compared to elders living in community settings, costing on average $13,150 per year. Additional health care cost includes utilization of prescription drugs, health insurance, alternative residential services, and veterans' services. The utilization of health care cost varies among older adults seeking health care services that include long-term care settings, hospice, in-patient hospitalization, home health care services, and prescription drugs.

In 2010, national health expenditures were $2.6 trillion, over ten times the $256 billion spent in 1980 (Kaiser, 2012). Further review of increased health care costs has identified such factors as the cost of improved technology, plus prescription drug use, which accounts for 10 percent of total health care expenditures among older adults; home health care, 3 percent; nursing home care, 5 percent; other health, residential, and personal care, 5 percent; hospital care, 31 percent; and physician services, 20 percent. These expenditures continue to rise with increases in the number of people with chronic disease, increased use of technology, and increases in prescription drug costs, plus the overall administrative costs of delivering health care to citizens. Given the toll this will take on economic as well as personal resources, it is not surprising that public health professionals are being called on to assist older adults in improving their quality of life and preventing or avoiding debilitating and expensive treatments (see figure 10.4).

The expected increased demand for health care services and subsequent increased costs is partially due to the fact that approximately one out of every three older adults has at least one chronic condition affecting his or her ability to function (Kaiser EDU, 2012).

Given population shifts, it is not surprising that the Centers for Disease Control has identified three areas that need to be addressed in our attempts to reach the elderly in the United States: adoption of a healthy lifestyle, one that incorporates physical activity, proper nutrition, and avoidance of

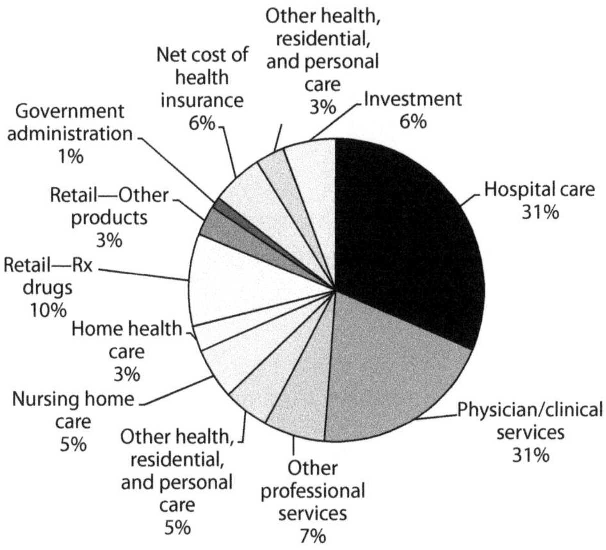

Figure 10.4 National Health Care Expenditures in the United States, 2012
Source: Kaiser EDU (2012).

tobacco products; the early detection of disease, including the use of diagnostic exams such as sigmoidoscopy, colonoscopy, and tests for colorectal cancer; and the use of specific immunizations, such as for flu, pneumonia, and shingles. Attention to these areas improves the likelihood of a happy and functional transition to retirement (Atchley & Barusch, 2004; Hillier & Barrow, 2010).

Suggestions for Working with Diverse Groups among the Aging Population

For those working with the aging population, knowledge of their unique cultural, social, psychological, and economic needs is critical (Yehieli et al., 2004). Health care practitioners should expand their knowledge in order to widen their perspective and address the needs of each age cohort in order to provide the services they need.

The foundation of aging programs, services, and community resources was laid in 1965 when President Lyndon Johnson signed into law the Older Americans Act (OAA). This legislation established the authority for grant distribution to states to address the increasingly diverse needs of the elderly through community planning and social services, research and development, and personnel training. Subsequently, the OAA legislation funded the Administration on Aging to administer federally funded projects for older individuals. The administration is charged with funding the majority of organizations, community-based programs, and social and nutrition services working with elderly groups. (Administration on Aging, 2012). In 2011 the Administration on Aging (AoA) published a training tool kit designed for groups serving diverse aging populations. The toolkit addresses four areas:

1. Assessments, including a self-assessment questionnaire to survey an individual provider's knowledge of services and identify training needs
2. Identifying community resources
3. Tailoring services
4. Program evaluation (Administration on Aging, 2012)

The goal of this tool kit is to provide care providers with a guide and a method that is respectful, inclusive, and sensitive to a diverse community and is grounded on a set of principles that address the following areas:

- Delivering outreach and other services based on a population's values and perceptions. This is the core of successful service delivery.
- Serving diverse populations is not a one-size-fits-all process. It requires asking the right questions to help address the population's needs and concerns.
- The meaning of diversity goes beyond race and ethnicity. It includes individuals with disabilities; lesbian, gay, bisexual, and transgender older adults; homeless seniors; older adult immigrants; and many other populations.
- Diversity is all around us. It is part of daily life and offers us opportunities to grow and learn about others.

The original Administration on Aging tool kit has been augmented with a series of ethnic-focused materials addressing African Americans, Asian and Pacific Islanders, and Hispanics. The kits provide materials aimed at family members dealing with issues that generally have not been previously addressed, such as elder abuse, mental health needs, legal services, and caregiving resources.

In 2012, the US Department of Health and Human Services reorganized the Administration on Aging, the Office on Disability, and the Administration on Developmental Disabilities into a single agency, the Administration for Community Living (ACL). The ACL has greater policy and program support for cross-cutting initiatives and efforts focused on the unique needs of individuals, including older adults. Its goal is to increase access to community support and full participation while focusing attention and resources on the unique needs of older Americans and people with disabilities (Administration for Community Living, 2012). All Americans, including people with disabilities and older adults, should be able to live at home with the supports they need and participate in communities that value their contributions (Administration for Community Living, 2012).

In addition, the World Health Organization, as a global health leader, encourages a framework to "provide strategies and ideas that will help policy makers implement the elements of interprofessional education and collaborative practice that will be most beneficial on their own jurisdictions" (World Health Organization, 2011). In 2011, in response to the need for a trained multidisciplinary workforce, the World Health Organization commissioned the development of a framework for action promoting collaborative work among health care colleagues around the world to share their expertise. This expansion of a global perspective on health and human resources provides a knowledge base for the next generation of health workers with capacity-building strategies bolstering a global health workforce.

In support of the Interprofessional Education and Collaborative Practice framework, a panel of health professional experts published a report encouraging a vision of interprofessional collaborative practice as the key to safe, high-quality, accessible, patient-centered care (Interprofessional Education Collaborative Expert Panel, 2011). The panel suggested that the training of educators in health interprofessional core competencies needs to move beyond profession-specific educational efforts to engage students of different disciplines. The practitioners ascertained that each profession's disciplinary competencies can be strengthened with competencies taught within their profession. Yehieli et al. (2004) address these in a pocket guide with practical resources for health care providers who are working with elder immigrants, refugees, and minorities in the United States. Another important point they outline is how the health condition of minority seniors is predominantly determined by broad differences in income, education, living conditions, lifestyle practices, insurance coverage, family support systems, and socioeconomic factors that can be changed and less by genetic differences that cannot be changed. Furthermore, the authors assert that an increasing number of diverse seniors are generally groups representing immigrants, refugees, and minorities.

Integrated health and educational policies require a workforce dedicated to health care and policymaking plans with integrated, interprofessional education and collaborative practice. Accordingly, the delivery of interprofessional education development has two themes:

1. Educator mechanisms: Academic staff training, champions, institutional support managerial commitment, and learning outcomes
2. Curricular mechanisms: Logistics and scheduling, programming content, compulsory attendance, shared objectives, adult learning principles, and contextual learning assessment

Once the specific training mechanisms are identified, the next step is to outline the three working parameters to elicit the systemic support needed:

- Institutional support mechanisms: Governmental process, structural protocols, common operating resources, personnel policies, and supportive management practice
- Working culture mechanisms: Communications strategies, conflict resolution policies, shared decision-making processes
- Environmental mechanisms: The built environment, facilities, space design (World Health Organization, 2010)

The challenges for partnerships in learning and collaborative efforts to develop effective educational venues require dealing with cultural limitations, social and economic constraints, health care access, and transportation barriers. Older adults' participation in and acceptance of community endeavors involves additional considerations, such as their willingness to accept community support, their personal financial constraints, and their lack of previous knowledge about community resources useful to them.

Health promotion programs targeting the elderly should be designed to promote well-being in old age and, more specifically, to promote productive, robust, and successful aging. To meet these criteria, health promotion and educational programs should take into account cognitive changes that people experience as part of the aging process, physiological changes and limitations, and the expectations of program participants (Flood & Scharer, 2006, see also Hooyman & Kiyak, 2010). Health promotion and aging programs focusing on older adults promote an early focus on disease prevention, injury and disability prevention, mental health, and physical health and should also encourage social engagement (Nakasato & Carnes, 2006).

Conclusion

The reality of an increasing aging population is upon us, bringing challenges and opportunities for practitioners in the areas of public health and aging to open a dialogue on developing a broad perspective on innovative public policies, program, services, and community resources to meet the challenges, barriers, and overall impact of living a long and productive live as an elder. This demographic transition is also bringing up changing perspectives facing older adults, for example, a culturally diverse older adult population dealing with socioeconomic limitations, a lack of affordable housing, and alternative transportation needs for those who have given up driving. There are as well changing perspectives that are more positive: improved health care technologies, improved overall health outcomes, limited disabilities experienced in later years, and a more productive and positive aging process.

As a result, new opportunities abound for health care professionals who will use the concepts addressed in this chapter to enhance the development of interprofessional conversations focusing on elders' life experiences and the changing dynamics of this population.

Points to Remember

- Thanks to medical advances, an increase in health care access, and decreased danger in workplaces, the life expectancy of Americans went up by an average of twenty-nine years between 1900 and 2000. Yet many public health professionals are not adequately prepared to provide preventive services to older Americans.
- Among the issues that the elderly face are ageism, loss of family and friends, reduction in socioeconomic status, loss of independence, and the development of one or more chronic diseases.
- Health educators should familiarize themselves with education techniques designed especially to reach the aging population. In particular, they should be prepared to overcome low levels of health literacy.
- Non-Hispanic whites are a majority of the older population, but the proportions of other ethnic and racial groups are growing rapidly. Health educators working with older adults need to become culturally competent.
- The context of the ethnogeriatrics model (see figure 10.3) relates ethnicity, aging, and health and thus provides a structure for building cultural competence for working with older adults. Ethnogeriatric materials are designed to contribute to the attainment of the Healthy People 2020 goal by increasing functional life expectancy.
- Health promotion and prevention programs for older adults may be best carried out by partnerships of state and local departments of public health in cooperation with state and local area agencies on aging, which include community-based programs focusing on older adult health issues as elders continue to age in place.

Case Study

Dave, a recent master's of public health graduate with a community health emphasis, has been hired by a rural community health center that works with older adults who represent the diverse ethnic groups that have lived in this rural community for more than five decades. Dave has been asked to develop a demographic profile and identify three to five objectives for meeting the needs of the elders he will be working with throughout the year and then develop and implement a National Institutes of Health and the National Institute on Aging (2001) Go4Life exercise program for older adults:

1. What resources will Dave have to use to develop a comprehensive demographic profile for the community?
2. What suggestions would you give him for developing a survey of community elders in this diverse rural community?
3. What goals and objectives should Dave incorporate as key health concerns for older adults who participate in the community health center?
4. Dave wants to learn more about older adults and their health care needs. What would you recommend as valuable resources Dave can use to expand his overall knowledge of older adults?
5. What strategies need to be implemented to establish the Go4Life exercise program for elders willing to participate in this weekly program?
6. What are Dave's options for meeting the diverse ethnic groups who attend the rural community center?

KEY TERMS

Ageism

Healthy aging

Health promotion

Interprofessional collaboration

Successful aging

References

Administration on Aging. (2012). *A profile of older Americans: 2012.* Retrieved from http://www.acl.gov/

Administration for Community Living. (2012). *A toolkit for serving diverse populations.* Retrieved from http://www.aoa.gov/AoARoot/AoA_Programs/Tools_Resources/DOCS/AoA_DiversityToolkit_full.pdf

Albert S. M., & Freedman, V. A. (2012). *Public health and aging maximizing function and well being.* New York, NY: Springer.

Alwin, D. F., McCammon, R. J., & Hofer, S. M. (2006). Studying boomer cohorts within a demographic and developmental context: Conceptual and methodological issues. In S. K. Whitbourne & S. L. Willis (Eds.), *The baby boomers grow up: Contemporary perspectives on midlife* (pp. 45–71). Mahwah, NJ: Erlbaum.

American Public Health Association. (2004). *Aging task force: Scope of Public Health and Aging.* Retrieved from http://www.apha.org.

Atchley, R. C., & Barusch, A. S. (2004). *Social forces and aging: An introduction to social gerontology.* Belmont, CA: Wadsworth.

Bahr, R. T. (1994). An overview of gerontological nursing. In M. O. Hogstel (Ed.), *Nursing care of the older adult* (3rd ed., pp. 2–25). Albany, NY: Delmar.

Bainbridge, L., Nasmith, L., Orchard, C., & Wood N. (2010). Competencies in interprofessional collaboration. *Journal of Physical Therapy Education, 24*(1), 6–11.

Bernstein, A. B., Hing, E., Moss, A. J., Allen, K. F., Siller, A. B., & Tiggle, R. B. (2003). *Health care in America: Trends in utilization.* Hyattsville, MD: National Center for Health Statistics.

Betancourt, J. R., Green, A. R., Carrillo, J. E., & Ananeh-Firempong, O. (2003). Defining cultural competence: A practical framework for addressing racial/ethnic disparities in health and health care. *Public Health Reports, 118,* 293–302.

Brown, D. R., Ludwig, R., Buck, G. A., Durham, D., Shurmard, T., & Graham, S. S. (2004). Health literacy: Universal precautions needed. *Journal of Allied Health, 33*(2), 150–155.

Centers for Disease Control and Prevention. (2004). *Healthy aging for older adults.* Retrieved from http://www.cdc.gov/aging/aginginfo/index.htm

Eggebeen, S., & Sturgeon, S. (2006). Demography of the baby boomers. In S. K. Whitbourne & S. L. Willis (Eds.), *The baby boomers grow up: Contemporary perspectives on midlife* (pp. 45–71). Mahwah, NJ: Erlbaum.

Federal Interagency Forum on Aging-Related Statistics. (2012). *Older Americans 2012: Key indicators of well-being.* Retrieved from http://www.agingstats.gov

Flood, M., & Scharer, K. (2006). Creativity enhancement: Possibilities for successful aging. *Issues in Mental Health Nursing, 27,* 939–959.

Greene, J., Hibbard, J., & Tusler, M. (2005). *How much do health literacy and patient activation contribute to older adults' ability to manage their health?* Washington, DC: AARP Public Policy Institute.

Gunderson, A., Tomkowiak, J., Menachemi, N., & Brooks, R. (2005). Rural physicians' attitudes toward the elderly: Evidence of ageism? *Quality Management in Health Care, 14*(3), 167–176.

Hagestad, G. O., & Uhlenberg, P. (2006, November). Should we be concerned about age segregation? Some theoretical and empirical explorations. *Research on Aging, 28*(6), 638–653.

Hillier, S. M., & Barrow, G. M. (2010). *Aging, the individual and society* (8th ed.). Belmont, CA: Wadsworth.

Hogson, T. A., & Chi, L. (2001). Medical care expenditures for hypertension, its complications, its comorbidity. *Medical Care, 396,* 599–615.

Hooyman N. R., & Kiyak H. S. (2010). *Social gerontology: A multidisciplinary approach*. Boston, MA: Pearson Education.

Interprofessional Collaboration Expert Panel (2011). *Core competencies' for interprofessional collaboration practice*. Washington, DC. Retrieved from http://www.asph.org/userfiles/CollaborativePractice.pdf

Kaiser EDU. (2012). *U.S. health care cost: Issue Module Background Brief.* Retrieved from http://www.kaiseredu.org/issue-modules/us-healthcare-costs/background/

Keller, C., & Fleury, J. (2000). *Health promotion for the elderly*. Thousand Oaks, CA: Sage.

Kemp, C. B. (2012). Public health in the age of health care reform. *Prevention Chronic Disease, 9*, 120–151. doi: http://dx.doi. org/10.5888/pcd9.120151

Kutner, M., Greenberg, E., Jin, Y., & Paulsen, C. (2006). The *health literacy of America's adults: Results from the 2003 National Assessment of Adult Literacy*. Hyattsville, MD: National Institutes of Health.

Lee, S., Gazmararian, J. A., & Arozullah, A. M. (2006). Health literacy and social support among elderly Medicare enrollees in a managed care plan. *Journal of Applied Gerontology, 25*(4), 324–337.

Moody, H. R. (2006). *Aging: Concepts and controversies* (5th ed.). Thousand Oaks, CA: Pine Forge.

Nakasato, Y., R., & Carnes, B. A. (2006, April). Health promotion in older adults: Promoting successful aging in primary care settings. *Geriatrics, 61*(4), 27–31.

National Institute on Aging. (2006). *Working with your older patient*. Retrieved from http://www.nia.nih.gov/HealthInformation/Publications/WorkingwithYourOlderPatient/default.htm.

National Institutes of Health and Institute on Aging. (2001). *Go4Life*. Retrieved from http://www.go4life.gov

Novak, M., (2012) *Issues in aging* (3rd ed.). Boston, MA., Pearson Education.

Osborne, H. (2005). *Health literacy from A to Z: Practical ways to communicate your health message*. Sudbury, MA: Jones & Bartlett.

Powell, C. K., Hill, E. G., & Clancy, D. E. (2007, January/February). The relationship between health literacy and diabetes knowledge and readiness to take health actions. *Diabetes Educator, 33*(1), 144–151.

Schiller, J. S., & Bernadal, L. (2004, May). Summary health statistics for the US population: National Health Interview Survey, 2002. *Vital and Health Statistics, 10*(220), 1–110.

Smith, J. (2003) *Education and public health: Natural partners in learning for life*. Alexandria, VA: Association for Supervision and Curriculum Development.

Stallard, J. M., Decker, I. M., & Sellers, B. J. (2002, April-June). Health care for the elderly: A social obligation. *Nursing Forum, 37*(2), 5–15.

Stanford Geriatric Education Center. (2012). *The context of ethnogeriatrics*. Retrieved from http://sgec.stanford.edu/resources/index.html

US Census Bureau. (2008). *International database.* Retrieved from http://www.census.gov/ipc.

US Census Bureau. (2010). *The next four decades: The older adult population in the United States 2010 2050.* Washington, DC: Author.

US Census Bureau. (2011). *Overview of race and Hispanic origin, 2010.* Retrieved from http://www.census.gov/population/www/socdemo/hispanic/hispanic.html

US Health and Human Services. (2012). *The Administration for Community Living (ACL) is part of the U.S. Department of Health and Human Services and is headed by the administrator, who reports directly to the Secretary of Health and Human Services (HHS). ACL's Principal Deputy Administrator serves as Senior Advisor to the HHS Secretary for Disability Policy.* Retrieved from http://acl.gov/About_ACL/Organization/Index.aspx

Vincent, C. K., Velkoff, V. A. (2010). *The Next four decades, the older population 2010 to 2050: Population estimations and projections.* Washington, DC: US Department of Commerce and US Census Bureau.

Wallace, S. P. (2005). The public health perspective on aging. *Generations, 29*(2), 5–10.

Winslow, C.E.A. (1920). The untilled field of public health. *Science New Series, 130,* 23–33.

World Health Organization. (2010). *The framework for action on interprofessional education and collaborative practice.* Retrieved from http://www.who.int/hrh/resources/framework_action/en/index.html

Yehieli, M., Grey, M., and Werff, A. V. (2004). *The caring for diverse seniors: A health provider's pocket guide to working with elderly minority, immigrant, and refugee patients.* Retrieved from http://www.Aoa/AOA/Programs

Yeo, G. (Ed.). (2000). *Curriculum in ethnogeriatrics.* Stanford Geriatric Education Center. Retrieved from http://www.stanford.edu/group/ethnoger/leftf.html

CHAPTER 11

CULTURE AND SEXUAL ORIENTATION

D. Kay Woodiel
Joan E. Cowdery

LEARNING OBJECTIVES

After completing this chapter, you will be able to

- Acknowledge the diversity within the gay cultures.
- Recognize health risks and common health concerns specific to lesbians and bisexual women, gay and bisexual men, transgender individuals, and racially and ethnically diverse LGBT people.
- Increase awareness of and sensitivity to health issues relevant to the LGBT culture.
- Demonstrate cultural competence when working with and addressing the LGBT culture.

Culture involves behaviors and beliefs characteristic of a particular social, ethnic, or age group. It can go beyond behaviors and beliefs and present a dynamic set of shared values, customs, communication patterns, and norms often influencing the behaviors and action of the group (Campinha-Bacote, 1999). This definition of culture provides ample evidence for the inclusion of a chapter about the lesbian, gay, bisexual, and transgender (LGBT) community in a multicultural health education book. A section on lesbian, gay, bisexual and transgender health is included for the first time in Healthy People 2020. In Healthy People 2010, the LGBT companion document (Gay and Lesbian Medical Association, 2001) highlighted the need for more research to address the social determinants that contribute to health disparities in the LGBT community.

Members of the LGBT community can share a culture regardless of their race or ethnicity in the same way that workers in the automobile industry share a culture regardless of race or ethnicity. So it is important for health educators to extend their definition of culture beyond race and ethnicity to include socioeconomic status, physical abilities and limitations, religious beliefs, and political affiliation, as well as sexual orientation. The LGBT culture is an undeniable fact, as evidenced by the symbol of the rainbow flag, pride parades, pride proms, and drag queens.

All health educators and health professionals should strive to provide culturally competent services. Yet the majority of LGBT people do not feel they are receiving culturally competent care (LGBT Medical Education

Research Group, 2011). The high profile assigned to human immunodeficiency virus (HIV) and acquired immunodeficiency syndrome (AIDS) has led many health educators and health professionals to conclude that this is the only health issue affecting the LGBT community. There is a lack of knowledge and appreciation for the extent of the problems facing this unique cultural group. This may be related to the fact that certain segments of the US population do not wish to recognize LGBT people as a cultural group. It is imperative that health educators and professionals recognize that the gay culture is made up of a collective of LGBT populations that are as diverse as their members.

Perhaps the most significant health disparity that the LGBT community faces is the comparative lack of research, especially in the area of transgender health. Previously several well-recognized health agencies have acknowledged that research on LGBT health is inadequate. The National Institute of Mental Health (US Department of Health and Human Services, National Institute of Mental Health, 2008), the Centers for Disease Control and Prevention (2011a, 2011b), the American Medical Association, and the Institute of Medicine (2011) have all released reports indicating that health care research in lesbian, gay, bisexual, and transgender communities is largely inadequate.

In spite of positive societal changes over the past decade, much remains unknown about the health status of the LGBT community. This research is complicated by the fact that lesbian, gay, bisexual and transgendered individuals are separate groups, and each has subgroups with unique needs (Institute of Medicine, 2011). The Institute of Medicine (2011) has given LGBT researchers and advocates a powerful new tool in its report, "The Health of Lesbian, Gay, Bisexual and Transgender People: Building a Foundation for Better Understanding," which recognized the previous tendency to treat all LGBT individuals as one homogeneous group. It details what is known about these individual groups at different stages of life. The report also proposes a research agenda and identifies the data needed to reduce disparities for the LGBT community. This document is considered to be historic because it is the first time the federal government laid out a blueprint of the health challenges of the LGBT culture and reframes the research from a scientific perspective.

This chapter addresses the health behaviors of the LGBT community. It explores cultural factors and myths, offering culturally sensitive information for health educators and health professionals who work with the community. We have included definitions for the key terms in this chapter in box 11.1. We hope this information will assist in decreasing the common confusion surrounding terminology for this culture.

BOX 11.1 DEFINITIONS OF KEY LGBT TERMS

Ally: Someone who advocates for and supports members of a community who are different from their own. A person who confronts homophobia, heterosexism, transphobia, and heterosexual privilege.

Bisexual: A man or a woman with a sexual and emotional orientation toward people of both sexes (US Department of Health and Human Services, Office on Women's Health, 2001).

Coming out: The process by which LGBT people acknowledge that they are not exclusively heterosexual. It may involve two phases: coming out to oneself and then coming out to others. This may occur over a short, intense period or gradually over time. Coming out is influenced by the person's comfort level and both internal and external influences.

Gay: Most commonly refers to men whose primary emotional and sexual attraction is to men but may also be used to refer to a homosexual person of either sex. Some lesbians identify as gay (Gay and Lesbian Medical Association, 2001).

Gender identity: A person's sense of self as being male or female. Gender identity does not always match biological sex. Unlike sex, which is biologically determined, gender is considered a social construct (Peterkin & Risdon, 2003; US Department of Health and Human Services, Substance Abuse and Mental Health Services Administration, 2000). Rejection of the traditional gender binary classification (Institute of Medicine, 2011).

Heterosexism: A belief that heterosexuality is the only "natural" sexuality and that it is inherently healthier than or superior to other types of sexuality (Shankle, 2006).

Homophobia: Irrational fear or hatred of lesbian, gay, bisexual, or transgender people (GLMA et al., 2001).

Homosexual: An outmoded term used primarily for diagnostic purposes, meaning *same-sexual* (Peterkin & Risdon, 2003).

Lesbian: A woman whose primary emotional and sexual attraction is to other women (Gay and Lesbian Medical Association 2001).

LGBT: Acronym for *l*esbian, *g*ay, *b*isexual, and *t*ransgender. (The preferred order of these four terms may vary, resulting in other acronyms in other books or articles.)

Queer: Once a derogatory term for gays and lesbians, this term is now being used with a sense of pride by members of the LGBT community, especially the younger members of LGBT communities (Peterkin & Risdon, 2003).

Questioning: Someone who is not sure of his or her gender identity or sexual orientation, or both.

Sexual identity: A chosen mode of self-presentation, based on social identity, sexual behavior, or both. A person may choose to publicly identify with a term that does not strictly conform to his or her sexual behavior (a self-termed "bisexual" woman may be intimate only with women). How one identifies is a personal choice (Peterkin & Risdon, 2003).

Sexual orientation: Includes behavior (activity), attraction (desire), and identity (personal and social) (Institute of Medicine, 2011). This term should replace *sexual preference*, which implies that these desires are a matter of choice rather than a result of one's nature (Peterkin & Risdon, 2003).

Transgender: A person whose gender identity or gender expression is not congruent with his or her biological sex. This term is sometimes used as an umbrella term encompassing transsexuals and cross-dressers (GLMA et al., 2001). "Trans" used as slang.

Transphobia: Irrational fear or hatred of transgender or transsexual individuals (GLMA et al., 2001).

Transsexual: An individual whose gender identity is that of the biologically opposite sex. There are female-to-male and male-to-female transsexuals. A transsexual may or may not have had sex reassignment surgery (Burrows, 2011; GLMA et al., 2001).

The LGBT Culture

Given that sexual orientation includes attraction, behavior, and identity and that patterns for all three can range along a continuum, attempts to estimate the size of this population can be challenging. One recent analysis by the Williams Institute (Gates, 2011) cross-compared a number of different population surveys and placed the number of LGBT individuals at approximately 3.5 percent of the population and transgender individuals at 0.3 percent. Recently the US Department of Health and Human Services (HHS) announced it would begin to collect data on sexual orientation and gender identity by 2013, partnering with the National Center for Health Statistics (Melby, 2011). This provides hope that more useful data can be collected to address health disparities in the LGBT culture.

It is important to realize that the LGBT community is a diverse group of people. They vary in sociodemographic characteristics such as ethnic or racial identity, age, education, income, and place of residence (Mayer, Bradford, Makadon, Stall, & Landers, 2008). This diversity extends to the degree to which they may or may not self-identify with the community. As a result, the community is referred to by a myriad of names. Terms such as *LGBT* and *GLBT* and *queer, homosexual, gay,* and *lesbian* are often used interchangeably. The terminology chosen will be specific to the individual's own personal identity and politics (Ferris, 2006). It is crucial that health educators and public health professionals not assume that any one term captures everyone who identifies as LGBT. For example, some lesbians may prefer the term *gay* to the term *lesbian*. Some members of the LGBT community, especially those born after 1970, may be very comfortable with the term *queer*, whereas many other members of the community find the term extremely offensive (Peterkin & Risdon, 2003). Although terminology is certainly not the foundation of any community, it can be relevant and helpful as health educators and health professionals address and target a community for disease prevention and health promotion (Ferris, 2006).

Health Issues of the LGBT Community

National data regarding LGBT health disparities are limited by the lack of population-based data collection systems that include items related to sexual orientation and gender identity. As a result, much of the epidemiological evidence comes from limited studies of specific populations within the LGBT community (GLMA, 2001). This research suggests that as with other marginalized groups, the LGBT community suffers multiple health disparities as a result of discrimination and homophobia. LGBT health disparities include a myriad of physical, mental, and social health issues including HIV/AIDS, substance abuse, depression, suicide, violence, and access to affordable care (Institute of Medicine, 2011; US Department of Health and Human Services, 2010).

Heterosexism and *homophobia* are the two most obvious social health issues for the LGBT community. Studies show that lesbian, gay, bisexual, and transgender populations have the same basic health needs as the general population but experience health disparities and barriers related to sexual orientation and gender identity or expression. Many individuals avoid or delay care or receive inappropriate or inferior care because of perceived or real homophobia and discrimination by health educators and health care professionals (Institute of Medicine, 2011; Shankle, 2006).

Recently more research has begun to focus on health issues affecting the LGBT community. This increased emphasis can be traced in part to the companion document for LGBT health that was released in conjunction with Healthy People 2010 and, more recently, the inclusion of a separate topic area and objectives as part of Healthy People 2020 (US Department of Health and Human Services, 2010). As a federal blueprint for building a healthier nation, the Healthy People objectives provide a framework for research and prevention activities, as well as helping to inform policymaking (GLMA et al., 2001; US Department of Health and Human Services, 2010).

In the past, the limited research in this area led to a lack of sensitive curricula and program policies that forced many gay youths to become the invisible minority (Anderson, 1997). When youth feel invisible, their health status will be negatively affected. LGBT youth are at increased risk for psychiatric disorders, including suicide, depression, and substance abuse (Mayer et al., 2008). In addition, this lack of research supports the existence of homophobia and heterosexism among health educators in the schools, which increases the invisibility of gay youths. It is impossible for gay youths to feel emotionally safe in schools if they feel invisible (Woodiel, Angermeier-Howard, & Hobson, 2003).

For example, one study revealed that one-third of health teachers indicated gay and lesbian rights are a threat to the American family and its values (Telljohann, Price, Poureslami, & Easton, 1995). In addition, more than half of the health teachers indicated that gay and lesbian support groups would not be supported by their school administrator (Telljohann et al., 1995). Another study looked at physical educators' confidence in teaching health education content areas and revealed that they felt least confident about teaching about sexual orientation (Larson, 2003). In another study, students who identified as gay or lesbian reported that the subject of homosexuality was virtually absent from classroom instruction (Lindley & Reininger, 2001). The same study revealed strong support for sexuality education, but homosexuality was the least-supported subject in the survey (Lindley & Reininger, 2001).

The Gay, Lesbian, and Straight Education Network (GLSEN) conducts the only annual survey to determine the school climate for LGBT youth. The 2011 National School Climate Survey indicates that 82 percent of gay youth are verbally harassed at school and 40 percent are physically harassed (Kosciw, Greytak, Bartkiewicz, Boesen, & Palmer, 2012).

One of the biggest issues common to LGBT communities is substance abuse, including smoking tobacco, drinking alcohol, and using drugs. US prevalence estimates are that approximately 20 percent of adults are smokers (Centers for Disease Control, 2011a). Smoking prevalence within the LGBT community is often much higher than the national average. Recent estimates show that gay men are up to 2.5 times more likely to smoke than straight men, and lesbians are twice as likely to smoke as straight women. Furthermore, at estimated rates between 30 and 40 percent, bisexual men and women have the highest smoking rate of any subgroup for which data are available (American Lung Association, 2010). Several factors contribute to this high rate of smoking, including participating in the "bar scene" in order to be part of an LGBT community and using smoking to deal with the stress of homophobia, transphobia, and LGBT discrimination and oppression (GLMA et al., 2001).

It is important to note that programs specifically tailored for the LGBT community have been successful. One study reported results from The Last Drag, a six-week, seven-session group education and support intervention tailored to LGBT smokers (Eliason, Dibble, Gordon, & Soliz, 2012). Sixty percent of the participants were smoke free at the end of the study and 40 percent remained smoke free six months later.

Peterkin and Risdon (2003) found that along with higher rates of smoking, lesbians and gay men have higher rates of alcohol consumption than heterosexual people do. As in the general population in the United States, substance abuse in the LGBT community is associated with myriad challenges, including HIV and AIDS, sexually transmitted diseases (STDs), violence (of particular concern are acts committed by and against the LGBT community), and chronic disease conditions.

Depression and mental health issues also affect LGBT people at a higher level than found among heterosexual people. Although homosexuality is no longer characterized by the American Psychiatric Association as a mental disorder, gender identity disorder (GID) was listed in the *Diagnostic and Statistical Manual of Mental Disorders, Volume Four* (*DSM-IV*) (1994). GID is the condition of significant discomfort with one's assigned gender (Peterkin & Risdon, 2003). Therefore, in order to receive health services, some transgender people were forced to identify themselves as having a mental illness. This was not true for lesbian, gay, and bisexual people who do not identify as transgender. The most recent edition of the DSM-5 has changed the GID diagnoses to Gender Dysphoria (GD) (APA, 2012). GD describes the emotional distress that can result from a marked incongruence between one's experienced/expressed gender and assigned gender.

Regardless, studies show cases of depression among LGBT populations (GLMA et al., 2001). Like substance abuse, this depression can be directly related to individuals' LGBT identification, which can involve navigating through the threat of hate crimes and violence, homophobic and transphobic laws and procedures, and coming out to family members, friends, and coworkers.

In addition to depression and substance abuse, domestic violence is problematic in LGBT communities. According to a 2001 study, 2,183 LGBT persons reported domestic violence to the National Coalition against Domestic Violence. Forty-three percent of the domestic violence survivors were lesbians, 49 percent were male, and 4 percent identified as transgender (National Coalition against Domestic Violence, 2003). Although domestic violence centers on power and control in LGBT relationships, as it does in heterosexual relationships, it also has unique elements when it occurs in LGBT relationships. One of the major ways that abusers control victims is through the victims' fear that their abusers will "out" them (disclosing their LGBT identity to family, friends, coworkers, and others). This results in LGBT people not reporting domestic violence. Another reason that LGBT people do not report domestic violence is fear of a homophobic and transphobic legal system where same-sex relationships are not afforded the same legal rights as opposite-sex relationships. This can become a tool used by the batterer, who may repeatedly tell the victim that he or she will never be helped by the legal system. There are several institutional barriers to obtaining domestic violence services as well. For example, crime victims' compensation programs provide services only to legally married couples. Because LGBT people cannot legally marry in the majority of the states in the United States, they are often denied these services (Baernstein et al., 2006).

Herek (2009) conducted a national probability sample of gay, lesbian, and bisexual adults. Twenty percent of the 662 participants reported a person or property crime based on their sexual orientation, and 50 percent reported being verbally abused. Along with domestic partner violence, external anti-LGBT violence and hate crimes also harm the health of LGBT people. Violence resulting from hate crimes, domestic violence, suicide, and other forms of physical, sexual, emotional, and environmental violence takes a heavy toll on the LGBT population.

Legal response to hate crimes is difficult to measure. Lack of reporting by authorities on the statistics of these crimes and underreporting by the victims themselves are reasons for the difficulty in measuring. Often victims do not report a crime because it will shed unwelcome light on their orientation and may invite more victimization (Stahnke et al., 2008).

In addition, not all state reporting systems use sexual orientation and gender identity as reporting categories for hate crimes. Therefore, it is hard to get accurate statistics about the rates of these crimes. However, we do know that anti-LGBT crimes do exist and that the threat of hate crimes can affect people's stress levels and mental health. This issue goes beyond the LGBT community and becomes everyone's responsibility. Hate crimes affect the mental health of the victim, his or her family, and all other societal members.

Health Issues of LGBT Youths

Adolescence is a difficult time regardless of sexual orientation, and a growing body of research on LGBT youths indicates that they have health problems and needs that are different from those of heterosexual youths (Heck, Flentje, & Cochran, 2011). The most prevalent health and social problems for gay teens are depression, family rejection, suicide, substance abuse, running away, homelessness, prostitution, truancy, victimization, violence, STDs, high-risk sexual behavior, and poor health maintenance (Peterkin & Risdon, 2003). In addition, these risk behaviors are more prevalent, begin at an earlier age, and are more frequently clustered together than are those common among heterosexual youths (Hunter, Cohall, Mallon, Moyer, & Riddle, 2006).

Many of the social and health issues that LGBT experience are interrelated. For example, recent research estimates that between 30 and 40 percent of homeless youth identify as LGBT (Corliss, Goodenow, Nichols, & Austin, 2011). Furthermore, the researchers report that LGBT homeless youth have greater risks and poorer outcomes than heterosexual homeless youth (Corliss et al., 2011). These risks include more physical and sexual victimization, sexual risk-taking behaviors, substance abuse, depression, and suicide (Corliss et al., 2011). Similarly, research has shown that LGBT youths' relationships with their families can have consequences for their physical and mental health. Youth who experience higher rates of family rejection tend to suffer poorer health outcomes, including depression, suicide, sexual risk taking, and substance abuse (Ryan, Huebner, Diaz, & Sanchez, 2009).

Unfortunately, schools often provide a hostile and unsafe environment for LGBT students (GLSEN, 2009). For instance, one report revealed that Boston's lesbian, gay, and bisexual youths were more likely than their heterosexual counterparts to be threatened or injured with a weapon in school. They were also found to be much more likely than heterosexual high school students to carry a gun or weapon and to be involved with a gang (National Coalition for LGBT Health & Boston Public Health Commission, 2002). The average high school student hears twenty-five anti-gay slurs each day. One out of three LGBT youths in Chicago had had an object thrown at him or her, and one out of five had been kicked, punched, or beaten because of his or her sexual orientation (Hunter et al., 2006). This victimization at school has been shown to be strongly linked to mental health issues and increased risk of STDs and HIV for LGBT youth (Russell, Ryan, Toomey, Diaz, & Sanchez, 2011).

LGBT youth use alcohol and other drugs for many of the same reasons as their heterosexual peers do: to experiment and assert independence, relieve tension, increase feelings of self-esteem and adequacy, and self-medicate for underlying depression or other mental health problems (GLMA et al., 2001). Although alcohol consumption has decreased in these communities throughout the past two decades, there is still widespread alcohol use among young gay and lesbian communities (GLMA et al., 2001).

Issues surrounding LGBT youths provide fuel for controversy in the schools, and for LGBT students nationwide, discrimination and harassment have become the rule, not the exception (Woodiel et al., 2003). Homophobia and heterosexism create a hostile environment that does not invite support from the other students and teachers in the school. Therefore, it becomes difficult for heterosexual students and teachers to be informed about and supportive of the special health issues of gay youths (Rienzo, Button, Sheu, & Li, 2006). A recent summary of current research on how teachers view their role in promoting safe schools for LGBT students concludes that schools tend to assume that everyone in the school community (teachers, staff, students) is or should be heterosexual and that few teachers are involved in countering the resultant heterosexism (Vega, Crawford, & Van Pelt, 2012). In order to create safe schools for LGBT students, teachers must be actively involved by addressing LGBT issues and topics (Vega et al., 2012). Health educators in the schools are uniquely positioned to assume leadership roles in addressing and combating the issues of homophobia and heterosexism in an effort to create safe school environments for LGBT students.

Access to adequate and affordable health care is an issue for many Americans. For LGBT youth, the problem can be compounded by the social issues they experience. For example, although youth can now be covered under their parents' health insurance policies up to age 26, the high proportion of LGBT youth who are not cared for by their families lack this coverage (Institute of Medicine, 2011). Furthermore, LGBT youths often have had negative experiences with health professionals (Garofalo & Katz, 2001). Adolescents in general are often reluctant to discuss sexuality and sexual behavior with health care providers. When they fear rejection, stigmatization, lack of confidentiality, and embarrassment, they are even more reluctant to seek health services, may avoid health education altogether, or do not reveal their sexual identity to the health professionals (Ginsberg et al., 2002). Homophobia and heterosexism play a distinct role in their rejection of health care and health education.

Health Issues of Lesbian and Bisexual Women

The health risks and health care needs of lesbians and bisexual women are similar to those of all women. However, lesbian and bisexual women experience additional risk factors and barriers to education and care, and these can affect their health. However, not enough research has focused solely on the concerns of both lesbian and bisexual women. The majority of the research in this field focuses on lesbian women, and there is a definite lack of information about the health concerns of bisexual women (Baernstein et al., 2006).

Among the main issues affecting lesbian and bisexual women are reproductive cancers. Although there is nothing biological to suggest that lesbian and bisexual women are more at risk than heterosexual women, lesbians are less likely to receive regular gynecological care, including regular Pap smears and breast exams (Matthews, Brandenburgh, Johnson, & Hughes, 2004; Institute of Medicine, 2011). Lesbians and bisexual women avoid regular visits to the gynecologist due to past negative experiences, placing them at higher risk of late diagnosis of cervical, ovarian, and endometrial cancers. Fewer pregnancies and decreased use of contraceptives also contribute to increased rates of ovarian and endometrial cancer, and human papillomavirus (HPV), which is associated with cervical cancer, can be transmitted by unclean sex toys (Baernstein et al., 2006).

According to the US Department of Health and Human Services' Office on Women's Health (2011), another reason lesbians are likely to receive inadequate treatment is that some health care providers falsely believe lesbians are immune to certain reproductive cancers, and they do not conduct the proper tests to screen for cancer. Still, lesbian and bisexual women, like all other women, need regular gynecological care and breast and STD screenings.

Along with cancer risks, lesbians and bisexual women are also at risk for obesity and heart disease. Heart disease continues to be the number one killer of women regardless of sexual orientation (US Department of Health and Human Services, Office of Women's Health, 2011). Due to their higher rates of obesity, smoking, and stress, lesbian and bisexual women are at increased risk for heart disease. There is evidence that lesbians are more likely to be overweight than their heterosexual counterparts, possibly because of cultural norms within the lesbian community and because lesbians may relate differently to, not accept, or not internalize mainstream notions of ideal beauty and thinness (Aaron et al., 2001). On average, lesbians have been found to have higher body mass indexes, which have been found to predict health status in regard to obesity (Baernstein et al., 2006).

Health Issues of Gay and Bisexual Men

Like other LGBT people, gay and bisexual men make up a diverse group of people who identify as different races, ethnicities, nationalities, and religions and represent multiple socioeconomic classes from various areas in the United States. These identities directly affect their health issues. However, we will focus on issues we see as the most common and relevant and are sometimes overlooked in gay and bisexual men's communities.

HIV, AIDS, and other STIs remain a major health concern among gay and bisexual men. Although overall the rate of HIV infection has remained relatively stable, it has continued to increase among young and African American men who have sex with men (MSM) (Centers for Disease Control, 2011b). Estimates are that gay and bisexual men make up approximately

2 percent of the US population yet account for over half of new and existing HIV cases (Centers for Disease Control, 2011b). Similarly, gay and bisexual men account for over 60 percent of US syphilis cases and are also at risk for HPV infection, which can lead to increased risk for anal and oral cancers (Centers for Disease Control, 2011c).

Substance use and abuse continues to be an issue among gay and bisexual men and has a significant impact on the health of this group (Hunt, 2012; Institute of Medicine, 2011). Reasons for the higher rates of substance abuse among gay and bisexual men compared to their straight counterparts include the stress of discrimination and victimization, a lack of cultural competency in the drug treatment and health care systems, and targeted marketing by alcohol and tobacco companies (Hunt, 2012). The use of club drugs, such as crystal methamphetamine (often referred to as *crystal meth*) and ecstasy, continues to be a concern in gay and bisexual male communities (GLMA et al., 2001; Halkitis, Palamar, & Mukherjee, 2007; Institute of Medicine, 2011). Crystal meth can cause erratic, violent behavior among its users. Effects also include suppression of appetite, interference with sleeping behavior, mood swings, tremors, convulsions, and an irregular heart rate. The long-term effects of the drug can include coma, stroke, or death (Partnership for a Drug-Free America, 2006). In addition, crystal meth, as is the case with many other club drugs and alcohol, can increase the risk of HIV transmission, as it lowers users' inhibitions, which can result in unsafe sex practices (Boone, Cook, & Wilson, 2013; Reuters, 2004).

Eating disorders and negative body image also affect gay and bisexual men. Research indicates that eating disorders occur more often among gay men than among heterosexual men (Feldman & Meyer, 2007; Meyer, Blissett, & Oldfield, 2001). Eating disorders such as anorexia (characterized by self-starvation) and bulimia (characterized by binging and purging food) can lead to kidney damage, cardiovascular disorders, dental damage, and even death. Although women with eating disorders still outnumber men with eating disorders, men's eating disorders often develop at a later age. One study suggests that for the general population, the average age for men developing an eating disorder is 21 compared to an age of 17 for women (Feldman & Meyer, 2007).

Health Issues of Transgender Communities

Transgender individuals remain the most misunderstood and underrepresented members of LGBT communities. Often the term *transgender* is confused with *transsexual*. *Transgender* is accepted as an umbrella term for a diverse group of individuals who cross culturally defined categories of gender. Transgender individuals can be any sexual orientation.

Transsexuals are born into one gender identity, but feel emotionally connected to another and may be transitioning to the other gender. Cross-dressers dress and take on mannerisms of the opposite gender but are often heterosexual. Drag kings and queens dress and act as the opposite gender for entertainment and can be gay, straight, or trans. Intersex individuals are also under this umbrella; they are born with some combination of both male and female genitalia. Finally, gender benders or androgynous individuals consider categories to be constraining and may exhibit both male and female characteristics.

Transgender individuals have a wide diversity of health care needs. The National Center for Transgender Equality (NCTE) and National Gay and Lesbian Task Force (NGLTF) recently presented the results of a national transgender discrimination survey (NCTE, 2010). The findings revealed significant discrimination and access routinely denied to transgendered individuals. There are high levels of postponing medical care due to discrimination and the lack of financial resources. Respondents reported over four times the national average of HIV infection (2.64 percent compared to 0.6 percent in the general population, with rates for transgender women at 3.76 percent, those who are unemployed at 4.67 percent, and those who have engaged in sex work at 15.32 percent) (NCTE, 2010).

An alarming 41 percent of respondents reported attempting suicide compared to 1.6 percent of the general population. In addition, respondents experienced twice the unemployment rate, especially in communities that are racially and ethnically diverse, significant adverse job outcomes, higher poverty levels, and instability in housing (Amnesty International USA, 2007).

In order to receive services from health care providers, transgender patients had to admit to having gender identity disorder (GID). This presented problems on several levels. First, it required that transgender people admit they had a psychiatric disorder, as GID was classified as such by the American Psychiatric Association. Also, there was a rather lengthy evaluation system that accompanied diagnoses of GID. Therefore, transgender people had to wait for extended periods of time before they could obtain services. Mental health providers would make decisions about who could obtain hormone therapy and sex reassignment surgery and who could not. This lengthy process and fear of being judged by mental health care providers often put transgender people in the position of either not taking advantage of services at all or going to the street to obtain hormones or surgery.

Fortunately, the revised DSM-5 will no longer use the term Gender Identity Disorder and being transgendered will no longer be classified as a mental disorder. The new manual will diagnose transgender people with "Gender Dysphoria," which communicates the emotional distress that can result from "a marked incongruence between one's experienced/expressed gender and assigned gender." This will allow for affirmative treatment and transition care without the stigma of disorder (APA, 2012).

Often the lack of access to health care options results in the practice of dangerous procedures. Many transgender women participate in injection silicone use (ISU): they inject silicone (or have someone else inject it) directly into their breasts. Studies in cities across the United States have indicated that as many as 33 percent of transgender women have reported participating in ISU. Among the health risks associated with ISU are the spread of viral infections such as HIV and hepatitis. It can also lead to systematic illness and disfigurement and even death in some cases. The use of hormones acquired illegally on the street is also extremely dangerous (National Coalition for LGBT Health, 2004). (Table 11.1 summarizes transgender health needs, and figure 11.1 depicts the transgender umbrella.)

Table 11.1 Transgender Needs

	Always Applicable	Before Hormones or Surgery	After Hormones	After Surgery
Male-to-female	Prostrate exams Sigmoidoscopies	Routine testicular examination	Breast exams Mammograms	Clinical vaginal examinations Pap smear
Female-to-male	Breast exams Mammograms Sigmoidoscopies	Examination of ovaries	Blood pressure Cholesterol Heart health	Breast exams (though not as often) Clinical penis exam

Source: Long (2005). Reprinted with permission of the author.

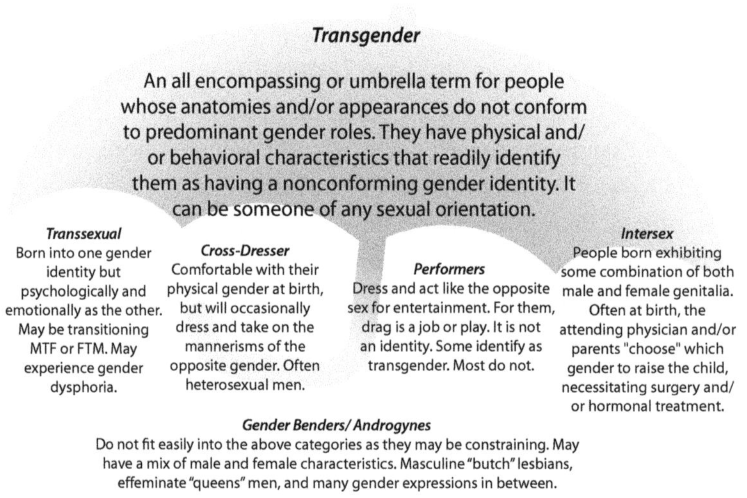
Transgender
An all encompassing or umbrella term for people whose anatomies and/or appearances do not conform to predominant gender roles. They have physical and/or behavioral characteristics that readily identify them as having a nonconforming gender identity. It can be someone of any sexual orientation.
Transsexual
Born into one gender identity but psychologically and emotionally as the other. May be transitioning MTF or FTM. May experience gender dysphoria.
Cross-Dresser
Comfortable with their physical gender at birth, but will occasionally dress and take on the mannerisms of the opposite gender. Often heterosexual men.
Performers
Dress and act like the opposite sex for entertainment. For them, drag is a job or play. It is not an identity. Some identify as transgender. Most do not.
Intersex
People born exhibiting some combination of both male and female genitalia. Often at birth, the attending physician and/or parents "choose" which gender to raise the child, necessitating surgery and/or hormonal treatment.
Gender Benders/Androgynes
Do not fit easily into the above categories as they may be constraining. May have a mix of male and female characteristics. Masculine "butch" lesbians, effeminate "queens" men, and many gender expressions in between.

Figure 11.1 The Transgender Umbrella

Health Issues of LGBT Racially and Ethnically Diverse Communities

While all LGBT individuals are subject to negative health outcomes, those who are racially and ethnically diverse are subject to cumulative negative health outcomes due to the combination of racism and the stigma of their orientation or identity. Research indicates that black and Latino/a LGBT people are more likely to be in poor health than their heterosexual and nontransgender counterparts within communities of color and their white counterparts within the LGBT community (National Coalition for LGBT Health and Boston Public Health Commission, 2002).

These disparities are influenced by limited access to health care and insurance, lower socioeconomic status, fear of bias from providers, a lack of provider competence, and the stress of managing multiple types of societal discrimination (Institute of Medicine, 2003) Perhaps the most significant concerns are the lack of access to health care and insurance coverage. It is estimated that the ratio of uninsured gay and lesbian adults to heterosexuals in the United States is two-to-one (Heck, Sell, & Gorin, 2006)

Racially and ethnically diverse LGBT people have some significant cultural factors contributing to their identity. Cultural factors influencing identity for African American and Latino LGBT individuals include the importance of family and traditional gender roles, conservative religious values, and widespread homophobia (Rosario, Scrimshaw, & Hunter, 2004). All of these factors influence the formation of an LGBT identity and the coming-out process. The recent endorsement of same-sex marriage by the NAACP (National Association for the Advancement of Colored People) can make great strides in the conservative African American religious values that have presented a significant barrier to the LGBT community (NAACP, 2012)

Another disparity for African American and Latino LGBT communities is the interaction of homophobia and racism. A case study in Boston found that African American and Latino/a LGBT people often encounter several forms of oppression and discrimination (National Coalition for LGBT Health & Boston Public Health Commission, 2002). The intersection of homophobia and race can lead to the outcome of violence, and a disproportionate number of victims of reported hate crimes are African American or Latino/a.

The last decade has brought much attention to LGBT families and LGBT families of color. An estimated 2 million children are being raised in LGBT families, and that number is expected to grow in the coming years. LGBT families are more racially and ethnically diverse than families headed by married heterosexual couples; 41 percent of same-sex couples with children identify as people of color compared to 34 percent of married different-sex couples with children. Both black and Latino/a same-sex couples are more likely to raise children than white same-sex couples (Movement Advancement Project, Family Equality Council and Center for American Progress, 2011).

Many LGBT families of color would like to adopt or foster children. A handful of states, however, still restrict or ban fostering by single people or unmarried couples (which by default restricts adoption by same-sex couples, who usually cannot marry in their state). For instance, in Utah, the law bans fostering by all unmarried cohabitors and gives preference to married couples. Same-sex couples can access second-parent or stepparent adoption in only nineteen states and the District of Columbia. In the thirty-one remaining states, neither of these options exists: children living in LGBT families of color lack legal ties to one parent (Movement Advancement Project, 2011).

Until questions about the intersection of race, ethnicity, sexual orientation, and transgender status are routinely included on health surveys, these cumulative disparities for racially and ethnically diverse communities will continue for LGBT people of color. The inclusion of lesbian, gay, bisexual, transgender health objectives in Healthy People 2020 provides hope for the future.

Increasing Cultural Sensitivity toward the LGBT Community

Some health educators may be invited to believe that the health care needs of the LGBT community are no different from those of the general population. Indeed everyone needs age-appropriate health education and treatment, as well as information about preventive measures for his or her health. However, the LGBT community has specific health needs that should be recognized and addressed. Studies show that LGBT populations, in addition to having the same basic health needs as the general population, experience health disparities and barriers related to the expression of their sexual orientation or their gender identity (Kaiser Permanente National Diversity Council and Kaiser Permanente National Diversity, 2004). Many avoid or delay care or receive inappropriate or inferior care as a result of perceived or real homophobia and discrimination on the part of health professionals and institutions.

In spite of the many differences that separate them, the members of the LGBT community have similar experiences of discrimination, rejection, shame, and violence. There are numerous ways that health educators and health professionals can reduce homophobia and heterosexism in their daily work. It is vital that all health educators and practitioners strive to provide a welcoming, supportive, and inclusive environment in addressing health promotion and disease prevention for the LGBT community.

Health educators must address their own attitudes and behaviors about gender identity and sexual orientation (Matthews, Lorah, & Fenton, 2006). Failure to be authentically affirming and accepting will invite the continuation of shame among this community. Consider the health educator who says things intended to show that he is affirming and accepting but also immediately increases the physical space between himself and his LGBT client. LGBT people will readily read such negative nonverbal and verbal cues and will feel validated in their distrust of the health educators and professionals.

We need to provide a physically welcoming environment. Members of the LGBT community will immediately scan our environments for clues that invite them to feel comfortable with a health care experience. Simple symbols such as rainbow flags, pink triangles, and LGBT–friendly stickers can be placed in offices, restrooms, or waiting areas (Dinkel, 2005). In addition, health educators and health professionals should consider using posters or brochures that display racially and ethnically diverse same-sex couples or transgender people. We can visibly display and provide a written copy of a nondiscrimination policy that addresses gender identity and expression, along with age, race, ethnicity, physical ability or attributes, religion, and sexual orientation (GLMA, 2006). And we can advocate for gender-inclusive (unisex) restrooms, which are safer and more comfortable for transgender people than single-sex restrooms.

We should use culturally sensitive language. Forms, assessments, and conversation should employ inclusive choices such as *partner* instead of *spouse* and *relationship status* instead of *marital status*. Adding the option of *transgender*, with selections for *male-to-female* and *female-to-male*, will encourage a feeling of acceptance by transgendered individuals. We can use the same language that the transgender person does to describe self, sexual partners, relationships, and identity. Remember that an individual may not define herself through a sexual orientation label, yet she may have sex with persons of the same sex or gender or with persons of both sexes. For example, men who have sex with men, especially African American and Latino men, may identify as heterosexual and have both female and male partners (GLMA, 2006).

We should not make assumptions about past, current, or future sexual behaviors. The fact that a woman identifies as a lesbian does not mean that she has never had a male sexual partner or never had children. We should include questions on violence as part of the screening or intake process.

LGBT people are not exempt from intimate partner and other domestic violence. However, the circumstances surrounding the violence and the process of helping the victim can be different because of LGBT individuals' fears of being outed to employers and or family.

Health educators and other health professionals are encouraged to participate in LGBT cultural competency training. The Sexuality Information and Education Council of the United States (SIECUS) works with the Centers for Disease Control and Prevention's Division of Adolescent and School Health to provide one-day training ("culturally competent HIV prevention and sexuality education") for health educators. SIECUS also offers free educator resources to assist health educators in exploring culture and sexual health. (SIECUS, 2011).

All of us can best achieve competency in this area by acquiring and applying skills in both simulated and actual settings. Training should be skill based and used with LGBT people. Empathy training could be a part of the work, so that we all come to better understand the stigmas and discrimination that LGBT people face. Finally, we can increase our knowledge of gay-affirming resources in our communities by finding and visiting those resources.

Conclusion

The *American Journal of Public Health* devoted its June 2001 issue to LGBT health issues. The demand was so great that this issue sold out—the first time in the journal's history that an issue had sold out. The decade following this publication has seen many positive changes for the LGBT community. The US Department of Health and Human Services (2000) has elevated sexual orientation from a noted disparity in their Healthy People 2010 (DHHS, 2000) objectives to a target group for concern and improvement in Healthy People 2020 (DHHS, 2010). The recent announcement of the US Department of Health and Human Services that it will begin collecting data in 2013 specific to the health concerns of sexual minorities gives new hope to the prospect of being able to target and address the health disparities of the LGBT community. However, health and politics are inextricably intertwined. The reality is that the progress of the past decade is precariously linked to the current political climate and could be instantly reversed.

In a pair of landmark decisions, the Supreme Court recently struck down the 1996 law blocking federal recognition of gay marriage, and it allowed gay marriage to resume in California by declining to decide a separate case. The court invalidated the Defense of Marriage Act, which denied federal benefits to gay couples who are legally married in their states, including Social

Security survivor benefits, immigration rights. and family leave. This was a powerful message that gay relationships deserve equal respect.

Without question, a celebration is warranted in the LGBT community. However, opponents have vowed to fight same-sex marriage in the states. Including California, thirteen states and the District of Columbia allow same-sex marriage. The Supreme Court rulings will help with the mental health issues associated with being gay. As health educators and health professionals, it is crucial that we continue to advocate for the legal rights of the gay community that are so closely linked to their mental and physical health.

Points to Remember

- Health educators and health professionals should acknowledge the LGBT community as a culture—one with health disparities similar to those associated with race, ethnicity, socioeconomic status, and gender.
- Health educators and health professionals should recognize and accept that there are more differences among the individuals within a culture than there are between cultures. For example, there is more diversity within the LGBT community than there is difference between the LGBT community and other cultural identity groups.
- When health educators and health care professionals deliver services to the LGBT community, it is important to remember that LGBT individuals may have experienced real or perceived homophobia and discrimination from others, including people in the field of health.
- Health educators and health professionals are encouraged to look for ways to provide a welcoming environment for the LGBT community. This includes using culturally sensitive language, not making assumptions, and respecting self-identity. For example, behavior does not always dictate identity. Men who have sex with men may not identify as gay.
- It is vital that health educators and health professionals explore their own homophobia, transphobia, and heterosexism and consider participating in training and workshops to increase their awareness and skills.

Case Study

Casey is a sixteen-year-old high school student. She is an exceptional athlete, playing on the volleyball team, and is an honor roll student. She has been nominated for homecoming queen. Two of her teammates are very jealous of the homecoming nomination, as they believe they should have been nominated instead of her. One day after an especially challenging practice, Casey is comforting her friend who was in tears because the coach had been especially hard on her. Casey was giving her a hug and telling her that everything would be better tomorrow. Her two jealous teammates observed this hug. That night, they went on Facebook and posted a message that said, "Vote for Casey if you want to be represented by a dyke."

The next day when Casey goes to school, she finds that everyone is avoiding her. Even her friends are whispering and laughing, and they walk away when she approaches them. She notices that flyers have been posted on the bulletin boards in school with her picture and "Vote for Casey the Dyke!"

1. What are the main issues in this case study?
2. Are the responsibilities of health educators different when someone is perceived as being gay versus actually being out?
3. What options does Casey have?
4. What could the school health educator do to assist Casey? How could the Coordinated School Health model be used in this case study?
5. What can the administration in the school do to address bullying and cyberbullying?

KEY TERMS

Ally
Bisexual
Coming out
Gay
Gender identity
Heterosexism
Homophobia
Homosexual
Lesbian
LGBT
Queer
Questioning
Sexual identity
Sexual orientation
Transgender
Transphobia
Transsexual

Resources

Centers for Disease Control and Prevention Lesbian, Gay, Bisexual and Transgender Health, http://www.cdc.gov/lgbthealth/links.htm

COLAGE—Children of Lesbian and Gays Everywhere, www.colage.org

Family Acceptance Project, http://familyproject.sfsu.edu/home

Fenway Institute—Fenway Community Health Center, http://www.fenwayhealth.org

Gay and Lesbian Medical Association, www.glma.org

GLSEN—Gay, Lesbian and Straight Education Network, www.glsen.org

Human Rights Campaign—Key LGBT Health Resources, http://www.hrc.org/resources/entry/key-lgbt-health-resources

National Coalition for LGBT Health, www.lgbthealth.net/

National Gay and Lesbian Task Force, http://www.thetaskforce.org/

National LGBT Cancer Network, http://www.cancer-network.org/

National LGBT Tobacco Control Network, http://www.lgbttobacco.org/

National Resource Center on LGBT Aging, www.lgbtagingcenter.org

Parents and Friends of Lesbian and Gays (PGLAG), www.pflag.org

UCSF Center for LGBT Health & Equity, http://lgbt.ucsf.edu/

References

Aaron, D. J., Markovic, N., Danielson, M. E., Honnold, J. A., Janosky, J. E., & Schmidt, N. J. (2001). Behavioral risk factors for disease and preventive health practices among lesbians. *American Journal of Public Health, 91*(6), 972–975.

American Lung Association. (2010). *Smoking out a deadly threat: Tobacco use in the LGBT community.* Retrieved from http://www.lung.org/about-us/publications/

American Medical Association. (2010). *Statement of the American Medical Association to the Institute of Medicine regarding LGBT Health Issues and Research Gaps and Opportunities*

American Psychiatric Association. (1994). *Diagnostic and statistical manual of mental disorders* (4th ed.). Washington, DC: Author.

American Psychiatric Association. (2012). *Diagnostic and statistical manual of mental disorders* (5th ed., text rev.). Washington, DC: Author.

Amnesty International USA. (2007). *Transgender day of remembrance.* Retrieved from http://www.amnestyusa.org/outfront/transgender_remembrance.html

Anderson, J. D. (1997). Supporting the invisible minority. *Educational Leadership, 54*, 65–68.

Baernstein, A., Bostwich, W. B., Carrick, K. R., Dunn, P. M., Goodman, K. W., Hughes, T. L.,. . . Smith, H. A. (2006). Lesbian and bisexual women's public health. In M. D. Shankle (Ed.), *The handbook of lesbian gay, bisexual, and transgender public health: A practitioner's guide to service* (pp. 87–117). New York, NY: Harrington Park Press.

Boone, M. R., Cook, S. H., & Wilson, P. (2013). Substance use and sexual risk behavior in HIV-positive men who have sex with men: An episode-level analysis. *AIDS and Behavior, 17*(5), 1883–1887. doi:10.1007/s10461–012–0167–4.

Burrows, G. (2011). Lesbian, gay, bisexual and transgender health part 2: Gender identity. *Practice Nurse, 41*(4), 22–25. Retrieved from http://ezproxy.emich.edu/login?url=http://search.proquest.com/docview/861503621?accountid=10650

Campinha-Bacote, J. (1999). A model and instrument for addressing cultural competence in health care. *Journal of Nursing Education, 38*(5), 203–207.

Centers for Disease Control and Prevention. (2011a). Vital signs: Current cigarette smoking among adults aged ≥ 18 years—United States, 2005–2010. *Morbidity and Mortality Weekly Report*, 60(33), 1207–1212.

Centers for Disease Control. (2011b). *HIV among gay and bisexual men*. Retrieved from http://www.cdc.gov/hiv/topics/msm/index.htm

Centers for Disease Control. (2011c). *Gay and bisexual men's health: Sexually transmitted diseases*. Retrieved from http://www.cdc.gov/msmhealth/STD.htm

Corliss, H. L., Goodenow, C. S., Nichols, L., & Austin, S. B. (2011). High burden of homelessness among sexual-minority adolescents: Findings from a representative Massachusetts high school sample. *American Journal of Public Health, 101*, 1683–1689.

Dinkel, S. (2005). Providing culturally competent care to lesbians. *Kansas Nurse, 80*, 10–12.

Eliason, M. J., Dibble, S. L., Gordon, R., & Soliz, G. B. (2012). The last drag: An evaluation of an LGBT-specific smoking intervention. *Journal of Homosexuality, 59*(6), 864–878.

Feldman, M. B., & Meyer, I. H. (2007). Eating disorders in diverse lesbian, gay, and bisexual populations. *International Journal of Eating Disorders, 40*(3), 218–226.

Ferris, J. (2006). The nomenclature of the community: An activist's perspective. In M. D. Shankle (Ed.), *The handbook of lesbian gay, bisexual, and transgender public health: A practitioner's guide to service* (pp. 3–10). New York, NY: Harrington Park Press.

Garofalo, R., & Katz, K. E. (2001). Healthcare issues of gay and lesbian youth. *Current Opinions in Pediatrics, 13*, 298–302.

Gates, G. (2011). *How many people are lesbian, gay, bisexual, and transgender?* Los Angeles: Williams Institute, UCLA School of Law.

Gay and Lesbian Medical Association. (2006). *Guidelines for care of lesbian, gay, bisexual, and transgender patients*. Retrieved September 9, 2006, from http://ce54.citysoft.com/_data/n_0001/resources/live/GLMA%20guidelines%202006%20FINAL.pdf

Gay and Lesbian Medical Association and LGBT Health Experts. (2001). *Healthy People 2010 Companion document for lesbian, gay, bisexual, and transgender (LGBT) health*. San Francisco, CA: Gay and Lesbian Medical Association.

Gay, Lesbian, and Straight Education Network. (2009). *National School Climate Survey: The school-related experiences of our nation's lesbian, gay, bisexual, and transgender youth*. New York, NY: Author.

Ginsberg, K. R., Winn, R., Rudy, B. J., Crawford, J., Zhao, H., & Schwarz, D. R. (2002). How to reach sexual minority youth in the health care setting: The teens offer guidance. *Journal of Adolescent Health, 31*, 407–416.

Halkitis, P. N., Palamar, J. J.,& Mukherjee, P. P. (2007). Poly-club-drug use among gay and bisexual men: A longitudinal analysis. *Drug and Alcohol Dependence, 89*, 153–160.

Heck, J. E., Sell, R., & Gorin, S. S. (2006). Health care access among individuals involved in same-sex relationships. *American Journal of Public Health, 96*, 1111–1118.

Heck, N. C., Flentje, A., & Cochran, B. N. (2011). Offsetting risks: High school gay-straight alliances and lesbian, gay, bisexual, and transgender (LGBT) youth. *School Psychology Quarterly, 26*, 161–174.

Herek, G. M. (2009). Hate crimes and stigma-related experiences among sexual minority adults in the United States. *Journal of Interpersonal Violence, 24*(1), 54–74.

Hunt, J. (2012). *Why the gay and transgender population experiences higher rates of substance use*. Center for American Progress. Retrieved from http://www.americanprogress.org/issues/2012/03/lgbt_substance_abuse.html

Hunter, J., Cohall, A. T., Mallon, G. P., Moyer, M. B., & Riddle, J. P. (2006). Health care delivery and public health related to LGBT youth and young adults. In M. D. Shankle (Ed.), *The handbook of lesbian gay, bisexual, and transgender public health: A practitioner's guide to service* (pp. 221–245). New York, NY: Harrington Park Press.

Institute of Medicine. (2003). *Unequal treatment: Confronting racial and ethnic disparities in health care*. Washington, DC: National Academies Press.

Institute of Medicine. (2011). *The health of lesbian, gay, bisexual, and transgender people: Building a foundation for better understanding*. Washington, DC: National Academies Press.

Kaiser Permanente National Diversity Council and Kaiser Permanente National Diversity. (2004). *A provider's handbook on culturally competent care: Lesbian, gay, bisexual, and transgender populations* (2nd ed.). Menlo Park, CA: Author.

Kosciw, J. G., Greytak, E. A., Bartkiewicz, M. J., Boesen, M. J., & Palmer, N. A. (2012). *The 2011 National School Climate Survey: The experiences of lesbian, gay, bisexual and transgender youth in our nation's schools*. New York: GLSEN.

Larson, K. L. (2003). Physical educators teaching health. *Journal of School Health, 73*(8), 291–292.

Lindley, L., & Reininger, B. (2001). Support for instruction about homosexuality in South Carolina public schools. *Journal of School Health, 71*(1), 17–22.

LGBT Medical Education Research Group. (2011). *Changing the face of medication education improve care to lesbian, gay, bisexual, and transgender patients*. Retrieved from http://med.stanford.edu/lgbt/

Long, E. (2005). Transgender: A health transition. *4 Our Health, 3*(1), 2.

Matthews, A. K., Brandenburgh, D. L., Johnson, T., & Hughes, T. L. (2004). Correlates of underutilization of gynecological cancer screening among lesbian and heterosexual women. *Preventive Medicine, 28*, 105–113.

Matthews, C. R., Lorah, P., & Fenton, J. (2006). Treatment experiences of gays and lesbians in recovery from addiction: A qualitative inquiry. *Journal of Mental Health Counseling, 28*, 111–122.

Mayer, K. H., Bradford, J. B., Makadon, H. J., Stall, R. S., & Landers, S. (2008). Sexual gender minority health: What we know and what needs to be done. *American Journal of Public Health, 98*, 989–995.

Melby, T. (2011). The nation's LGBT health check-up. *Contemporary Sexuality, 45*, 1–6.

Meyer, C., Blissett, J., & Oldfield, C. (2001). Sexual orientation and eating psychopathology: The role of masculinity and femininity. *International Journal of Eating Disorders, 29*(3), 314–318.

Movement Advancement Project, Family Equality Council and Center for American Progress. (2011). *All children matter: How legal and social inequalities hurt LGBT families* (Full Report). Movement Advancement Project, Denver, CO. Retrieved from http://www.lgbtmap.org/all-children-matter-full-report

NAACP. (2012). *NAACP passes resolution in support of marriage equality.* Retrieved from http://www.naacp.org/press/entry/naacp-passes-resolution-in-support-of-marriage-equalit

National Center for Transgender Equality and the National Gay and Lesbian Task Force. (2010). *National Transgender Discrimination Survey.* Retrieved from http://2fwww.thetaskforce.org/downloads/resources_and_tools/ntds_report_on_health.pdf

National Coalition against Domestic Violence. (2003, March 24). *Domestic violence among the gay, lesbian, bisexual and transgender communities.* Retrieved from http://www.ncadv.org

National Coalition for LGBT Health and Boston Public Health Commission. (2002, June 28). *Double jeopardy: How racism and homophobia impact the health of black and Latino lesbian, gay, bisexual, and transgender (LGBT) communities.* Retrieved from http://www.lgbthealth.net/downloads/research/BPHCLGBTLatinoBlackHealthDispar.doc

National Coalition for LGBT Health. (2004, August). *An overview of U.S. trans health priorities: A report by the Eliminating Disparities Working Group.* Retrieved from http://www.spectrumwny.org/info/HealthPriorities.pdf

Partnership for a Drug-Free America. (2006). *Crystal meth.* Retrieved from http://www.drugfree.org/Portal/drug_guide/Crystal_Meth

Peterkin, A., & Risdon, C. (2003). *Caring for lesbian and gay people: A clinical guide.* Toronto: University of Toronto Press.

Reuters. (2004, June 7). *Crystal meth linked to AIDS in New York.* Retrieved from http://www.msnbc.msn.com/id/5158153

Rienzo, A. A., Button, J. W., Sheu, J., & Li, Y. (2006). The politics of sexual orientation issues in American schools. *Journal of School Health, 76*(3), 93–97.

Rosario, M., Scrimshaw, E. W., & Hunter, J. (2004). Ethnic/racial differences in the coming-out process of lesbian, gay, and bisexual youths: A comparison of sexual identity development over time. *Cultural Diversity and Ethnic Minority Psychology, 10*, 215–228.

Russell, S. T., Ryan, C., Toomey, R. B., Diaz, R. M., & Sanchez, J. (2011). Lesbian, gay, bisexual, and transgender adolescent school victimization: Implications for young adult health and adjustment. *Journal of School Health, 81*, 223–230.

Ryan, C., Huebner, D., Diaz, R., & Sanchez, J. (2009). Family rejection as a predictor of negative health outcomes in white and Latino lesbian, gay, and bisexual young adults. *Pediatrics, 123*, 346–352.

Sexuality Information and Education Council of the United States (SIECUS) (2011, March 11). *SIECUS's Programs in Action*. Retrieved July 10, 2013 from http://www.cdc.gov/healthyyouth/partners/ngo/siecus.htm

Shankle, M. D. (Ed.). (2006). *The handbook of lesbian, gay, bisexual and transgender public health: A practitioner's guide to service*. New York, NY: Harrington Park Press.

Stahnke, T., LeGendre, P., Grekov, I., Petti, V., McClintock, M., & Aronowitz, A. (2008). *Violence based on sexual orientation and gender identity bias: 2008 Hate Crime Survey*. New York, NY: Human Rights First.

Telljohann, S. K., Price, J. H., Poureslami, M., & Easton, A. (1995). Teaching about sexual orientation by secondary health teachers. *Journal of School Health, 65*(1), 18–22.

US Department of Health and Human Services. Office of Disease Prevention and Health Promotion. (2010). *Healthy People 2020*. Washington, DC. Retrieved from http://healthypeople.gov/2020/topicsobjectives2020/overview.aspx?topicid=25

US Department of Health and Human Services, Office on Women 's Health. (2001, November 2). *Lesbian health fact sheet*. Retrieved from http://www.4woman.gov/owh/pub/factsheets/lesbian1.pdf

US Department of Health and Human Services, Office on Women's Health (2011). *Lesbian and bisexual health*. Retrieved from http://womenshealth.gov/publications/our-publications/fact-sheet/lesbian-bisexual-health.cfm#c

US Department of Health and Human Services, Substance Abuse and Mental Health Services Administration. (2000). *A provider's introduction to substance abuse treatment for lesbian, gay, bisexual, and transgender individuals*. Rockville, MD: Author.

US Department of Health and Human Services, National Institute of Mental Health. (2008). *Strategic plan* (NIH Publication No. 08–6368). Washington, DC: US Government Printing Office.

Vega, S., Crawford, H., & Van Pelt, J. (2012). Safe schools for LGBTQI students: How do teachers view their role in promoting safe schools? *Equity and Excellence in Education, 45*, 250–260.

Woodiel, K., Angermeier-Howard, L., & Hobson, S. (2003). School safety for all: Using the coordinated school health program to increase safety for LGBTQ students. *American Journal of Health Studies, 18*(2/3), 98–103.

CHAPTER 12

CULTURAL COMPETENCY AND HEALTH EDUCATION

A Window of Opportunity

Raffy R. Luquis
Miguel A. Pérez

LEARNING OBJECTIVES

After completing this chapter, you will be able to

- Understand and explain the importance of cultural and linguistic competence in health promotion and education.
- Discuss ways to integrate cultural and linguistic competence into health promotion and education programs.
- Discuss strategies to promote cultural and linguistic competence in order to work effectively with the individuals or communities served by your organization and address their health needs successfully.

Demographic estimates suggest that US racial and ethnic populations, such as the populations of African Americans, Hispanics, Asians, Pacific Islanders, and others, will continue to grow in the next few decades. Estimates show that by 2050, the percentage of non-Hispanic whites will be only half the total US population (US Census Bureau, 2009). This increasing racial and ethnic diversification is making it essential to incorporate the concept of cultural and *linguistic competence* into every aspect of the planning, implementation, and evaluation processes of *health education* and promotion programs (Luquis & Pérez, 2005, 2006; Luquis, Pérez, & Young, 2006; Marin et al., 1994; Pérez, Gonzalez, & Pinzon-Perez, 2006). Moreover, leading public health organizations, including the Institute of Medicine (2004) and the Office of Minority Health (2001), have advocated for a workforce capable of delivering culturally competent and linguistically appropriate services to an ever more diverse US population.

What do these changes have to do with health educators? The field of health education is predicated on the belief that providing health information and skills through planned learning experiences will enable the individuals, groups, and communities receiving that education to make informed choices that will assist them in making quality health decisions and attaining optimal health.

linguistic competence
The capacity of an organization and its personnel to communicate effectively and convey information in a manner that is easily understood by diverse audiences including persons of limited English proficiency, those who have low literacy skills or are not literate, individuals with disabilities, and those who are deaf or hard of hearing

health education
Any combination of planned learning experiences using evidence-based practices and sound theories that provide the opportunity to acquire the knowledge, attitudes, and skills needed to adopt and maintain healthy behaviors

health promotion
Any planned combination of educational, political, environmental, regulatory, or organizational mechanism that supports actions and conditions of living conducive to the health of individuals, groups, and communities

health disparities
A particular type of health difference that is closely linked with a social, economic, or environmental disadvantage

Similarly, *health promotion* is based on the belief that providing a combination of educational, political, environmental, regulatory, and organizational mechanisms can support the actions and conditions of living conducive to the health of individuals, groups, and communities. However, these foundational beliefs often fail to address the reality that given the current diversity of the population in the United States, health education and promotion interventions found to be effective in one racial or ethnic group might not be equally effective with another group. Thus, in order to be effective, health education and prevention strategies must address each group's unique culture, experiences, language, age, gender, and sexual orientation and be culturally and linguistically appropriate.

This chapter provides some final thoughts on the importance of cultural and linguistic competence and discusses how to integrate these concepts into health education and health promotion programs. This chapter also discusses some strategies for promoting cultural and linguistic competence that can assist health education specialists in working with individuals or communities effectively and addressing their health needs successfully. Finally, this chapter discusses standards to promote cultural and linguistic competence in health education.

The Need for Cultural and Linguistic Competence

The professional literature discussed in the previous chapters reveals that non-whites in the United States are less likely than their non-Hispanic white counterparts to have access to health insurance and take advantage of preventive services, are more likely to experience disproportionate levels of morbidity and mortality rates based on leading health indicators, and are more likely to postpone obtaining health services until it may be too late for effective treatment. These differences have been called *health disparities*.

Healthy People 2020, based on the accomplishments of previous Healthy People initiatives, and its indicators continue to provide a directive for improving the health status of all ethnic and racial groups in the United States. One of the four overarching goals of Healthy People 2020, "to achieve health equity, eliminate disparities, and improve the health of all groups," expands on previous goal for the nation (US Department of Health and Human Services, 2012). Thus, now more than ever, there is a pressing need to address the health of all groups.

While several studies have provided excellent suggestions for improving the health status of underrepresented groups, the elimination of health disparities is a challenge as there is no single cause of the problem (Health Resources and Services Administration, 2002). Health disparities are caused by a myriad of factors, including lack of health information; lack of health insurance; individuals' beliefs and attitudes about accessing health care; a shortage of diverse health care providers; comorbidity involving other serious health problems such as addiction and mental illness; and poverty. There are, however, several unifying factors that have been identified in the literature, including income, race and/or ethnicity, and language competence. The overwhelming evidence suggests that cultural and linguistic competencies play a significant factor in decreasing health disparities. For example, lack of background information about different ethnic groups, lack of culturally competent health care providers and health educators, a small percentage of racial and ethnic minorities working in the health care and health promotion fields, an inadequate number of health professionals with diverse skills, and culturally biased health care services have been identified as detrimental factors for the health status among non-white populations (Brach & Fraser, 2000; King, Sims, & Osher, n.d.; US Department of Health and Human Services, 2003).

Similarly, the National Center for Cultural Competence (NCCC) (Cohen & Goode, 1999, revised by Goode & Dunne, 2003) has suggested a variety of reasons that cultural and linguistic competence are required at the health care provider and patient levels. For example, beliefs about health and their perceptions of disease and illnesses vary by cultural groups. Individuals' cultural groups also influence their help-seeking behaviors and their attitudes toward health care providers, and they play a role in their use of traditional and complementary healing practices. Box 12.1 displays six of the salient reasons identified by the NCCC that highlight the critical importance of cultural and linguistic competence in health care.

BOX 12.1 SIX REASONS THAT WE NEED CULTURAL AND LINGUISTIC COMPETENCE IN HEALTH CARE AND HEALTH EDUCATION

1. *To respond to current and projected demographic changes in the United States.* Significant population increases are occurring among racially, ethnically, and culturally and linguistically diverse groups in the United States. Health care organizations and programs must implement systemic change in order to meet the health needs of this diverse population.

2. *To eliminate long-standing disparities in the health status of people of diverse racial, ethnic, and cultural backgrounds.* Although there has been progress in the overall health of the nation, African Americans, Hispanics, Native Americans, Asians, and Pacific Islanders still have poorer health in many areas than the US population as a whole does. In response to these disparities, the federal government has aggressively targeted and committed resources to

six areas: cancer, cardiovascular disease, infant mortality, diabetes, HIV/AIDS, and child and adult immunizations (see Centers for Disease Control, n.d.).

3. *To improve the quality of services and health outcomes.* The delivery of accessible, effective, cost-efficient, and high-quality primary health care calls for health care practitioners who have a deep understanding of the sociocultural backgrounds of their patients and their patients' families and who are also aware of the environments in which their patients live. Culturally and linguistically competent health services facilitate encounters with more favorable outcomes, increase the potential for a more rewarding interpersonal experience, and increase the satisfaction of the individuals receiving health care and disease prevention services.
4. *To meet legislative, regulatory, and accreditation mandates.* Title VI of the Civil Rights Act of 1964 mandates that "no person in the US shall, on ground of race, color, or national origin, be excluded from participation in, be denied the benefits of, or be subjected to discrimination under any program or activity receiving Federal financial assistance." In addition, in 2001, the Office of Minority Health (OMH) published the National Standards for Culturally and Linguistically Appropriate Services in Health Care (CLAS Standards). In April 2013, the OMH released the enhanced National CLAS Standards, which "are intended to advance health equity, improve quality, and help eliminate health care disparities by establishing a blueprint for individuals as well as health and health care organizations to implement culturally and linguistically appropriate services" (OMH, n.d., p. 1). Accreditation bodies such as the Joint Commission on Accreditation of Healthcare Organizations, the Liaison Committee on Medical Education, and the National Committee for Quality Assurance support these standards.
5. *To gain a competitive edge in the marketplace.* The current health care environment is concerned with issues of health care cost and quality, the cost effectiveness of services delivery, and the marketing of such services. Health care organizations that incorporate culturally competent policies, structures, and practices into their services for people with diverse ethnic, racial, cultural, and linguistic backgrounds are well positioned in the current marketplace and for the future as the diversity of the US population continues to increase.
6. *To decrease the likelihood of liability or malpractice claims.* Lack of awareness about race, ethnicity, and cultural differences and failure to provide culturally and linguistically appropriate services may result in liability in several ways. For example, health care organizations might potentially be challenged with claims that the failure on the part of their health care providers to understand and appropriately respond to the beliefs, practices, and behaviors of patients breaches professional standards of care. In addition, the practices of offering effective communication in languages other than English and addressing the communication needs of persons with disabilities and those with low or no literacy have been shown to be effective in reducing the likelihood of malpractice claims.

Source: Adapted from Cohen and Goode (1999); revised by Goode & Dunne (2003).

The recommendations listed in box 12.1 for incorporating cultural and linguistic competency in the health care practice apply to health educators just as they do to health care providers. Our work is an essential ally of health care services, and if that work is to fulfill all its functions, we must join forces with health care and other health allied professionals in the elimination of health disparities to accomplish the goals enumerated in Healthy People 2020.

Cultural Competence

To become culturally competent, health educators and health promoters need to understand the complexity of cultural competence. Recall that *cultural competence* is "a developmental process defined as a set of values, principles, behaviors, attitudes, and policies that enable health professionals to work effectively across racial, ethnic, and linguistically diverse groups" (Joint Committee on Health Education and Promotion Terminology, 2012, p. 11). A similar definition is provided by the Office of Minority Health (2005): "Cultural and linguistic competence is a set of congruent behaviors, attitudes, and policies that come together in a system, agency, or among professionals that enables effective work in cross-cultural situations" (para. 1). Although this definition provides a basic understanding of the concept, it does not go beyond defining the capability of the individual to work with the existing racially, ethnically, and culturally diverse population. Some of the chapter authors for this book have provided other definitions of cultural competence. Cross, Bazron, Dennis, and Isaacs (1989) define *cultural competence* as "a set of congruent behaviors, attitudes, and policies that come together in a system, agency, or among professionals that enables this system, agency, or those professionals to work effectively in cross-cultural situations" (p. 4). Thus, in keeping with these definitions, Luquis and Pérez (2003) have suggested that in the field of health education, we define *cultural competence* as "the capacity of an individual and organization to understand, behave, and respect the values, attitudes, and beliefs of different cultural groups, and to incorporate these differences in the development and implementation and evaluation of policies and health education and promotion programs" (p. 113).

cultural competence
A developmental process defined as a set of values, principles, behaviors, attitudes, and policies that enable health professionals to work effectively across racial, ethnic, and linguistically diverse groups

Health educators must also realize that the process of becoming culturally competent does not happen overnight; it is a lifelong journey. The 2011 report of the Joint Committee on Health Education Terminology (2012) defines this journey as "cultural confidence," which includes a self-reflection on biases and prejudice as well as a motivation to expand their limited understanding of complex issue. At the organization level, the process of acquiring cultural competence requires a comprehensive and coordinated plan that specifies interventions at many levels: policymaking, infrastructure building, program administration and evaluation, the delivery of service and enabling support, and the individual (Goode & Sockalingam, 2000). At the personal level, individuals must examine both their own cultural values and their awareness and acceptance of the cultural values and beliefs among other diverse groups. In addition, the individual must make a commitment to honor and respect the beliefs and values of other cultures. Working toward cultural competence must also include acquiring the ability to develop, adapt, and implement practices and skills that fit the cultural context of the individuals being served. Therefore, given the cultural diversity of the United States, developing cultural competence must be seen as a complex process rather than an end point, and it is unrealistic for an organization to expect to serve all cultural groups in a competent manner; rather, it must create an environment that supports an ongoing process of becoming culturally competent.

At the organization level, the process for cultural competence requires a comprehensive and coordinated plan, which includes interventions at different levels of policymaking, infrastructure building, program administration and evaluation, the delivery of service, and enabling support for the individual (Goode & Sockalingam, 2000). According to the NCCC's *Conceptual Concepts/Models, Guiding Values and Principles* (n.d.b, para. 4), Cultural competence requires that organizations:

- Have a defined set of values and principles and demonstrate behaviors, attitudes, policies, and structures that enable them to work effectively cross-culturally.
- Have the capacity to (1) value diversity, (2) conduct self-assessment, (3) manage the dynamics of difference, (4) acquire and institutionalize cultural knowledge, and (5) adapt to diversity and the cultural contexts of the communities they serve.
- Incorporate the above in all aspects of policy making, administration, practice, service delivery and involve systematically consumers, key stakeholders and communities. (NCCC, n.d.b)

Therefore, given the cultural diversity of the United States, cultural competence becomes a complex process rather than an end point, and it is unrealistic for an organization to serve all cultural groups in a competent manner; rather, the organization must create an environment that supports an ongoing process of cultural competence.

Acquiring Linguistic Competence

Health educators need to understand the intricacy of linguistic competence in order to become linguistically competent. The NCCC *Conceptual*

Concepts/Models, Guiding Values and Principles (n.d.b) defines *linguistic competence* as "the capacity of an organization and its personnel to communicate effectively, and convey information in a manner that is easily understood by diverse audiences including persons of limited English proficiency, those who have low literacy skills or are not literate, and individuals with disabilities" (para. 9). As discussed in chapter 8, it is crucial for health educators to exemplify how health practitioners communicate and interact with racial and ethnic diverse populations in order to provide them with adequate health information to assist them in making decisions concerning their health and health care.

Linguistic competence includes the use of (1) bilingual and bicultural or multilingual and multicultural staff; (2) cross-cultural communication approaches; (3) foreign language interpretation services, including distance technologies; (5) sign language interpretation services; (6) multilingual telecommunication systems; (7) print materials in easy-to-read, low-literacy, picture and symbol formats; (8) materials in alternative formats (e.g., audiotape, Braille, enlarged print); (9) materials developed and tested for specific cultural, ethnic, and linguistic groups; (10) translation services; and (11) ethnic media in languages other than English (e.g., television, radio, newspapers). It requires that individuals and organizations have the capacity to respond effectively to the health literacy needs of the populations served. The organization must have policies, structures, practices, procedures, and dedicated resources that support this capacity.

Cultural and Linguistic Competence in Health Education

In 1994, the American Association for Health Education (AAHE) became a leader in promoting cultural sensitivity among health educators when it published *Cultural Awareness and Sensitivity: Guidelines for Health Educators.*[1] Although the recommendations released at that time were accurate and still serve as a starting point for working with diverse groups, today's health educators need to be more than just sensitive to cultural groups; they need to be culturally and linguistically competent as well. The approach to the cultural competence process has continued to evolve, and in 2006, AAHE published an official position paper on cultural competency and health education (this document is reproduced in appendix A). This position statement acknowledges the fact that due to cultural differences, health promotion interventions found to be effective in one ethnic or racial group cannot be assumed to be equally effective with another group. Prevention strategies must be culturally appropriate and group specific if they are to effectively serve each of various underserved populations.

In 2002, the Society for Public Health Education published "SOPHE's Resolution to Eliminate Racial and Ethnic Health Disparities: Process and Recommendations for Accountability," which not only identified the health disparity problem but also explored lessons learned and offered recommendations for decreasing health disparities. In 2005, SOPHE invited some eighty-five researchers and practitioners to its Inaugural Summit to Eliminate Racial and Ethnic Health Disparities, with the purpose of developing a research agenda focused on eliminating health disparities by promoting research dealing with cultural issues (Airhihenbuwa, 2006).

Although the field of health education has made some progress in addressing cultural and linguistic competence, the fields of medicine, nursing, and social work have taken active steps to address health care disparities and provide culturally appropriate services (Dana, Dayger Behn, & Gonwa, 1992; Goode, Jones, & Mason, 2002). In addition, several models for addressing cultural competence in the field of health care, as described in previous chapters, have been developed in the past two decades (Campinha-Bacote, 2007; Purnell, 2009). However, the field of health education continues to lag in addressing cultural and linguistic competence for its people. To our knowledge, only two models have been developed to address the impact of culture in health promotion and disease prevention (Airhihenbuwa, 2007) and to address culture when planning health promotion programs for multicultural groups (Huff & Kline, 2007). In addition, as reflected throughout the sources cited in this book, materials related to cultural and linguistic competence and specifically developed for health educators are limited; most of the materials and textbooks used in health education to address cultural issues were written for other fields.

Moreover, our field's lack of focus on cultural issues is evident in the fact that none of the seminal documents in health education (e.g., the report produced by the Role Delineation Project and the research agenda of the Society for Public Health Education) specifically address diversity in health education. The recent National Health Educator Competencies Update Project (National Commission for Health Education Credentialing, Society for Public Health Education, & American Association for Health Education, 2006) also fails to address cultural and linguistic competence as a core competency for health educators. In fact, the new Competencies Update Project competency-based hierarchical model only briefly addresses (in four of the subcompetencies for entry-level health educators) diversity, cultural sensitivity, and the use of appropriate language (National Commission for Health Education Credentialing et al., 2006). Thus, the profession of health education would benefit from the development of discipline-specific standards that address culturally and linguistically competent health education programs. The development and implementation of cultural and linguistic competence standards across the health education field would encourage the development and implementation of culturally and linguistically appropriate health education programs (Luquis & Pérez, 2005, 2006; Luquis et al., 2006). Moreover, professional accreditation bodies such as the AAHE-National Council for Accreditation of Teacher Education, the Council on Education for Public Health, SOPHE-AAHE Baccalaureate Program Approval Committee, and the National Commission for Health Education Credentialing should establish cultural and linguistic competence requirements to ensure standardized objectives and content areas throughout the professional preparation of health educators, health promoters, and public health professionals (Luquis et al., 2006).

Public Law 111–148, also known as the Patient Protection and Affordable Care Act (ACA), signed into law on March 23, 2010, and amended by the Health Care and Education Reconciliation Act of 2010, provides new opportunities for health educators to become leaders in terms of designing, delivering, and evaluating cultural and linguistically appropriate programs. Among its provisions, the ACA amends the Public Health Services Act and directs all health programs and population surveys that receive federal monies "to collect and report data on race, ethnicity, primary language, and other demographic characteristics identified as appropriate by the Secretary of Health and Human Services (HHS) for reducing health disparities" (Andrulis, Siddiqui, Purtle, and Duchon, 2010, p. 2; GPO, n.d.).

The ACA also provides the collection and dissemination of data on health professionals, funding for professional training in cultural competency and diversity, and funding for community health workers who deliver programs using CLAS standards. It is important to note that while health educators are not specifically listed in the ACA, health professional such as behavioral and mental health professionals, public health professionals, allied health professionals, and community health workers are specifically listed in the ACA. Thus, health educators who are or will be practitioners within these professional categories must learn to work within the parameters of the ACA. Finally, section 5307 of the ACA also provides for the development and evaluation of model cultural competent curricula and directs the OMH, which it elevates to the level of institute, to disseminate that information through a website (Healthcare.gov, 2012; Health Resources and Services Administration, n.d.).

Strategies to Incorporate Cultural and Linguistic Competence into Health Education

In a multicultural and diverse society, health educators and other health professionals alike must strive to achieve cultural and linguistic competence and incorporate cultural competence training into health education and promotion programs. In order to accomplish this goal, health educators do not need to become experts on every racial, ethnic, cultural, and diverse group residing in the United States, but they do need to be cognizant of differences, which may affect their ability to reach target populations, and be proficient in using techniques to bridge cultural divisions (Luquis & Pérez, 2003). Health educators can begin to acquire these abilities by pursuing some of the following strategies.

First, health educators must learn to recognize the importance of culture and respect diversity. Culture influences many aspects of our lives, our families, and our communities and also how we operate in society. It may be characterized by factors such as national origin; customs and traditions; length of residency in the United States; language; age; generation; gender and sexual orientation; religious beliefs; political beliefs; perceptions of family and community; perceptions of health, well-being, and disability; physical ability or limitations; socioeconomic status; educational level; geographical location; and family and household composition (US Department of Health and Human Services, 2003). Thus, health educators need to understand all the factors surrounding culture and diversity and how they affect different groups' views of health and health education. For example, the REACH initiative has identified culture and history as one of its key principles in the development of effective community-based strategies and interventions (Centers for Disease Control, 2007).

Second, health educators should maintain a current profile of the cultural composition of their community of interest. One of the most important steps in the development of health education programs is performing the needs assessment. By maintaining a current profile of the population they serve (see the case study in chapter 1, for example), health educators will be prepared to identify the culturally related needs of the community, such as learning style and education, language and interpreter services needed, level of health literacy, housing availability, and other health-related services. Information included in this community profile should be updated frequently, because given ongoing demographic changes, such data can change rapidly (US Department of Health and Human Services, 2003).

Third, health organizations, community-based organizations, schools, work sites, and other health-related agencies should provide ongoing cultural and linguistic competence training to health educators and other health staff. As stated throughout this book, the development of cultural and linguistic competence is an essential element in the professional preparation of health educators. In previous studies, the chapter authors found that health educators who attended cultural diversity training or education programs had achieved a higher level of cultural competence than those who had not attended a similar program (Luquis & Pérez, 2005, 2006). This training should include basic cultural competence principles, concepts, terminology, and frameworks and discussion about cultural values and traditions, family values, linguistics and literacy, help-seeking behavior, and cross-cultural outreach techniques and strategies, among other issues (US Department of Health and Human Services, 2003).

Fourth, health educators must involve cultural brokers from the targeted racial and ethnic groups during the development of health education programs. These cultural brokers can include community leaders and organizations representing diverse cultural groups. Collaborating with organizations and leaders who are knowledgeable about the community is the most effective way of gaining information about the community and assists health educators in assessing needs, creating community profiles, gaining trust with community members, and ensuring that strategies are culturally and linguistically appropriate (US Department of Health and Human Services, 2003). In addition, community leaders and key organizations can act as catalysts for change in the community, including forging unique partnerships, which may be essential in the development of effective health education and promotion programs (Centers for Disease Control, 2007).

Fifth, health educators must ensure that health education programs and services are culturally and linguistically appropriate. For example, language can be a major barrier in the provision of health promotion and disease prevention services. Health educators must ensure that written health information is translated into one or more languages, as appropriate for the community to be served, and must consider the health literacy level of the target population when developing written health-related materials (US Department of Health and Human Services, 2003). Chapter 8 discussed the importance of culturally and linguistically appropriate health communication and described strategies for addressing this issue in health education and promotion. The chapter also points out that effective communication is foundational for the health education profession. Clearly it is essential for health promotion specialists to learn to communicate across cultures, following the recommendations throughout this book.

Finally, health educators must continuously assess and evaluate the level of cultural and linguistic competence in programs that are under way as well as the organizations where they work. Self-assessment, process, and organization evaluation are keys to ensuring that health education programs are as effective as possible. In a study designed to ascertain cultural competence training needs in a health services system in California, Pérez, Gonzalez, and Pinzon-Perez (2006) "found that administrators reported participating in activities related to cultural awareness twice as often as staff" (p. 106). The researchers concluded that "while this commitment to cultural competence is commendable, it is at the same time disturbing that the people most likely to come in contact with diverse populations are less trained" (p. 106).

Self-assessment will measure how health practitioners and health organizations are serving diverse populations (NCCC, n.d.a). The NCCC's *Tools and Processes for Self-Assessment* (n.d.a) provides several tools and processes for self-assessment that determine the level of cultural and linguistic competence of both the organization and the individuals working within it. Box 12.2 contains a selected list of tools identified by the NCCC to conduct those self-assessments. Health educators should become familiar with and use these tools to ensure that they and their organizations are effective in serving the diverse population in the United States.

BOX 12.2 SELF-ASSESSMENT TOOLS

- Cultural and Linguistic Competence Assessment for Disability Organizations (CLCADO): Assessment and Guide
- Cultural and Linguistic Competence Family Organization Assessment (CLCFOA) Guide for Using the CLCFOA
- Cultural and Linguistic Competence Organizational Assessment Instrument for Fetal and Infant Mortality Review Programs (CLCOA-FIMR)
- Cultural and Linguistic Competence Policy Assessment (CLCPA)
- Curricula Enhancement Module Series: Cultural Self-Assessment
- A Guide to Planning and Implementing Cultural Competence Organizational Self-Assessment
- Innovative Self-Assessment and Strategic Planning: Addressing Health Disparities in Contra Costa County
- Promoting Cultural and Linguistic Competency Self-Assessment Checklist for Personnel Providing Services and Supports in Early Intervention and Early Childhood Settings. This tool is available in Spanish.
- Promoting Cultural and Linguistic Competency Self-Assessment Checklist for Personnel Providing Primary Health Care Services
- Promoting Cultural Diversity and Cultural Competency Self-Assessment Checklist for Personnel Providing Services and Supports to Children with Disabilities and Special Health Needs and Their Families. This tool is available in Spanish.
- Promoting Cultural Diversity and Cultural Competency: Self-Assessment Checklist for Personnel Providing Behavioral Health Services and Supports to Children, Youth and Their Families
- Promoting Cultural Diversity and Cultural Competency Self-Assessment Checklist for Personnel Providing Services and Supports to Individuals and Families Affected by Sudden Infant Death Syndrome and Other Infant Death (SUID). This tool is available in Spanish.

Source: National Center for Cultural Competence. (n.d.a).

Standards for Cultural and Linguistic Competence in Health Education

The CLAS standards are designed to provide cultural and linguistic goals for health care providers. Cultural and linguistic competence in health education focuses on the key issues of a trained workforce and health education and prevention programs. The following standards proposed for health educators are based on an extensive review of the professional literature, many years of work experience, and our own experiences.

A Workforce Trained for Cultural and Linguistic Competence

- Professional preparation programs in health education must offer cultural competence courses that transmit and discuss the history, traditions, values, belief systems, acculturation, and language of the major racial and ethnic groups in the United States. These programs must include awareness-based, knowledge-based, and skills-based objectives in their required courses to prepare students to become culturally competent professionals.
- Professional health educators must participate in continuing education designed to develop their ability to become culturally and linguistically competent and to update the skills they learned in classroom training and their work experience. In order to promote continued professional development among Certified Health Education Specialists (CHES) and Master Certified Health Education Specialist (MCHES), the NCHEC should set a minimum number of continuing education contact hours (CECHs) in the area of cultural and linguistic competence as part of the seventy-five CECHs needed over the five-year certification period.

Health Education Programs Designed for Cultural and Linguistic Competence

- Health educators must conduct needs assessments that collect racial, ethnic, or cultural group–specific demographic characteristics including age, gender, social class, education and literacy, religion and spirituality, and language preferences, among others, in order to properly assess the needs for health education programs and then to incorporate the local meaning and understanding of the health-illness continuum as well as the differences of symptom expression in the prevention messages that they deliver.
- Health educators must use culturally and linguistically appropriate tools to collect data that will help them understand the attitudes and beliefs and also the educational, social, and economic conditions in the community. They then can incorporate this information when

developing, implementing, and evaluating health education and prevention programs.

- Health educators must work with members of their target communities and make them integral members of the program team during the development, implementation, and evaluation of health education and prevention programs.
- Health educators must use the targeted racial, ethnic, or cultural group's preferred language during the development, implementation, and evaluation of a health education and prevention program. Health educators should not use health education and prevention messages that are simply translated literally from the English language because they may not convey the intended message in the group's preferred language.
- A priority of health educators must be to empower racial, ethnic, and cultural communities to ensure that health education and prevention programs are long-lasting and self-sustaining.
- Health educators must ensure that health education and prevention programs are accessible, appropriate, and equitable to all racial, ethnic, and cultural groups in the community.

Conclusion

The increasing racial and ethnic diversification of the US population is making it very clear that we need to incorporate the concept of cultural and linguistic competence into every aspect of the planning, implementation, and evaluation process of health education and promotion programs. It has also become clear that cultural and linguistic competence can help to eliminate health disparities among the diverse segments of the population. Throughout this book, the chapter authors have explored strategies to incorporate cultural and linguistic competence into the development and implementation of materials, programs, and learning opportunities that take into account the specific needs of different racial, ethnic, and cultural groups.

Points to Remember

- Health educators need to understand that cultural and linguistic competence are an integral part of the development, implementation, and evaluation of health education and promotion programs.
- Health educators need to promote cultural and linguistic competence in order to work effectively with the individuals or communities served by their organizations and to address these individuals' or communities' health needs.

- We already know a number of good strategies for incorporating cultural and linguistic competence into health education.
- It is time for our profession to develop standards that address cultural and linguistic competence in health education programs and in the preparation of health education professionals. This chapter offers an initial set of such standards.

KEY TERMS

Cultural competence

Health disparities

Health education

Health promotion

Linguistic competence

Note

1. In fall 2011, the American Alliance for Health, Physical Education, Recreation, and Dance board of governors unanimously voted to approve the release of the American Association for Health Education (AAHE) as part of its reorganization. In spring 2013, AAHE aligned its programs and resources with the Society for Public Health Education to strengthen the health education profession. Thus, AAHE as an organization has ceased to exist.

References

Airhihenbuwa, C. O. (2006). The inaugural SOPHE summit on eliminating racial and ethnic health disparities. *Health Promotion Practice, 3*, 293–295.

Airhihenbuwa, C. O. (2007). On being comfortable with being uncomfortable: Centering an Africanist vision in our gateway to global health. *Health Education and Behavior, 34*(1), 31–42.

American Association for Health Education. (1994). *Cultural awareness and sensitivity: Guidelines for health educators.* Reston, VA: Author.

Andrulis, D. P., Siddiqui, N. J., Purtle, J. P., & Duchon, L. (2010). *Patient Protection and Affordable Care Act of 2010: Advancing health equity for racially and ethnically diverse populations.* Retrieved from http://www.jointcenter.org/hpi/sites/all/files/PatientProtection_PREP_0.pdf

Brach, C., & Fraser, I. (2000). Can cultural competency reduce racial disparities? A review and conceptual model. *Medical Care Research and Review, 57*(Suppl. 1), 181–217. http://mcr.sagepub.com/cgi/content/abstract/57/suppl_1/181

Campinha-Bacote, J. (2007). *The process of cultural competence in the delivery of healthcare services: A culturally competent model of care* (5th ed.) Retrieved from http://www.transculturalcare.net/Cultural_Competence_Model.htm

Centers for Disease Control and Prevention. (2007). *REACHing across the divide: Finding solutions to health disparities.* Atlanta, GA: Author.

Centers for Disease Control and Prevention. (n.d.). *Racial and ethnic approaches to community health: REACH US* Retrieved from http://www.cdc.gov/reach/index.htm

Cohen, E., & Goode, T. D. (1999). Revised by Goode, T. D., & Dunne, C. (2003). *Policy brief 1: Rationale for cultural competence in primary Care.* Washington, DC: National Center for Cultural Competence, Georgetown University Center for Child and Human Development.

Cross, T. L., Bazron, B. J., Dennis, K. W., & Isaacs,. M. R. (1989). *Toward a culturally competent system of care: A monograph on effective services for minority children who are severely emotionally disturbed.* Washington, DC: Georgetown University Child Development Center, Child and Adolescent Service System Program.

Dana, R. H., Dayger Behn, J., & Gonwa, T. (1992). A checklist for the examination of cultural competence. *Research on Social Work Practice, 2*(2), 220–233.

Goode, T., Jones, W., & Mason, J. (2002). *A guide to planning and implementing cultural competence organization self-assessment.* Washington, DC: National Center for Cultural Competence, Georgetown, University Child Development Center. Retrieved from http://ww11.georgetown.edu/research/gucchd/nccc/documents/ncccorgselfassess.pdf

Goode T., & Sockalingam, S. (2000). Cultural competence: Developing policies to address the health care needs of culturally diverse clientele. *Home Health Care Management and Practice, 12*(5), 49–55.

GPO. (n.d.). An act entitled the Patient Protection and Affordable Care Act. Retrieved from http://www.gpo.gov/fdsys/pkg/BILLS-111hr3590enr/pdf/BILLS-111hr3590enr.pdf

Healthcare.gov. (2012). *Health disparities and the Affordable Care Act.* Retrieved from http://www.healthcare.gov/news/factsheets/2010/07/health-disparities.html

Health Resources and Services Administration, HIV/AIDS Bureau. (2002). *HRSA Care ACTION: Mitigating health disparities through cultural competence.* Retrieved from http://hab.hrsa.gov/publications/august2002.htm

Health Resources and Services Administration. (n.d.). *Culture, language, and health literacy.* Retrieved from http://www.hrsa.gov/culturalcompetence/index.html

Huff, R. M., & Kline, M. V. (2007). The cultural assessment framework. In R. M. Huff & M. V. Kline (Eds.), *Health promotion in multicultural populations: A handbook for practitioners and students* (2nd ed., pp. 125–145). Thousand Oaks, CA: Sage.

Institute of Medicine. (2004). *In the nation's compelling interest: Ensuring diversity in the health care workforce.* Retrieved from http://www.iom.edu/report.asp?id=18287

Joint Committee on Health Education and Promotion Terminology. (2012). Report of the 2011 Joint Committee on Health Education and Promotion Terminology. [Special Supplement Issue]. *American Journal of Health Education, 43*(2), 1–19.

King, M., Sims, A., & Osher, D. (n.d.). *How is cultural competence integrated in education?* Retrieved from http://cecp.air.org/cultural/Q_integrated.htm

Luquis, R., & Pérez, M. (2003). Achieving cultural competence: The challenges for health educators. *Journal of Health Education, 34*(3), 131–138.

Luquis, R., & Pérez, M. A. (2005). Health educators and cultural competence: Implications for the profession. *American Journal of Health Studies, 20*(3/4), 156–163.

Luquis, R., & Pérez, M. (2006). Cultural competency among school health educators. *Journal of Cultural Diversity, 13*(4), 218–222.

Luquis, R., Pérez, M. A., & Young, K. (2006). Cultural competence development in health education professional preparation programs. *American Journal of Health Education, 37*(4), 233–241.

Marin, G., Burhansstipanov, L., Connell, C. M., Gielen, A. C., Helitzer-Allen, D., Lorig, K., . . . Thomas, S. (1994). A research agenda for health education among underserved populations. *Health Education and Behavior Quarterly, 22*(3), 346–364.

National Center for Cultural Competence. (n.d.a). *Tools and processes for self-assessment.* Retrieved from http://nccc.georgetown.edu/foundations/assessment.html

National Center for Cultural Competence. (n.d.b). *Conceptual concepts/models, guiding values and principles.* Retrieved from http://nccc.georgetown.edu/foundations/frameworks.html

National Commission for Health Education Credentialing, Society for Public Health Education, & American Association for Health Education. (2006). *A competency-based framework for health educators—2006.* Whitehall, PA: Author.

Office of Minority Health. (2001). *National standards on culturally and linguistically appropriate services (CLAS).* Retrieved from http://www.omhrc.gov/templates/browse.aspx?lvl=2&lvlID=15

Office of Minority Health. (n.d.). *National CLAS Standards: Fact sheet.* Retrieved from https://www.thinkculturalhealth.hhs.gov/pdfs/NationalCLASStandardsFactSheet.pdf.

Office of Minority Health. (2005). *What is cultural competency?* Retrieved from http://minorityhealth.hhs.gov/templates/browse.aspx?lvl=2&lvlID=11

Pérez, M. A., Gonzalez, A., & Pinzon-Perez, H. (2006). Cultural competence in health care systems: A case study. *California Journal of Health Promotion, 4*(1), 102–108.

Purnell, L. D. (2009). *Guide to culturally competent health care.* (2nd ed.) Philadelphia, PA: F. A. Davis.

US Census Bureau. (2009). *Table 5. Percent distribution of the projected population by net international migration series, race, and Hispanic ORIGIN for the US: 2010–2050.* Retrieved from http://www.census.gov/population/projections/data/national/2009/2009comparisonfiles.html

US Department of Health and Human Services. (2003). *Developing cultural competence in disaster mental health programs: Guiding principles and recommendations.* Rockville, MD: US Department of Health and Human Services, Substance Abuse and Mental Health Services Administration, Center for Mental Health Services.

US Department of Health and Human Services. (2012). *Healthy people 2020: About Healthy People.* Retrieved from http://healthypeople.gov/2020/about/

APPENDIX A

SELECTED LIST OF WEB RESOURCES FOR HEALTH DISPARITIES

Agency for Health Care Research and Quality: National Health Disparities Report	http://www.ahrq.gov/qual/Nhdr05/nhdr05
American Medical Association	https://www.ama-assn.org/ama/pub/physician-resources/public-health/eliminating-health-disparities.page
American Psychological Association	http://www.apa.org/topics/health-disparities/initiative.aspx
California Department of Health Service: Multicultural Health Disparities	http://www.dhs.ca.gov/hisp/chs/OHIR/Publications/OtherReports/MHD051703.pdf
Community health and elimination of health disparities	http://www.calendow.org/Category.aspx?id=308&ItemID=208
Community health and health disparities	http://www.preventioninstitute.org/healthdis.html
Eliminating health disparities	http://www.amsa.org/disparities
Eliminating racial and ethnic health disparities	http://www.cdc.gov/omhd/Topic/HealthDisparities.html
Federal collaboration on health disparities research	http://minorityhealth.hhs.gov/fchdr/
Fogarty International Center	http://www.nih.gov/fic/
Healthy People 2020	http://www.healthypeople.gov/2020/about/disparitiesAbout.aspx
Institute of Medicine	http://www.iom.edu/
Indian Health Services	http://www.ihs.gov/index.cfm
Kaiser Family Foundation: A weekly look at health care disparities	http://www.kaiserhealthnews.org/Topics/Health-Disparities.aspx
National Alliance for Hispanic Health	http://www.hispanichealth.org/
National Association of School Psychologists	http://nasponline.org/resources/culturalcompetence/index.aspx
National Cancer Institute	http://www.cancer.gov/cancertopics/disparities
National Center for Cultural Competence	http://www11.georgetown.edu/research/gucchd/nccc/
National Center for Complementary and Alternative Medicine	http://nccam.nih.gov/

National Center for Research Resources	http://www.ncrr.nih.gov/
National Library of Medicine	http://www.nlm.nih.gov/
National Information Center on Health Services Research and Health Care Technology	http://www.nlm.nih.gov/hsrinfo/disparities.html
National Institute of Allergy and Infectious Diseases	http://www.niaid.nih.gov/topics/minorityhealth/pages/disparities.aspx
NIH Program of Action: Addressing Health Disparities	http://healthdisparities.nih.gov
National Institute of Minority Health and Health Disparities	http://www.nimhd.nih.gov/default.html
Office of AIDS Research	http://www.nih.gov/od/oar/index.htm/
Office of Behavioral and Social Sciences Research	http://www1.od.nih.gov/obssr/obssr.htm/
Office of Disease Prevention	http://odp.od.nih.gov/
Office of Minority Health and Health Equity	http://www.cdc.gov/minorityhealth/omhhe.html
Office of Research on Minority Health	http://www1.od.nih.gov/ORMH/main.html/
Prevention Institute	http://preventioninstitute.org/component/jlibrary/article/id-91/127.html
Public Health Reports	http://www.publichealthreports.org/user-files/117_5/117426.pdf
State profiles: Minority health and health equity offices	http://www.ncsl.org/issues-research/health/disparities-state-profiles.aspx
Substance Abuse and Mental Health Services Administration	http://samhsa.gov/about
US DHHS, OMH: Think Cultural	http://www.thinkculturalhealth.org/
US Surgeon General	http://www.surgeongeneral.gov/initiatives/prevention/strategy/elimination-of-health-disparities.html
Warren Grant Magnuson Clinical Center	http://www.cc.nih.gov/

APPENDIX B

SUMMARY OF SELECTED HEALTH DISPARITIES

Cancer

- African American men are over twice as likely to die from prostate cancer as whites.
- Vietnamese American women have a higher cervical cancer incidence rate than any other ethnic group in the United States—5 times that of non-Hispanic white women.
- American Indian women are 1.7 times as likely to die from cervical cancer as compared to white women.
- Asian/Pacific Islander men and women have higher incidence and mortality rates for stomach and liver cancer.
- Hispanic women are twice as likely as non-Hispanic white women to be diagnosed with cervical cancer.

Diabetes

- American Indian/Alaska Native adults were over twice as likely as white adults to be diagnosed with diabetes.
- In Hawaii, Native Hawaiians are more than 5.7 times as likely as whites living in Hawaii to die from diabetes.
- Mexican American adults were 1.8 times more likely than non-Hispanic white adults to have been diagnosed with diabetes by a physician.

Gender

- Men (18.4/100,000) are 4 times more likely to die by suicide than women are (4.8/100,000).
- In 2007, the rate of new AIDS cases was almost three times as high for men (21.6/100,000) as for women (7.5/100,000).

HIV/AIDS

- African American males have 7.6 times the AIDS rate of white males.
- American Indian/Alaska Native women have three times the AIDS rate of non-Hispanic white women.
- Hispanic females have 4 times the AIDS rate of non-Hispanic white females.
- Native Hawaiian/Pacific Islanders are 2.2 times as likely to be diagnosed with AIDS as the white population.

Hypertension

- African American women and men aged 45 to 74 years had much higher death rates from congestive heart disease than women and men of the three other races.
- Hypertension is more prevalent in non-Hispanic blacks (42 percent) than whites (28.8 percent).
- American Indian/Alaska Native adults are 1.3 times as likely as white adults to have high blood pressure.
- Mexican American women are less likely than non-Hispanic white women to have high blood pressure.

Immunization

- In 2009–2010, lower influenza vaccination coverage was observed for non-Hispanic black and Hispanics compared to non-Hispanic whites among people age 5 and older.
- American Indian/Alaska Native adults aged 18 to 64 years are as likely as their non-Hispanic white counterparts to have received the influenza (flu) shot in the past twelve months.
- In 2010, both Hispanic and Asian American adults over age 65 were less likely to have ever received a pneumonia shot as compared to non-Hispanic whites of the same age group.
- In 2010, Asian/Pacific Islander children aged 19 to 35 months reached the Healthy People goal for immunizations for hepatitis B, MMR (measles-mumps-rubella), polio, and chicken pox.

Income and Poverty

- In 2005, the mammography rate for poor women was about two-thirds that for high-income women (48.5 percent compared with 75.3 percent).
- Income disparity in noncompletion of high school was greatest for those with family income below the federal poverty level (poverty income ratio less than 100 percent).

Insurance Coverage

- In 2010, 11.7 percent of the non-Hispanic white population was not covered by health insurance.
- In 2010, 20.8 percent of African Americans in comparison to 11.7 percent of non-Hispanic whites were uninsured.
- In 2010, 29.2 percent of American Indians/Alaskan Natives had no health insurance coverage.
- In 2010, 30.7 percent of the Hispanic population was not covered by health insurance.

Infant Mortality

- The highest infant mortality rate in 2006 was for non-Hispanic black women, with a rate 2.4 times that of non-Hispanic white women.
- American Indian/Alaska Natives have 1.6 times the infant mortality rate of non-Hispanic whites.
- Puerto Rican infants were twice as likely to die from causes related to low birth weight compared to non-Hispanic white infants.
- The infant mortality rate is 1.7 times greater for Native Hawaiians than for non-Hispanic whites.

Obesity

- In 2010, African American women were 40 percent more likely to be obese than non-Hispanic white women.
- Native Hawaiian/Pacific Islanders are 2.7 times more likely to be obese than the overall Asian American population.
- In 2009–2010 Mexican American children between the ages 6 and 17 were 60 percent more likely to be overweight than non-Hispanic white children.
- American Indian/Alaskan Natives are 70 percent more likely to be obese than non-Hispanic whites.

Oral Health

- In general, American Indian/Alaska Natives populations have much greater rates of dental caries and periodontal disease in all age groups than the general US population.
- Mexican American children aged 2 to 5 years, especially those from lower-income households, were more likely than their African American and white counterparts to have one or more decayed primary teeth.
- African American males have the highest incidence rate of oral cavity and pharyngeal cancers in the United States compared with women and other racial/ethnic groups.

Sources

Agency for Healthcare Research and Quality. (2009). *National healthcare disparities report.*

Blake, G., Zhu, J., Moonsinghe, R. (2011). Diabetes—United States, 2004 and 2008. *Morbidity and Mortality Weekly Reports, 60,* 90–93. http://www.cdc.gov/mmwr/preview/mmwrhtml/su6001a20.htm?s_cid=su6001a20_w#tab1

Centers for Disease Control and Prevention. (2011). *Health disparities and inequities report—US 2011.* http://www.cdc.gov/minorityhealth/CHDIReport.html

Centers for Disease Control and Prevention. (n.d.). *Eliminate disparities in cancer screening and management.* http://www.cdc.gov/omhd/AMH/factsheets/cancer.htm

Centers for Disease Control and Prevention. (2012, August). *Overweight and obesity.* http://www.cdc.gov/obesity/data/adult.html

Kenan, A., Shaw, K. (2011). Coronary heart disease and stroke deaths—United States, 2006. *Morbidity and Mortality Weekly Reports, 60,* 62–66. http://www.cdc.gov/mmwr/preview/mmwrhtml/su6001a13.htm?s_cid=su6001a13_w

Office of Minority Health. (2012, June). *Cancer data/statistics.* http://minorityhealth.hhs.gov/templates/browse.aspx?lvl=3&lvlid=4

Office of Minority Health. (2012, July). *Heart disease data/statistics.* http://minorityhealth.hhs.gov/templates/browse.aspx?lvl=3&lvlid=6

Office of Minority Health. (2012, July). *Infant mortality/SIDS data and statistics.* http://minorityhealth.hhs.gov/templates/browse.aspx?lvl=3&lvlid=8

Office of Minority Health. (2012, August). *Diabetes data/statistics.* http://minorityhealth.hhs.gov/templates/browse.aspx?lvl=3&lvlid=5

Office of Minority Health. (2012, November). *HIV/AIDS data/statistics.* http://minorityhealth.hhs.gov/templates/browse.aspx?lvl=3&lvlid=7

CULTURALLY AND LINGUISTICALLY APPROPRIATE SERVICES STANDARDS

Principal Standard

1. Provide effective, equitable, understandable, and respectful quality care and services that are responsive to diverse cultural health beliefs and practices, preferred languages, health literacy, and other communication needs.

Governance, Leadership and Workforce

2. Advance and sustain organizational governance and leadership that promotes CLAS and health equity through policy, practices, and allocated resources.
3. Recruit, promote, and support a culturally and linguistically diverse governance, leadership, and workforce that are responsive to the population in the service area.
4. Educate and train governance, leadership, and workforce in culturally and linguistically appropriate policies and practices on an ongoing basis.

Communication and Language Assistance

5. Offer language assistance to individuals who have limited English proficiency and/or other communication needs, at no cost to them, to facilitate timely access to all health care and services.
6. Inform all individuals of the availability of language assistance services clearly and in their preferred language, verbally and in writing.
7. Ensure the competence of individuals providing language assistance, recognizing that the use of untrained individuals and/or minors as interpreters should be avoided.
8. Provide easy-to-understand print and multimedia materials and signage in the languages commonly used by the populations in the service area.

Source: The National CLAS Standards are available at https://www.thinkculturalhealth.hhs.gov/Content/clas.asp.

Engagement, Continuous Improvement, and Accountability

9. Establish culturally and linguistically appropriate goals, policies, and management accountability, and infuse them throughout the organization's planning and operations.
10. Conduct ongoing assessments of the organization's CLAS-related activities and integrate CLAS-related measures into measurement and continuous quality improvement activities.
11. Collect and maintain accurate and reliable demographic data to monitor and evaluate the impact of CLAS on health equity and outcomes and to inform service delivery.
12. Conduct regular assessments of community health assets and needs and use the results to plan and implement services that respond to the cultural and linguistic diversity of populations in the service area.
13. Partner with the community to design, implement, and evaluate policies, practices, and services to ensure cultural and linguistic appropriateness.
14. Create conflict and grievance resolution processes that are culturally and linguistically appropriate to identify, prevent, and resolve conflicts or complaints.
15. Communicate the organization's progress in implementing and sustaining CLAS to all stakeholders, constituents, and the general public.

NAME INDEX

Page references followed by *t* indicate a table; followed by *b* indicate a box.

C

G

H

N

O

P

SUBJECT INDEX

Page references followed by *fig* indicate an illustrated figure; followed by *t* indicate a table; followed by *b* indicate a box.

B

C

D

I

J

K

L

N

O

R

S

Lightning Source UK Ltd.
Milton Keynes UK
UKHW031258291119
354452UK00007B/14/P

9 781118 347492